Veterinary Practice Management

M000250075

For Saunders:

Commissioning Editor: Mary Seager
Project Development Manager: Zoë Youd
Project Manager: Gail Wright
Design Direction: George Ajayi

Veterinary Practice Management

A Practical Guide

Maggie Shilcock BSc Post Grad Dip Lib CMS
Veterinary Practice Project Manager, Norfolk, UK; Veterinary Practice Management and Support Staff Training Consultant; Editor, *Veterinary Management for Today*; President, Veterinary Practice Management Association

and

Georgina Stutchfield BSc CVPM
Experienced Veterinary Practice Manager; Veterinary Computer Consultant, Windermere, UK; Honorary Treasurer, Veterinary Practice Management Association

SAUNDERS

SAUNDERS
An imprint of Elsevier Science Limited

© 2003, Elsevier Science Limited. All rights reserved.

No part of this publication may be reproduced, stored in a retrieval system, or transmitted in any form or by any means, electronic, mechanical, photocopying, recording or otherwise, without either the prior permission of the publishers (Permissions Manager, Elsevier Science Ltd, Robert Stevenson House, 1–3 Baxter's Place, Leith Walk, Edinburgh EH1 3AF), or a licence permitting restricted copying in the United Kingdom issued by the Copyright Licensing Agency, 90 Tottenham Court Road, London W1T 4LP.

First published 2003

ISBN 0 7020 2696 4

British Library Cataloguing in Publication Data
A catalogue record for this book is available from the British Library

Library of Congress Cataloging in Publication Data
A catalog record for this book is available from the Library of Congress

Note
Management is constantly changing. As new information becomes available, changes in procedures become necessary. The authors and the publishers have taken care to ensure that the information given in this text is accurate and up to date. However, readers are strongly advised to confirm that the information, especially with regard to employment and health and safety, complies with the latest legislation and standards of practice.

ELSEVIER SCIENCE your source for books, journals and multimedia in the health sciences
www.elsevierhealth.com

The publisher's policy is to use **paper manufactured from sustainable forests**

Printed in China by RDC Group Limited

Contents

Preface ix

Abbreviations xi

1 THE STRUCTURE OF VETERINARY PRACTICE 1
- The buildings 3
- The types of veterinary practice 4
- Ownership 5
- The services 6
- The veterinary staff 7

2 FACTORS AFFECTING THE CHANGE IN STRUCTURE OF VETERINARY PRACTICE 11
- External factors 11
- Internal factors 14

3 THE MANAGEMENT OF VETERINARY PRACTICES 17
- Management of practices in the twentieth century 17
- The veterinary practice as a business 19
- Management of practices in the twenty-first century 19

4 WHAT IS A VETERINARY PRACTICE MANAGER? 23
- Today's practice managers 23
- The role of a practice manager 24
- Real-life managers 27
- The changing role of the practice manager 28

5 MANAGING YOURSELF 31
- Managing your job 31
- Managing your time 34
- Yourself 42

6 BUSINESS PLANNING 47
- Where are we now? 47
- Where do we want to go? 52

7 MANAGING HUMAN RESOURCES – THE IMPORTANCE OF STAFF, RECRUITMENT AND DISCIPLINE 57
- Why are staff important? 57
- What do you want from your staff? 58
- What do your staff want from you? 59
- Recruitment 61
- Discipline 68

8 PRINCIPLES OF EMPLOYMENT LAW 75
- Discrimination 75
- Maternity rights 76
- Rights for working parents 77
- The right to time off for family emergencies 77
- Part-time work 77
- Human rights 77
- National minimum wage 77
- Working Time Regulations 78
- Redundancy 78
- Dismissal 78

9 HUMAN RESOURCES – TEAMWORK, COMMUNICATION AND MANAGING CHANGE 81
Teamwork *81*
Communication *85*
Managing change *90*

10 HUMAN RESOURCES – TRAINING AND APPRAISALS 93
Training *93*
Appraisals *102*

11 CLIENT CARE 111
What does the client want? *111*
How to provide good client care *112*
Measuring and maintaining client care *114*
Dealing with client complaints *116*
Dealing with difficult clients *117*
Excellence in customer service *118*

12 SALES AND MARKETING 119
What is sales and marketing and what's the difference? *119*
Why do we need it? *120*
General marketing principles *121*
The marketing plan *124*
Marketing of products *124*
Marketing services *127*
Marketing the practice *128*
Marketing tools *129*

13 UNDERSTANDING FINANCIAL ACCOUNTS 135
Why have financial accounts? *135*
Accounting basics *136*
What is a profit and loss account? *136*
What is a balance sheet? *139*
Interpreting financial accounts *141*

14 MANAGEMENT ACCOUNTS AND FINANCIAL PLANNING 147
Management accounts *147*
Figures derived from the financial accounts *149*
Figures derived from income analysis *149*
Other figures *150*
Financial management *151*
Budgeting for profit – will we make any money? *152*
Budgeting for cash – can we stay afloat? *154*
Budgeting for capital expenses – can we afford to buy? *156*

15 STOCK MANAGEMENT 161
Where are you now? *162*
Where do you want to be? *163*
How are you going to get there? *164*
Legislation and stock control *170*

16 PRICING OF FEES AND PRODUCTS 171
Pricing of products *172*
Dispensing and injection fees *175*
Fee setting *176*
Effects of changing selling price *180*
Discounts *181*
Surcharges *182*
Problems arising from prices *183*

17 INFORMATION TECHNOLOGY 185
The use of computers in veterinary practice *186*
Choosing and evaluating a system *191*
Contingencies *195*
Associated legislation *197*

18 OFFICE MANAGEMENT 199
Record keeping *199*
Credit control *201*
Office equipment *204*
Telecommunications *205*
Premises management *207*
Security *209*

19 HEALTH AND SAFETY 211
Why be concerned with health and safety? *211*
Health and safety legislation *211*
Enforcing bodies *212*
Responsibility for health and safety *213*
The practice health and safety policy *213*
Risk assessments *213*

Control of substances hazardous to health (COSHH) *220*
Staff training *221*

20 PHARMACY AND DISPENSING 225
Drug storage and management *226*
Health and safety *228*
Dispensing *228*

21 STATUTORY AND ETHICAL ASPECTS OF PRACTICE 233
Insurance and pensions *233*
Taxes *235*
Business structure *236*
Ethics *237*

22 WHO SHOULD DO THE MANAGING? 239
Resistance to employing managers *239*
Spreading the load *240*
Does your veterinary practice need a practice manager? *241*
The pitfalls *243*
Well, who should do the managing? *244*

23 WHERE DO WE GO NOW? 245
Management training *245*
Management roles *246*
The effective use of staff *246*
Adaptation to change *247*
Specialization *247*
Diversification *247*
Reviewing and revising practice policy and procedure *248*
Strategic planning *248*

APPENDIX: USEFUL CONTACTS 249

INDEX 253

Preface

In a rapidly changing business world the efficient and effective management of any business is crucial to its success. Veterinary practices are no exception. In order to survive and prosper, they must not only produce excellent clinical services, but also manage and deliver those services in a highly professional manner.

Many veterinary owners and partners have found juggling clinical and management roles increasingly difficult, and have employed practice managers and administrators to help them run their businesses.

This book is intended as a guide for all those involved in the management of veterinary practices: managers, administrators, partners and owners. Those who work closely with practices, such as professional advisors and suppliers, will also find it a valuable insight into the structure, operation and management of veterinary practice.

This book is a practical guide to management techniques and processes, covering all aspects of veterinary practice management. It will be valuable both to newcomers to the field, as well as to more experienced individuals, and is intended to be used as a practical tool for help and guidance in the day-to-day management of veterinary practice.

We have many years' experience as veterinary practice managers in mixed and small animal practice. We felt there was a need for a veterinary management book that was practical, realistic and would enable managers to put theory into practice.

We would like to thank all our friends and colleagues within the world of veterinary practice for their help, support and guidance over the years. Veterinary practice management is constantly developing and presenting the manager with new challenges. There is always something new to learn. We hope this book will be as valuable to others as the help we have received has been to us.

Anmer and
Windermere 2002

Maggie Shilcock
Georgina Stutchfield

Abbreviations

ARR	Accounting rate of return
BACS	Bankers Automated Clearing Service Ltd
BSAVA	British Small Animal Veterinary Association
BSE	Bovine Spongiform Encephalitis
BVA	British Veterinary Association
BVNA	British Veterinary Nursing Association
CD	Controlled drugs
CHIP2	The Chemical (Hazard Information and Packaging for Supply) Regulations
COSHH	Control of substances hazardous to health
CPD	Continuing professional development
CVPM	Certificate in Veterinary Practice Management
FDI	Fort Dodge Indices
FMD	Foot and Mouth Disease
FSB	Federation of Small Businesses
GSL	General Sales List (medicines)
HSC	Health and Safety Commission
HSE	Health and Safety Executive
IP	Income protection insurance
IPT	Insurance premium tax
L/A	Large animal
LLP	Limited liability partnership
MAT	Moving annual total/Moving annual turnover
MSDS	Manufacturer's safety data sheet
NIC	National Insurance contributions
NPV	Net present value
OFGEM	Office of Gas and Electricity Markets
PAYE	Pay as you earn
PDSA	Peoples Dispensary for Sick Animals
PHI	Permanent health insurance
PML	Pharmacy and Merchants List (medicines)
PMS	Practice Management System
POM	Prescription Only (medicines)
PPE	Personal protective equipment
RCVS	Royal College of Veterinary Surgeons
RIDDOR	Reporting of Injuries, Diseases and Dangerous Occurrences Regulations 1995
ROCE	Return on capital employed
ROE	Return on equity
ROI	Return on investment
RPA	Radiation Protection Advisor
RPS	Radiation Protection Supervisor
RPSGB	Royal Pharmaceutical Society of Great Britain
RRP	Recommended retail price
RSPCA	Royal Society for the Prevention of Cruelty to Animals
SIPP	Self-investment pension plan
SMP	Statutory Maternity Pay
SPP	Statutory Paternity Pay
SPVS	Society of Practising Veterinary Surgeons
UPS	Uninterruptible power supply
VBD	Veterinary Business Development
VCU	Veterinary Computer Users group
VDS	Veterinary Defence Society
VMD	Veterinary Medicines Directorate
VN	Veterinary nurse
VPMA	Veterinary Practice Management Association

CHAPTER CONTENTS

The buildings 3

The types of veterinary practice 4

Ownership 5

The services 6

The veterinary staff 7
Veterinary surgeons 7
Support staff and nurses 7
Managers 8
The clients 8

1

The structure of veterinary practice

Veterinary medicine has been practised in some form for 1000 years, but it is only in the last 50–100 years that significant changes have really taken place, and these have been generally of a clinical nature. Changes over the last 20 years have had a real impact on the structure and management of veterinary practice and it is likely that the next 20 years will see the most dramatic changes yet.

The first veterinary book to be printed in England was probably *Proprytees and Medicynes of Hors* in 1497, which was followed by numerous texts on the treatment of horses and farriery. In 1791 the London Veterinary College was founded, but it was not until 1844 that a Royal Charter established the Royal College of Veterinary Surgeons (RCVS), the first veterinary college in Great Britain.

Veterinary science at this time was very much in its infancy, with no real understanding of infectious disease until 1876, when Louis Pasteur in France and Robert Koch in Germany independently proved that anthrax was spread by a bacillus, and the science of bacteriology was born.

In the early twentieth century veterinary treatment was still fairly basic, and concentrated mainly on the care of horses which played a vital role in the farming industry. The veterinary surgeons were the 'car mechanics' of today, and treatment consisted chiefly of the use of home-made medicines, magnesium sulphate for purging and a considerable degree of hope. The major factor changing the face of veterinary medicine was the introduction from the early 1940s of antibiotics for animal treatment.

The decline in the use of horse power in the 1930s and 1940s reduced dramatically the major species of animal that veterinary surgeons treated, but alongside this decline came the increase in intensive farming practices which required more veterinary intervention.

In 1957 the British Small Animal Veterinary Association was formed, illustrating the increase in numbers of domestic pets being treated by veterinary surgeons. With the 1960s and 1970s came the real pet explosion and by the end of the twentieth century there were an amazing 15 million pet owners in the UK.

The last years of the twentieth century and the beginning of the twenty-first have seen a series of catastrophes in the farming industry, Bovine Spongiform Encephalitis (BSE), Swine Fever, Foot and Mouth Disease (FMD), together with a general recession in agriculture associated to a large extent with European Union (EU) agricultural policy. The farming crisis has seriously impacted on the large animal side of veterinary practice and led to a reduction in the amount of large animal work in favour of companion animal. Recent figures from the Forte Dodge Indices now suggest that the numbers of cats and dogs kept in the UK is declining, a trend which if sustained will have a serious effect on small animal veterinary practice.

The structure of the veterinary practice has to change with a changing environment and clientele if the business is to survive. The veterinary practice of the twenty-first century is a very different business from that of the early twentieth century; this is illustrated in Figures 1.1 and 1.2.

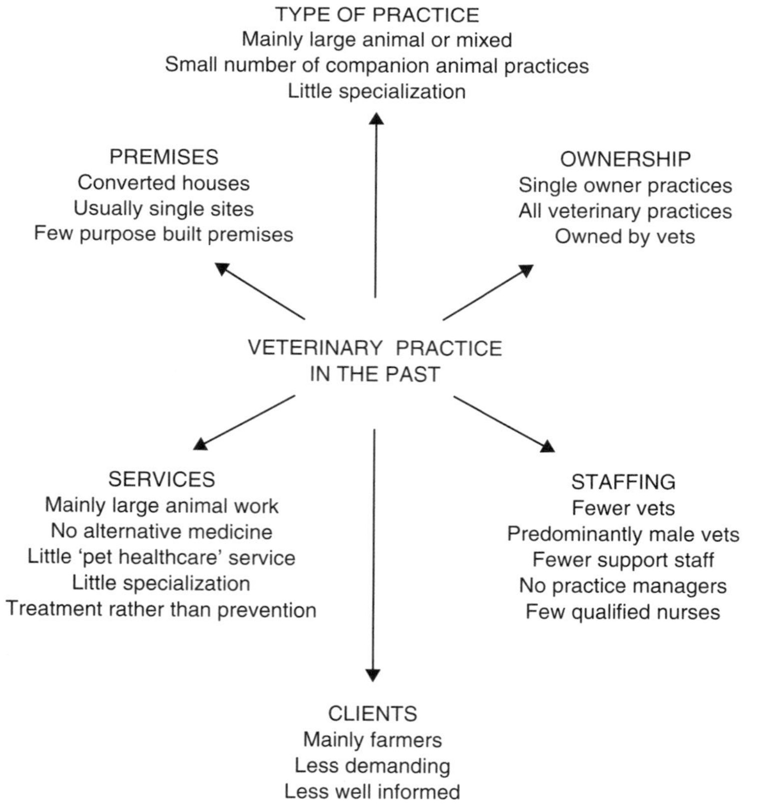

Figure 1.1 Structure of veterinary practice in the past.

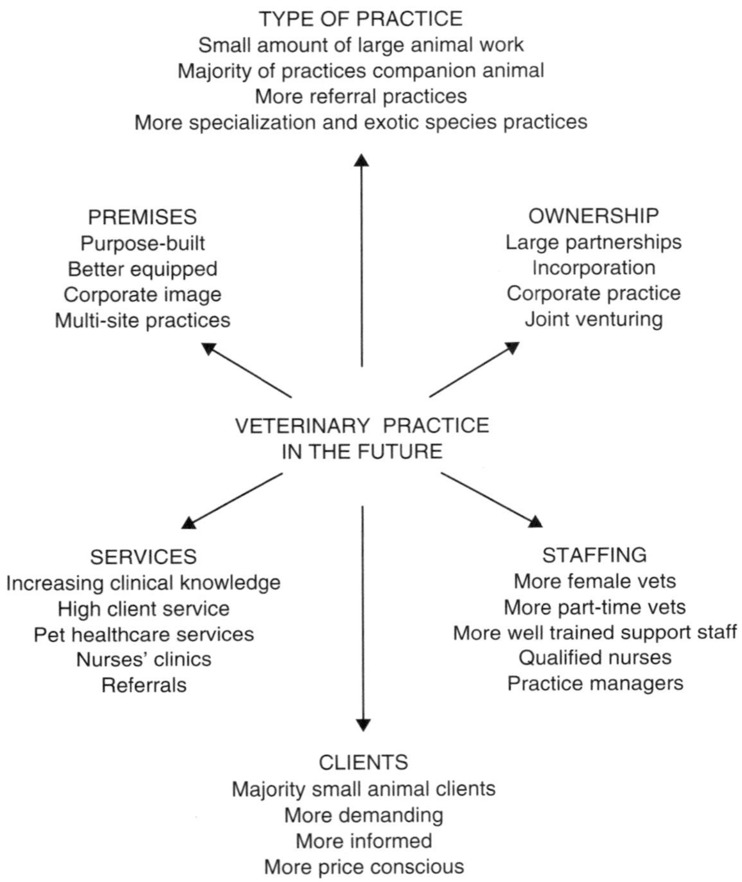

Figure 1.2 Structure of veterinary practice in the future.

Veterinary practice structure comprises:

- the buildings – the premises where the veterinary surgeon and staff work
- the type of practice – large animal, mixed, small animal, equine, exotic, referral, etc.
- ownership – the type of ownership, sole principal, partnership, Charity, Corporate, etc.
- the services – the veterinary services and treatment the practice provides for its clients
- the staff – those working in the practice and the roles they have
- the clients – who they are and what their requirements are.

THE BUILDINGS

In the first half of the twentieth century the vast majority of veterinary practices consisted of a room or rooms in the veterinary surgeon's house. There would be a waiting room for clients and a consulting room where animals were examined and occasionally operated on. Most veterinary work was large animal and the veterinary surgeon was out for the majority of the day visiting farms. Only a small proportion of clients actually visited the surgery with animals.

By the 1950s and 1960s veterinary surgeries were being set up in other accommodation, usually converted shops and offices. But some were already being purpose-built and the first

Veterinary Hospitals which complied with the British Veterinary Hospital Association (BVHA) standards were established in the late 1960s.

Present-day veterinary buildings are a far cry from the typical 'James Herriot' practice of the 1940s. Increasingly practices are purpose-built on sites which provide parking for clients, or existing buildings are being completely renovated to accommodate the Practice needs. Buildings are larger, incorporating a number of consulting rooms as well as operating suites and preparation rooms, X-ray rooms, modern kennelling facilities and dedicated dispensaries. Waiting rooms are larger and more client-friendly and there are offices, staff rooms and training or meeting rooms reflecting the increased number of veterinary support staff and training needs.

Such is the enthusiasm for practice building and refurbishment that journals such as the Veterinary Business Journal regularly feature practice profiles of mouth-watering state-of-the-art veterinary practices in the UK and USA.

THE TYPES OF VETERINARY PRACTICE

The horse was the main animal treated by veterinary surgeons until the 1930s. Farmers depended upon horses for pulling the plough and other machinery and it was vital that they were fit and well cared for. Farm animals came very much second in veterinary attention, with farmers carrying out a great deal of home treatment in the form of drenches and potions purchased from the local pharmacy; the vet was usually called as a last resort.

As tractors took over from horses, and farm animals began to be reared more intensively, veterinary care started to become more important and the farm or large animal practice came into being. Large animal practices gradually evolved into mixed practices as pet keeping (mainly cats and dogs) became more popular and clients became more able or willing to afford veterinary care. The horse vet remained, but his clients changed and he was now dealing with horses used for hunting, racing and recreation.

Large numbers of practices were still single-handed, with perhaps a non-veterinary assistant who helped the vet and did the books. The purely small animal practice was rare and would only be seen in larger towns. As pet keeping increased in the 1960s and 1970s, practices gradually increased in size, partnerships were established and the numbers of branch surgeries increased, a smaller surgery in a nearby town or village being seen as a way of making the practice more accessible to distant clients as well as hopefully encouraging the growth of new clientele.

Towards the end of the twentieth century the size of practices had increased considerably and practices with ten or more veterinary surgeons were not uncommon, but despite this the single-handed veterinary practitioner had not disappeared.

The Quo Vadis Survey of 1998 provided the following statistics on practice type:

- large animal 8%
- mixed 50%
- small animal 39%
- equine 3%.

The number of veterinary surgeons employed by practices varied widely:

- 1–2 veterinary surgeons – 21% of practices
- 3–4 veterinary surgeons – 25% of practices
- 5–6 veterinary surgeons – 25% of practices
- 7–9 veterinary surgeons – 17% of practices
- 10–19 veterinary surgeons – 9% of practices
- 20+ veterinary surgeons – 2% of practices.

The number of sites practices had also varied:

- 1 site, 47%
- 2 sites, 26%
- 3 sites, 15%
- 4+ sites, 11%.

Hospital status had been granted to 14% of veterinary practices.

The farming crisis at the end of the 1990s and in particular FMD in 2001 has severely affected large animal and mixed practices. Many large animal practices are struggling and some have merged in order to survive, while many mixed practices have had to look to the small animal sector to supplement their income.

OWNERSHIP

The single-handed veterinary surgeon was still the norm halfway through the twentieth century and today there remains a significant number (22%) of single-handed practices. However, the single-handed practice of today will employ a larger number of support staff.

By the 1950s practices were becoming larger, small animal work was beginning to increase, and owners were beginning to take on veterinary assistants, who over time would often move into partnership with the existing owner.

The size of practices and partnerships grew until by the end of the twentieth century there were many practices with partnerships of 3–6 vets, while the occasional larger practice would have more than six partners. Animal charities such as the Royal Society for the Prevention of Cruelty to Animals (RSPCA) and People's Dispensary for Sick Animals (PDSA) own veterinary practices, and in the case of the RSPCA, Wildlife Hospitals, which employ veterinary surgeons. Until recently these practices were the only ones not owned by veterinary surgeons.

The late 1990s saw the beginning of a significant change in veterinary practice ownership when it was established that the RCVS would allow, or at least could not prevent, non-veterinary ownership of veterinary practices. Initially a small number of non-veterinary surgeons, generally marital partners or practice managers, bought into partnerships, but before too long the change in ownership status attracted corporate practice.

With the backing of venture capital provided by the large financial institutions, individuals (veterinary surgeons and non-veterinary surgeons) have been able to set up Corporate Practice Enterprises, buying existing or setting up new veterinary practices to establish a network/chain of 'branded' practices locally or nationally. Corporate practices are still in their infancy but are likely to increase rapidly in number in the next 5–10 years, mirroring the growth of companies such as Specsavers who established in the USA, and later the UK, large numbers of branded chains of high-street opticians. The structure of corporate practices varies; some buy out existing practices, some set up new green-field sites and some set up practices within pet superstores, and some may do all three. In essence their aim is to establish a chain of practices which will benefit from central management, buying power and resources. Increasingly corporate practices are offering Joint Venturing Schemes to veterinary surgeons, allowing them to buy their own practices for a modest financial commitment, in a close relationship with the parent company, enabling them to take advantage of corporate benefits and support. They are of course also subject to any corporate constraints.

The new generation of veterinary surgeons graduating from veterinary schools has different expectations and ambitions from their predecessors; many do not want the responsibility, financial commitment and mobility constraints of a partnership. The expectations and lifestyle of some of these 'new' veterinary surgeons is far more in line with the type of veterinary work and offers of joint venturing available from the Corporates. This may be seen by the veterinary surgeon to provide the best of both worlds, lower financial input, a level of ownership, a degree of clinical freedom and mobility. In the future graduates are likely to be looking to three main areas for veterinary employment:

- veterinary assistant – concentrating on clinical work with the option of specializing and gaining veterinary certificates
- owner/partner – in a 'traditional' veterinary practice
- joint venture ownership – in a corporate environment

Partnerships have been the traditional business medium for veterinary surgeons for a number of generations, and the partners of the practice have been personally liable for all the business debts. The Limited Liability Partnership Act of 2000 now allows the formation of a Limited Liability Partnership (a hybrid between a limited company and a partnership, which allows the practice to benefit from limited liability status). As practices increase in size, so does the potential debt that partners could be responsible for should the business fail. Incorporation may be seen as the best method of safeguarding their personal assets in the face of business failure and may allow partners to dispense with their unlimited joint liability whilst maintaining their existing taxation treatment.

It can be seen that the ownership of veterinary practice in the twenty-first century is more varied than it has ever been, but the single-handed veterinary surgeon is still surviving in a world which seems to be increasingly dominated by multi-site and corporate practice. The future and success of corporate practice is still to be seen, as is the final effect of the corporate on the small practice.

THE SERVICES

The services provided today to clients of veterinary practices have changed and improved dramatically compared with only two or three decades ago. Clinically veterinary surgeons are able to provide an upwardly spiralling service as new advances are made in veterinary medicine and surgery. This service has its cost, and veterinary fees parallel this increasing ability to treat cases which in the past would have been considered hopeless. Drugs and surgical equipment are constantly improving and allowing the veterinary surgeon to provide a higher level of treatment. At the same time there has been a rise in the popularity and practice of alternative and holistic veterinary medicine. Acupuncture in particular is increasing in use as an alternative method of treating a variety of animals, and the Association of British Veterinary Acupuncturists (ABVA) now has over 100 members. The practice of homeopathic medicine is also on the increase, as is the use of herbal medicines, very popular with some veterinary clients.

An increasing number of veterinary surgeons take certificates and diplomas in their chosen specialization, enabling their practices to offer specialist services such as dermatology, radiology, orthopaedics, cardiology, etc., and some practices now only provide referral services.

The treatment of exotics such as birds, fish, reptiles and insects has also increased, while there are also a small number of single species clinics, notably feline.

Veterinary surgeons are obliged to provide a 24-hour emergency service, but the old system of 'on call' is changing at least in urban areas. Specialist emergency night clinics now exist, and as with the medical profession, it is now quite common practice for groups of veterinary practices in cities to pool resources to share night duty commitments.

All this is a far cry from the clinical services veterinary surgeons supplied only a matter of 50 years ago. But even greater changes have been made in the other customer services veterinary practices now provide. The most notable of these is the provision of nurses' clinics, where clients may take their pets for preventative healthcare advice such as weight control, nutrition, flea and worm control, to name just a few. The qualified nurse is playing a far more significant role in veterinary practice than ever before and is set to increase her participation in the future as the Schedule 3 amendment to the Veterinary Surgeons Act 1966 allows more clinical freedom for the veterinary nurse.

Veterinary practices are under pressure to increase client services as a way of retaining and bonding clients. Just a few of the client services now provided are:

- booster reminders
- client newsletters
- client evenings
- information leaflets
- practice brochures
- healthcare packages
- pet insurance information
- transport of pets to and from the surgery
- pet food and pet products
- client loyalty schemes.

In the veterinary marketplace client service in the twenty-first century is seen to be the key to success. An increase in these services combined with ever-improving clinical care would seem to be the only road forward for the future.

THE VETERINARY STAFF

Veterinary surgeons

The number of veterinary surgeons per practice has steadily increased, and by the end of the twentieth century the Quo Vadis Survey quoted 2% of practices with 20+ veterinary surgeons.

The RCVS Manpower Survey 1998 provided an insight into the shape and structure of the veterinary profession, identifying trends of employment, hours of work and career objectives. The Quo Vadis Survey took the Manpower Survey even further by looking at the veterinary profession's attitudes, beliefs and lifestyle objectives from the point of veiw of the profession as well as veterinary clients. The survey was designed to answer questions such as how the veterinary surgeons perceived their relationship with their clients, how clients perceived their veterinary surgeons, and how the commitment and attitude of the veterinary surgeon was changing. The project gathered data from over 4,500 respondents including pet owners, clients with business income from animals, and veterinary surgeons. Information was gathered by means of face-to-face or telephone interviews, with the longest and most detailed interviews taking place with veterinary surgeons.

More details are shown in Table 1.1.

Traditionally the great majority of veterinary surgeons were male. Today there is an increasing proportion of female veterinary surgeons. In 2000, 34% of all veterinary surgeons were female, but this trend varies considerably depending upon age; 61% of veterinary surgeons aged 30 or under in 2000 were female while only 10% aged 60 or over were female. The dramatic increase in female veterinary surgeons (the 2001 intake of veterinary students to Bristol Veterinary School was 80% female) is likely to have a major impact on the management of veterinary practices. This will be discussed in more detail in Chapter 2, Factors affecting the change in structure of veterinary practice.

Table 1.1 Number of veterinary surgeons employed in practices (from Quo Vadis Survey 1998)

Number of vets employed in the practice	Percentage of practices
1–2	21
3–4	25
5–6	25
7–9	17
10–19	9
20+	2

Support staff and nurses

When the majority of veterinary practices were large animal or predominantly mixed, a relatively small number of support staff were required and many practices would consist of one or two veterinary surgeons, a nurse/receptionist and perhaps an administrative assistant. As veterinary practices became larger in size and small animal work increased, more support staff were needed to provide the services required by the small animal client. These support staff were multi-skilled members of the veterinary practice, working as receptionist, nurse and also carrying out many administrative duties. Their training was in-house and geared to the specific needs of the individual veterinary practice.

It was not until 1961 that a recognized training and examination programme was established for veterinary nurses by the RCVS and in 1963 the first qualified nurses, Registered Animal Nursing Auxiliaries (RANA), appeared and 1965 saw the formation of the British Animal Nursing Auxiliaries Association (BANAA). The title 'nurse' was at this time protected by law under the Nurses, Midwives and Health Visitors Act and it was not until 1984 that the RCVS was able to change the RANA title to Veterinary Nurse (VN). In the following year the BANNA became The British Veterinary Nursing Association (BVNA).

Veterinary nursing has gone from strength to strength and the BVNA membership is now over

2000. The VN role in veterinary practice is continually increasing in complexity and responsibility. The Schedule 3 amendment to the Veterinary Surgeons Act allowed nurses to carry out certain minor medical and surgical treatments to companion animals under the direction of a veterinary surgeon. In many practices nurses hold Pet Healthcare Clinics and some nurses now specialize in specific areas of veterinary nursing and take nursing diplomas – a far cry from the days of the nursing assistant and the single-handed veterinary surgeon.

The role of non-nursing staff has increased as veterinary practices have become larger, computerized and offered new and varied services. Theirs is a vital role in client care and communication and their value and potential is now far more appreciated than in the past. Non-nursing staff are also involved in the whole spectrum of veterinary support roles ranging from administration, bookkeeping, dispensing and secretarial work, to of course reception work, and while in the past veterinary practices would have employed only small numbers of these support staff, today the ratio of support staff to veterinary surgeons is usually in the region of 3 : 1.

Managers

Until the late 1980s, practices were generally managed by the owner or a partner. Support staff may have taken on basic administrative tasks and larger practices may have had bookkeepers, but the business and management side of the practice was the sole province of the veterinary surgeon.

As the world of business and commerce became more complicated, some larger practices began to employ Practice Managers and Administrators to take on the daily management tasks. This allowed the veterinary surgeon/owner to continue with their clinical responsibilities while delegating some management tasks but retaining ultimate control of the business.

In 1992 the Veterinary Practice Management Association (VPMA) was formed to promote quality management in veterinary practices and to provide an effective means of communication and interaction between those managing practices. The Association has blossomed over the last ten years and now has a membership of over 500.

The number of veterinary practices employing a manager or administrator has significantly increased over the last decade. Today few large or medium-sized practices are without some form of manager/administrator, responsible for the daily organization of the practice. The Quo Vadis Survey of 1998 recorded the presence of practice managers in veterinary practices. Four years on and the figures will have increased significantly. This is shown in Table 1.2.

We are living in an increasingly complex business and technical world: legislation, information technology, staffing and client needs all require considerable management. If veterinary practices are to thrive in the twenty-first century the only way forward will be through efficient and effective management strategies.

The clients

The structure of veterinary practice is dependent upon the clientele. Veterinary practice was established on a large animal client base, but as pet keeping increased and the farming recession deepened, the client base has altered to that of a companion animal-owning clientele with very

Table 1.2 The presence of practice managers in veterinary practices (from Quo Vadis Survey 1998)

	1–2 Vet practice	3–5 Vet practice	6+ Vet practice	Total
% with no practice manager	80	64	43	60
% with part-time practice manager	8	15	14	13
% with full-time practice manager	11	20	42	27

different needs and expectations from their veterinary surgeon. These new clients regard their pets as part of the family and are often willing to spend large sums of money for the treatment and service they require.

The explosion in pet keeping probably reached its peak in the late 1990s and we are now seeing a small but significant reduction in the number of companion animals in the UK. The increase in small animal veterinary practices in itself produced greater competition in the marketplace and now as the pet population is reduced so this competition will become more fierce and the needs and demands of clients will be the driving force in structuring the service the veterinary practice must provide. The days when clients looked upon the veterinary surgeon as the 'fount of all knowledge' have gone, the proliferation of veterinary TV programmes, websites and the internet have increased clients' knowledge and awareness of veterinary procedures and services. Clients of today and the future have and will have far greater demands on the profession than their parents or grandparents. Their expectations will be higher, both in clinical and customer service, and our veterinary practices will have to adapt and change to meet these needs. In addition those farming clients who do remain after the recession and BSE and FMD have taken their toll will continue to be even more cost-conscious, requesting discounts on drugs, something almost unheard-of before the late 1990s.

CHAPTER CONTENTS

External factors 11
Pet owners 11
The farming recession 12
The media 12
The pet industry 13
Legislation 13
Technology 13
Litigation 14
Competition 14

Internal factors 14
Veterinary knowledge 14
Attitudes of younger veterinary surgeons 14
Women in the profession 15
Support staff 15
Stress 15
Management skills 16

2

Factors affecting the change in structure of veterinary practice

There is no doubt that veterinary practice is changing, and we have already looked at the main structural changes there have been. The reasons for change are very complex and interconnected and although certain forces have played an important part, change has come about due to a combination of both internal and external factors, as shown in Figure 2.1.

EXTERNAL FACTORS

Pet owners

A new breed of pet-owning client has emerged over the last two decades, owners who see their pet as part of the family, who are more affluent, better informed and willing to spend relatively large amounts of money on their pet's health. The annual expenditure on veterinary fees in 1999 was £796 million and has been forecast to rise to £844 million by 2003.

This is a far cry from the pet owner who only brought their sick or injured pet to the veterinary surgeon and often requested euthanasia if the bill was going to be too high. The new generation of clients are more demanding and have higher expectations of veterinary care and service. This is often reinforced by the numerous veterinary TV programmes showing complex procedures and operations on clients' pets. Clients are more aware of pet healthcare and more discriminating about the service they receive. Veterinary practice has had to respond to this change by looking at the services it provides,

Figure 2.1 Factors affecting veterinary practice.

by increasing opening times, improving communication and employing well-trained support staff as well as delivering excellent clinical care.

The farming recession

BSE, which began in the 1980s and continued throughout the 1990s, seemed to set the trend for the downturn in livestock farming in the UK. Implementation of EU legislation on animal welfare cost the British farmer dear in the 1990s and almost every sector of livestock farming had begun to go into recession by the end of the twentieth century; 2001 then saw the recurrence of Foot and Mouth Disease, last seen in mainland UK in 1967. Many farmers could not sustain these economic strains and simply sold up or went out of business. The crisis in the farming industry had a great impact on large animal veterinary practice and many, seeing their clientele and income permanently reduced, turned to small animal work to supplement or replace their previous large animal income. This has resulted in an increase in the number of practices offering small animal services and consequently increased competition for a now static or declining pet market.

The media

The public's obsession and/or love of all things veterinary probably started with the James Herriot books of the 1960s and the TV series in the 1970s and 1980s. It has since blossomed with the help of numerous TV veterinary programmes and newspaper articles. Veterinary surgeons such as Trude Mostue have turned into superstars, and celebrities such as Rolf Harris host veterinary programmes. Veterinary practice now has a much higher profile than ever before and the 'real life' vet has to somehow live up to or live down this media coverage while

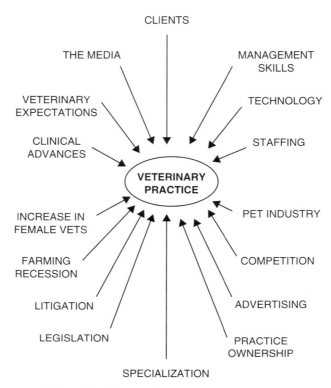

providing the kind of service the client now expects as the norm.

The pet industry

Over the last ten years pet superstores have proliferated and the pet food product sections of supermarkets have expanded. Gone are the days when two or three brands of cat and dog food were all that were to be seen on the shelves. Today choice is the watchword and pet owners are bombarded with shelves of colourful tins and packets of pet food as well as TV adverts extolling the virtues of specialist foods.

The internet is hosting an increasing number of on-line pet shops, all competing for what is still a relatively small market of internet users. Most small animal practices now provide pet care products in the form of prescription or lifestyle diets, pet toys, worming and flea products, books, shampoos and training toys. Some practices have pet healthcare centres attached to their premises with dedicated staff to advise clients on purchases while others have a more limited supply of products displayed and for sale in their reception areas.

The market for pet supplies is enormous, and although opinion differs among veterinary practitioners as to whether the sale of pet products in veterinary practices is unprofessional or an essential part of providing a total healthcare service to clients, the fact remains that it can be a great income generator.

Legislation

Veterinary practices like all other businesses are continually bombarded with new legislation from both the UK and the EU.

Since the 1970s there has been a constant stream of new legislation affecting both employers and employees. Veterinary practice administrators must keep up to date with and implement all new legislation and have in place procedures for legally complying with such areas as:

- contracts of employment
- race discrimination
- sex discrimination
- disability discrimination
- statutory sick pay and rights
- statutory maternity pay and rights
- redundancy procedures
- dismissal procedures
- minimum wage regulations
- working time regulations
- health and safety at work.

Complying with new legislation involves time, people and money. Setting up procedures and policies is very time-consuming, and also very costly in the case of health and safety legislation which involves carrying out risk assessments, ensuring employee health and safety, implementing COSHH (The Control of Substances Hazardous to Health Regulations), and ensuring safe waste disposal. Implementing such legislation is a specialist role and is one usually designated to the practice managers as part of their job description.

Technology

The technology revolution has had a profound effect on veterinary practice. The use of computers in the veterinary practice for client records, appointments, accounting and payroll administration is now widespread, and there are an increasing number of veterinary computer suppliers providing constantly more sophisticated versions of software packages for use in the practice.

Computer technology has revolutionized the use of data in veterinary practice and supplies the tools for providing vast quantities of information for use in marketing. Quality, computer-generated, in-house production of leaflets and literature, newsletters and displays is now commonplace and few adverts for veterinary staff do not have a requirement for computer skills. The typewriter is now virtually redundant and word processing is used for all letter and document production.

The internet has provided a new and fast way of communicating with clients, suppliers and colleagues. Many practices now have their own websites advertising the practice, its services and products, with some having an attached on-line 'pet shop' from which clients may order pet food and products. Clients can now be e-mailed about pet information and booster reminders, and in turn can e-mail the practice with queries. Increasingly, computers and the internet are being used for the provision of CPD (Continuing Professional Development). A variety of CD Roms are now on the market and the internet is becoming a huge source of clinical information as well as being used directly for veterinary and support staff training. For a profession where finding time for training is always problematical, this aspect of IT growth has been revolutionary.

Litigation

We are sadly now in a world where litigation is becoming more common. The 'blame' factor seems to predominate in society and this is reflected in veterinary clientele. The Veterinary Defence Society (VDS) dealt with 700 claims against veterinary practices in 1999 and the number of veterinary surgeons telephoning for advice rose threefold between 1999 and 2001. One of the major concerns now voiced by new graduates is their fear of being sued by clients.

Suing for a perceived or real lack of clinical care is still the commonest area for litigation, but injury to clients on the practice premises is also now becoming an issue. Clients who slip on wet floors or trip in the practice car park are far more likely to claim against the practice public liability insurance.

Competition

Veterinary practice is experiencing greater competition for clients than ever before. The increase in small animal practices and reduction in the pet population has meant more practices competing for fewer clients. Added to this is the emergence of corporate and large group practices, many of which are financed by non-veterinary investment. These may be perceived or real threats, but have resulted in many practices rapidly re-thinking and improving their marketing and advertising strategies. The professional attitude to advertising is quickly changing as competition begins to bite; not many years ago the only 'advertising' carried out by the majority of practices would have been an advert in Yellow Pages, and real marketing was deemed unnecessary. Today, marketing and new ways of advertising are on the mind of every managing partner or practice manager.

INTERNAL FACTORS

Veterinary knowledge

The rapid increase in clinical knowledge, surgical techniques, treatment and drugs makes keeping up to date time-consuming, and CPD essential. As knowledge increases there is a trend towards specialization, mirroring the medical profession consultants and general practitioners.

The availability of new drugs and techniques makes it possible to prolong the life of a sick or injured animal, but at a financial cost to the client and sometimes to the quality of life for the pet. New clinical knowledge has brought with it the dilemma of the two-tier treatment system: basic treatment and life saving at a basic price, or the complete medical or surgical package, blood tests, X-rays, operations, and expensive medication at a much higher cost to the client. This choice can be very difficult to make both for clients with limited funds and for vets who wish to do all that is possible for the pet.

Attitudes of younger veterinary surgeons

New and recently qualified graduates have very different expectations from a career in veterinary practice than their older colleagues. Younger vets are looking for quality time to spend with family and friends and wish to pursue outside interests away from the veterinary practice. Nor are the traditional high levels of on-call and night duty any longer acceptable. Another important change is the attitude of younger vets towards partnerships and a financial commitment to a practice. The modern graduate is generally less likely to want, or be able to afford, a traditional partnership in veterinary practice. Add to this the desire for more job mobility, especially as partners/spouses are also likely to have career choices to make, and today's young vet can be seen as having a very different set of requirements to those of even ten years ago.

The emergence of corporate practices and their offers of joint venturing to veterinary surgeons may be one of the more attractive paths that the new generation of vets, wishing to make a degree of realistic commitment to a practice, may take.

Women in the profession

Figures quoted earlier illustrate the dramatic increase in the number of qualifying female veterinary surgeons. Figures show that female vets have significantly different requirements from their employment than their male counterparts, the three main requirements being:

- a preference for part-time working
- more career breaks
- earlier retirement.

This poses a challenge for veterinary practice. A larger part-time workforce makes it more difficult to maintain continuity of service and organize out-of-hours rotas, as well as there being additional labour costs per hour worked and an increase in administration. More career breaks and early retirement can lead to staffing shortages and recruitment difficulties. The staffing requirements will rise as the profession becomes increasingly female and part-time work becomes the norm. As the number of female vets rises so the number of graduates required to satisfy the veterinary workload will also increase. Christine Sheild, in her talk at the SPVS, VBD, VPMA Management Day at BSAVA in April 2001, estimated that for a 75% female veterinary profession an extra 40% new graduates would be required in order to supply the staffing needs resulting from part-time work.

Support staff

Veterinary support staff are now appreciated as important members of the veterinary practice team. Nurses are becoming more highly qualified, and Schedule 3 has enabled them to take a greater role in the clinical and medical aspects of animal care. Receptionists can make or break the relationship of clients with a practice; their role is critical to the efficient and effective running of the veterinary surgery and the need for good receptionist training programs is now recognized.

Veterinary practices employ many more support staff than they used to even 20 years ago, due to the increase in small animal work and the recognition of the value of the non-veterinary staff member. Well-trained and qualified support staff are a great asset to veterinary practice and can improve the standards of client care dramatically. However, good quality staff come at a financial cost to the practice and support staff salaries are now a significant part of the practice salaries bill.

Stress

Veterinary surgeons now have the highest suicide rate of all the professions. They work in a stressful environment and have to contend with the constant pressures of clinical work and demands from owners. The combination of a busy day's consulting or surgery together with the ever-increasing administration involved in working in a veterinary surgery can become just too stressful for some. Add to this the young graduate's worry of litigation, the financial pressure on a partner or the stress of the large animal vet dealing with farmers experiencing financial problems and the loss of their stock, and it is not surprising that veterinary stress levels are high. In many cases it is for these reasons that partners have taken on Practice Managers who can deal with the administrative and management aspects of the practice, removing at least this area of stress.

Work-related stress is now recognized as a health and safety risk by the Health and Safety

Executive. There is no such thing as a stress-free job and some pressures can be a good thing, but an individual's ability to deal with pressure varies and must be assessed and danger signals monitored. The RCVS now runs a confidential Veterinary Helpline for veterinary surgeons who have emotional, addictive or financial problems or for vets worried about colleagues who have.

Management skills

One of the results of these internal and external factors affecting veterinary practice has been the increase in the quality of veterinary practice management. Veterinary practices are small and medium-sized businesses, in many cases turning over £1 million plus a year, and this demands efficient and effective management.

As the business environment has become increasingly complex and as competition has increased, it has become increasingly difficult for partners with clinical roles in their practice to fulfil the practice management needs as well. The mid 1980s saw the appointment of the first practice managers and in 1992 the Veterinary Practice Management Association was established to aid and promote quality management in veterinary practice. Today the VPMA has a membership comprising vets, managers and administrative and nursing staff, all of whom play a role in the management of veterinary practice.

The success of veterinary practices in the future will depend as much on the skills of the people managing them as the clinical skills of the veterinary surgeons. Management skills such as communication, marketing, strategic planning, client care and human resource management will need to be practised alongside the clinical skills of the veterinary surgeon.

Veterinary practitioners are facing some of the greatest changes to their profession ever experienced, whether it be client pressure to open later, new computer systems to install and websites to set up, more legislation to contend with, the purchase of new state-of-the-art veterinary equipment or the competition from a new corporate practice. Change needs to be understood and managed and turned into opportunity, rather than perceived as a threat. It can seem very threatening and resistance is natural, but the veterinary practice needs to be a proactive not reactive business and flexible enough to accept and respond positively to the veterinary challenges of the twenty-first century.

CHAPTER CONTENTS

Management of practices in the twentieth century 17

The veterinary practice as a business 19

Management of practices in the twenty-first century 19

3

The management of veterinary practices

MANAGEMENT OF PRACTICES IN THE TWENTIETH CENTURY

Business management is a concept which has come late to many in the veterinary world, but veterinary practices have always been 'managed' consciously or unconsciously by the veterinary surgeons who own them.

It is only relatively recently that large multi-site practices have emerged on the veterinary scene. Historically most practices were single-site or perhaps with one or two part-time branch surgeries. The management of these single-site practices was usually undertaken by the owner or senior partner, with some delegation of tasks to support or administrative staff. Traditionally these tasks would have been those such as book-keeping, banking, payroll, client accounts, etc. as shown in Figure 3.1.

In the larger practices with perhaps one or two branch surgeries a little more formal management was often employed. In these practices partnerships were more common and in many cases each, or at least some, of the partners would take responsibility for a certain area of practice management, such as drug purchase and stock control, mentoring assistant veterinary surgeons, the branch surgeries, etc., while the senior partner acted as the main managing partner delegating tasks to an administrative assistant who latterly, as they took on more responsibilities, began to be called a practice manager. This is illustrated in Figure 3.2.

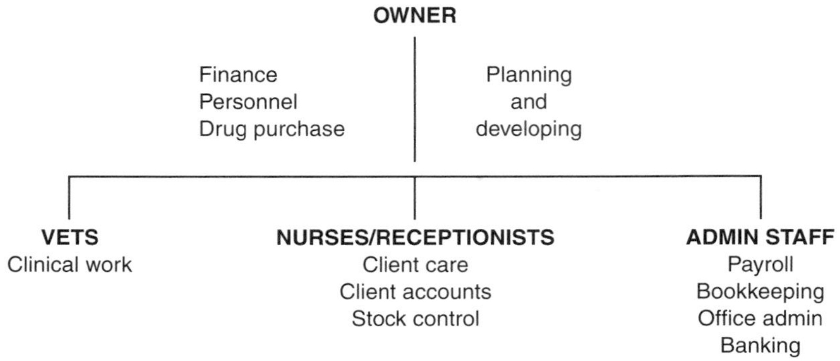

Figure 3.1 Traditional management in a small veterinary practice.

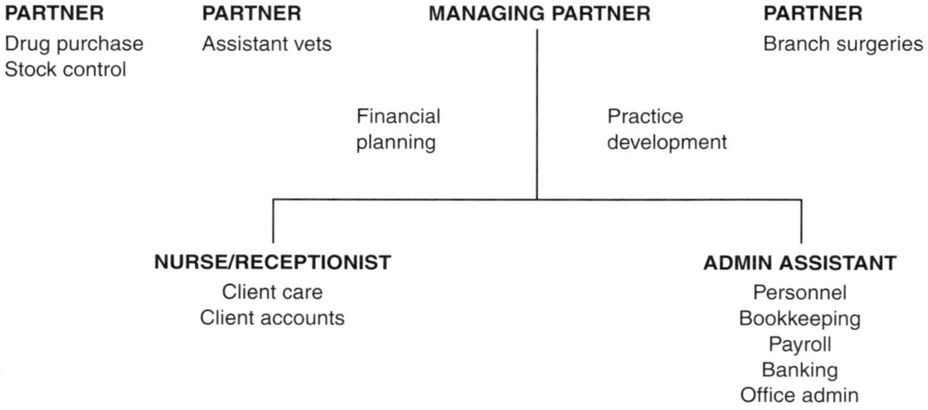

Figure 3.2 Traditional management in larger veterinary practices.

These systems of practice management were generally successful for the following reasons:

- Clients were less demanding of the practice.
- Most emphasis was placed on clinical skills and services, an area where the owner/partner was clearly highly qualified.
- Practices were smaller with fewer staff to manage.
- The size of the practice and its low staff numbers enabled good communication and teamwork.
- The owner/partner was able to remain fully in touch with the daily running of the practice.
- Complying with health and safety and other legislation was not so onerous.
- No serious marketing plans or sales strategies were required, as at that time practices to a very large extent simply sold themselves and there was less competition for clients.
- The complex world of IT had not yet arrived.
- Most practices were financially successful regardless of the management techniques adopted, and although they could probably have been more profitable if some of today's marketing skills had been employed, they still provided a more than adequate living for the owners.

THE VETERINARY PRACTICE AS A BUSINESS

As Veterinary Practice Management emerged as a distinct activity within the profession, it was often claimed that 'Veterinary practice is just a business and should be managed like any other'. Many within the profession disagreed, however, and 'That won't work in veterinary practice' was a frequent comment on the initial introduction of business management techniques.

It is now recognized that many aspects of business management are common to most organizations. Many areas of veterinary practice management have similarities with various trade and professional groups, such as:

- healthcare professions (dentists, opticians, GPs)
- other professions (accountants, lawyers, architects)
- service industries (hotels, hairdressers)
- retail outlets (pet shops, agricultural merchants)
- emergency/service trades (motor mechanic, plumber).

These similarities encompass aspects of general business management such as business structure, client care, stock control, employment, marketing, and financial management, as well as more specific issues such as pharmacy management, coping with client grief, and out of hours work.

Another issue, which challenged the place of management in veterinary practices, was whether it is appropriate for a 'caring' profession to be concerned with profits. Business ethics is an issue which concerns all organizations, from large multinationals down to sole traders. Finding the correct balance between the needs of the business owners, employees, customers, competitors, suppliers and the environment is not always easy.

Whilst the core purpose of veterinary practices is the treatment and alleviation of suffering of animals under the veterinary surgeon's care, the generation of profits is essential for the continued success of this objective. It is a fact of life in the business world that most things come down to money in the end. Failure to manage the business properly will have a detrimental effect on employees' working conditions and standards of premises and equipment. Ultimately this will compromise patient care. Poor profitability leads to lack of reinvestment in the business, or closure of the business altogether.

Profits only become unethical when they become out of proportion to the amount of time and investment spent generating them, or are made for the sole benefit of the business owners with no regard or concern for others. The combination of free competition in the marketplace, veterinary ethics and consumer group pressure should be sufficient to guard against this happening in the veterinary world. It will be a long time before we see veterinary practice owners targeted as 'industrial fat cats'.

MANAGEMENT OF PRACTICES IN THE TWENTY-FIRST CENTURY

Twenty-first century practice management is by necessity more focused on specific areas of management. The veterinary business world is more complex and competitive, and the need for effective and efficient management is of greater importance than in the past and the concepts of 'everyone manages' and delegation with empowerment are becoming more common.

Broadly speaking, today's veterinary management can be divided into:

- information technology
- human resources
- finance
- marketing and sales
- general office management
- health and safety.

Each of these areas is becoming increasingly complex and time-consuming for whoever has the responsibility of management in the practice. If we take just one of the above examples – human resources – we can see in Table 3.1 how management input in this area has changed.

Add to this the fact that for most practices there has been a significant increase in staff numbers, which in itself engenders extra work, and it can be seen how the management burden has increased.

Table 3.1 Human resource management

Past management input	Present management input
Recruitment	Recruitment
Training on the job	Induction training
Rotas	Lifelong learning/training
Discipline	Appraisals
Salaries	Employment legislation
	CDP
	Discipline
	Job descriptions
	Contracts of employment
	Staff health and safety
	Rotas
	Coaching and mentoring

Although the traditional small practices with owner managers are still relatively common, there is a trend towards the empowerment of managers and administrators to oversee daily, general and often specific areas of veterinary practice management.

In the small practice the owner is still taking responsibility for many of the management tasks, while delegating many of the new management roles such as health and safety to administrative assistants. Owners are much more aware of the need to actively and pro-actively manage their practices, and increasingly find that practice management roles take up more and more of their clinical time, as shown in Figure 3.3.

Larger practices are increasingly employing a practice manager or administrator who has experience in the management of a veterinary practice or other small business. This allows the partners to continue to practise veterinary medicine rather than spend less financially-productive time as managers. The manager is responsible for the daily management of the practice, often delegating a significant number of administrative tasks to other members of the practice, as illustrated in Figure 3.4. This delegation serves to reinforce the present day concept of 'everyone manages' – i.e. everyone has a share in the management/administration of the practice as well as carrying out their other daily routine tasks.

Multi-site practices have grown too large to enable management control by a single manager and the management format shown in Figure 3.5 is often employed, where there is a specific manager for each management area who is responsible for all the practice sites. This system allows expertise in each management area and consistency in business planning.

At the time of writing the management of the corporate veterinary practice is still uncertain but the scenario in Figure 3.6 is a likely one. Here the veterinary surgeons who have invested in joint venturing schemes run and manage their practices on a daily basis, while sourcing

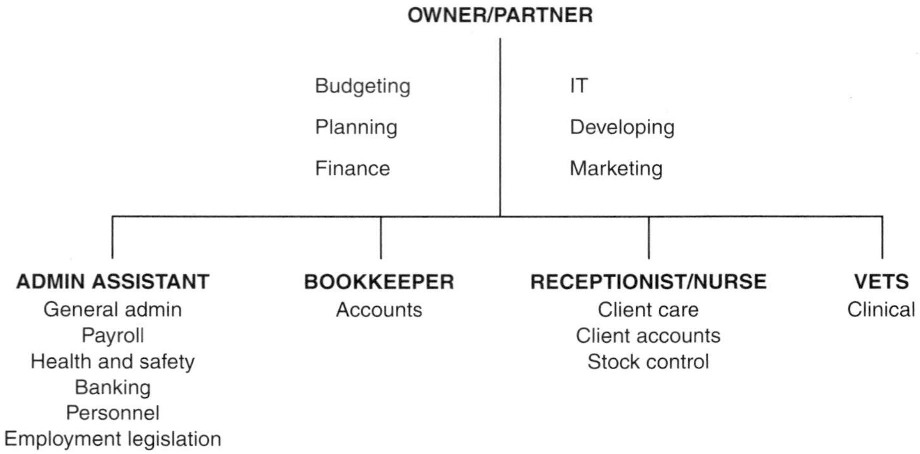

Figure 3.3 Present-day management of a small veterinary practice.

management skills from the corporate body. The main advantage to the individual vet of this system is that the purchase of management expertise should be cheaper when bought from the corporate than purchased individually, and is easily available.

There are of course many variations on the types of management systems just described, but what is for certain is that in the twenty-first century all veterinary practices will need to be effectively managed if they are to survive in today's more competitive marketplace.

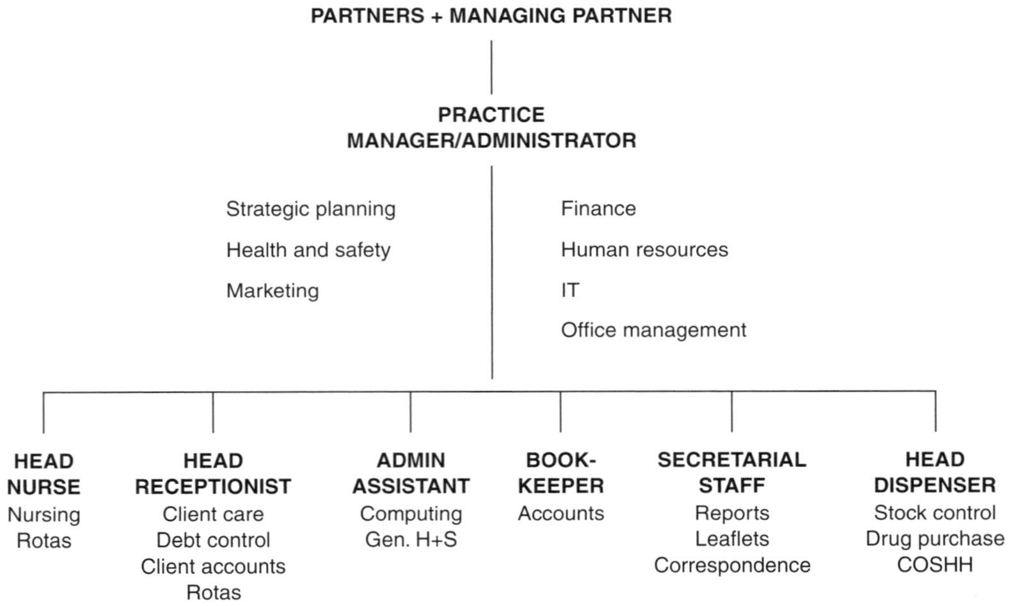

Figure 3.4 Present-day management of a large practice.

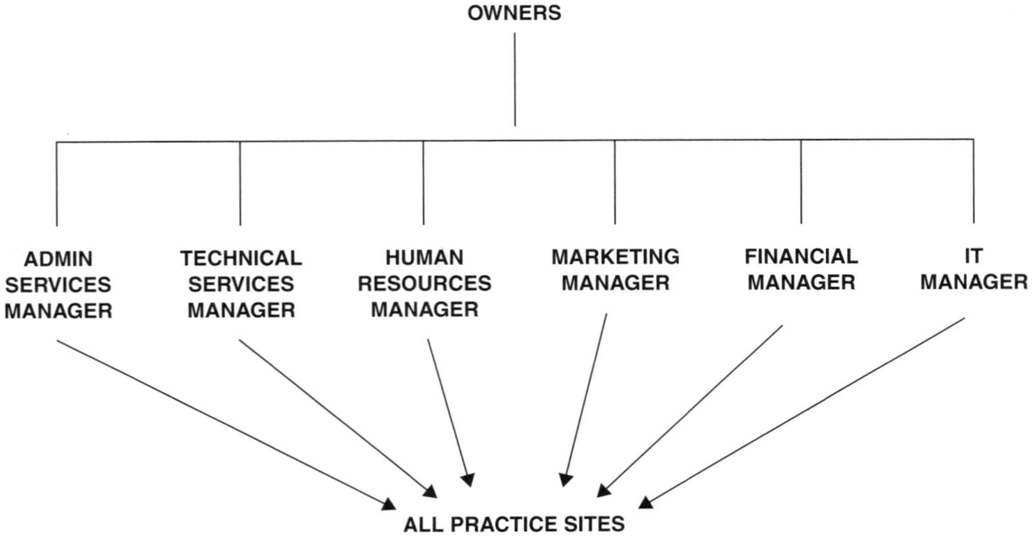

Figure 3.5 Present-day management of a large multi-site practice.

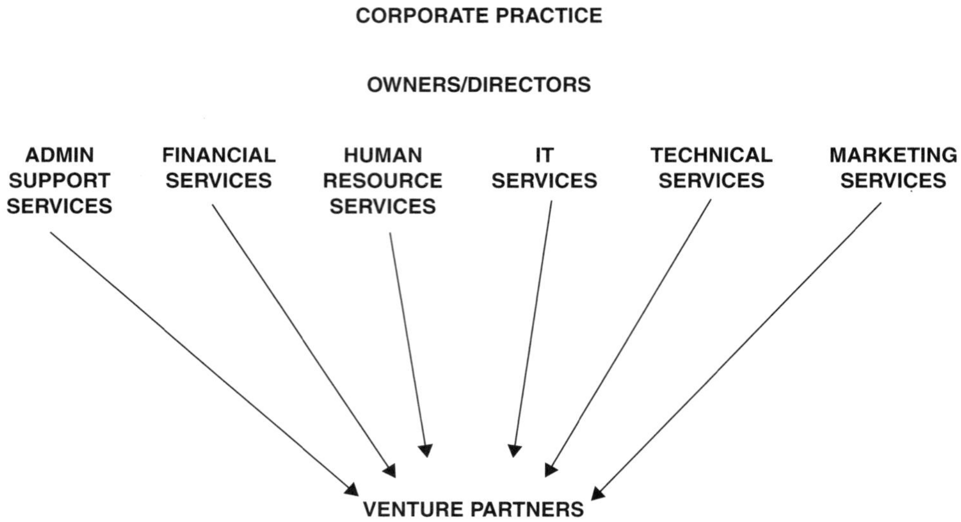

Figure 3.6 Likely management of corporate/joint venture practices.

CHAPTER CONTENTS

Today's practice managers 23

The role of a practice manager 24
General management 25
Human resource management 25
Financial management 26
Health and safety management 26
IT management 26
Marketing, services and sales management 27

Real-life managers 27

The changing role of the practice manager 28

4 What is a veterinary practice manager?

This is a much more difficult question than it might at first appear. Managers in most small and medium-sized businesses have a clearly defined role and anyone applying for a post as a manager would have a good understanding of the tasks of job he/she is applying for before they receive the job description. This is often not the case in veterinary practice. The manager's role varies greatly between practices, and the title Practice Manager can cover a multitude of sins. This is however changing, and the manager's role becoming better defined as the part a manager can play in the practice becomes better understood.

In this chapter we will look at:

1. who today's practice managers are and their backgrounds
2. what role a practice manager can take in veterinary practice
3. what some real-life managers actually do in their practices
4. how the role of practice manager is changing.

TODAY'S PRACTICE MANAGERS

Practice managers in veterinary practice today come from a variety of backgrounds. The practice may be managed by the owner or senior partner, who have had years of experience running their veterinary practice. These managers take overall responsibility for both the clinical aspects and management of the business.

In some cases the manager comes from a nursing background and may have been a Head Nurse who has been promoted to a management role, taking responsibility for human resources, stock control, health and safety and so on.

In many instances a long-standing member of the administrative or office staff is given an increasing management workload and promoted to become a Practice Manager, overseeing the daily running of the practice and taking responsibility for human resources, accounts, office management, etc.

Some practices recruit a practice manager from outside the profession or from the small but growing band of managers holding the Certificate in Veterinary Practice Management (CVPM). These managers will usually take on full responsibility for management of the practice, including strategic and financial planning, and delegate many of the general administrative tasks to others.

The qualifications and experience of practice managers varies tremendously, from those who have years of experience in veterinary practice administration but few academic or professional qualifications, to the highly-qualified manager with a certificate, diploma or degree in management. In between these two is the whole spectrum of education and experience.

Practice management in veterinary practice is a relatively new discipline, with little career structure or recognized/agreed qualifications, and to a large extent this is why the qualifications of managers are so variable at the present time.

THE ROLE OF A PRACTICE MANAGER

The role of a practice manager is to enable the good management of the veterinary practice so that the owner or partners can continue to carry out their clinical functions without the need to devote too much expensive time to management.

There is an old phrase, 'What's in a name?' and it certainly applies to those who manage veterinary practices in the UK. Below are just a few of the job titles given to those who have this responsibility:

- Practice Manager
- Practice Administrator
- Practice Secretary
- Office Manager
- Administration Manager
- Clinic Manager
- General Manager
- Group Administrator
- Operations Manager
- Practice Co-ordinator
- Practice Development Manager
- Business Manager.

In essence all these individuals will carry out a very similar role, but the variation in their titles is confusing, especially for those looking for employment in veterinary management.

There is also still a certain degree of confusion in the profession as to the role of a Veterinary Practice Manager and there are many individuals who have the title of 'manager' but the responsibilities of an administrator.

Everyone in the practice has a role to play in its administration; it may be the nurse who draws up rotas, the Head Receptionist who supervises reception services, the Head Nurse who organizes nursing services to the veterinary team, the person responsible for drug selection, the bookkeeper who does the accounts or the receptionist who deals with debt control. The list is almost endless. These are the administrators. The manager organizes and oversees many of these tasks and the people carrying them out. Generally the difference between the administrator and the manager is that the administrator does the task while the manager organizes its doing.

The practical role of the Veterinary Practice Manager can be divided into six main areas:

- general management
- human resource management
- financial management
- health and safety management
- IT management
- marketing services and sales management.

A full-time practice manager in a medium-sized practice may well have responsibility for all these areas, while in a very large multi-site practice there may be managers for each area.

The responsibilities involved in these six areas of management may include a wide variety, as listed below.

General management

• *Daily office organization:* managing the day-to-day running of the office/admin tasks of the practice, organizing paperwork, the provision of office equipment such as the faxes, telephone systems and franking machines, dealing with incoming post, etc.

• *General purchasing:* purchasing office equipment and stationery, and stock control of office supplies. Ordering protective clothing, uniforms and domestic items. Controlling petty cash.

• *Equipment lease, purchase, hire, maintenance and servicing:* researching and organizing leasing and hiring agreements for equipment and cars. Organizing servicing of equipment and maintenance contracts.

• *Building fabric:* building maintenance and repairs, car park, gardens, fabric of building and fixtures and fittings.

• *Banking:* organizing/overseeing cashing-up procedures, ensuring money is banked on banking days, maintaining banking records.

• *Client accounts:* overseeing the production and sending of client accounts.

• *Debt control:* responsibility for administering practice debt control policy. Overseeing the administration of debt control either internally or externally if debt collection agencies are used. Putting into place procedures to reduce client debtors.

• *Client complaints:* dealing with client complaints received by letter, by telephone or in person, and handling complaints passed on from reception. Clinical complaints would be referred on to a veterinary surgeon.

• *Policies, protocols and procedures:* drafting of practice policies, protocols and procedures and their distribution to staff. Monitoring how well policies and protocols are followed.

• *Staff manual:* production and maintenance of staff manual.

• *Internal communications:* ensuring good internal staff communications by use of appropriate communication methods such as staff newsletters, meetings, memos, etc.

• *Rotas:* production and maintenance of staff rotas.

• *Ethical and statutory requirements:* sound knowledge and administration of relevant veterinary ethics (professional conduct, confidentiality, etc.) statutory requirements (relevant government legislation applying to the veterinary profession, e.g. Medicines Act, Health and Safety Act, animal movements, etc.).

• *Security:* ensuring building security (burglary and fire) and drug security for scheduled drugs.

Human resource management

• *Implementing employment legislation:* knowledge of current employment legislation and responsibility for putting this into practice.

• *Staff recruitment and selection:* advertising, interviewing and selecting new staff.

• *Job descriptions:* production of job descriptions for all staff and keeping job descriptions up to date.

• *Contracts of employment:* drawing up contracts of employment for staff.

• *Staff induction:* designing and implementing induction training for all new staff.

• *Appraisals:* designing appraisal schemes for practice staff, implementing and monitoring appraisals.

• *Staff training:* design and provision of staff training schemes. Monitoring and evaluating training on a regular basis.

- *Staff motivation and teamwork:* encouraging and developing staff motivation and teamwork.
- *Staff discipline:* monitoring staff discipline, carrying out disciplinary proceedings and maintaining appropriate records.
- *Payroll:* administration of staff payroll, payment of salaries and record keeping.
- *Sickness/holiday monitoring:* monitoring staff holiday, sickness and absence leave, keeping records and reviewing staff absence rates.

Financial management

- *End of year accounts:* production of end of year accounts as computerized or manual records for practice accountants.
- *Monthly financial report production:* generation of monthly financial reports such as profit and loss for use in financial monitoring and planning.
- *Financial and business planning:* acting with the partners to produce financial and business plans for the practice.
- *Financial trend analysis:* analysing financial information to identify practice trends.
- *Cash flow and bank account management:* monitoring and controlling cash flow, managing the practice bank accounts.
- *Administering practice insurances, vehicle, premises and personnel:* liaising with insurance companies to obtain the best insurances for the practice. Administering insurance claims.
- *Drug purchase:* control of drug purchase, ensuring best drug discounts, liaising with drug wholesalers and drug companies.
- *Stock control:* maintenance of drug stock control applying efficient stock control methods; stock taking.
- *Monitoring/controlling equipment purchase:* using financial information and planning to monitor and control the cost of purchasing new equipment.
- *Liaising with practice accountant, bank, insurers and solicitors:* keeping up to date with accounting, banking, insurance and legal situation of the practice by liaising with the relevant companies.

Health and safety management

- *Implementation of all health and safety legislation:* maintaining up-to-date knowledge of all current health and safety legislation and requirements. Implementing the necessary legislation.
- *COSHH:* administering COSHH, monitoring and reviewing procedures and systems.
- *Carrying out risk assessments:* responsible for carrying out risk assessments in the required health and safety areas. Monitoring and reviewing procedures and systems.
- *Fire regulations:* ensuring all fire regulations are adhered to and necessary equipment provided.
- *First aid and RIDDOR:* ensuring first aid training and provision, complying with RIDDOR and maintaining a practice accident book.
- *Drawing up and implementing safe working procedures:* production of safe working procedures for practice staff.
- *Waste disposal:* ensuring practice compliance with waste disposal regulations.
- *Health and safety staff training:* organizing and implementing health and safety training for all staff on an on-going basis.

IT management

- *Organization and maintenance of the practice computer systems:* overall responsibility for the operation, maintenance and use of the practice computer system.
- *Working knowledge of hardware and software:* good general knowledge of veterinary software and the type of hardware required by the practice.

• *IT troubleshooting:* ability to carry out basic computer trouble shooting maintenance and solve simple problems associated with the practice computer system.

• *Assessment of veterinary software programs:* working knowledge of types of veterinary software programs and providers so that assessment and comparison of software available can be made.

• *Website production and maintenance:* setting up or organizing the setting up and maintenance of a practice website.

• *Generation and management of computerized and financial information:* design of input of financial information. Ability to generate relevant financial details from the computer database to use for practice planning.

• *Liaising with software and hardware companies:* general liaison with computer companies, for purchasing, back-up and helpline.

• *Computer training:* organizing computer training for practice staff. Assessment of training needs.

Marketing, services and sales management

• *Developing marketing strategies:* together with the partners, planning, developing and implementing new strategies for marketing the practice and its services.

• *Target marketing planning:* identification of target markets within the practice and exploiting their potential.

• *Setting up/overseeing new services:* designing and planning new services the practice can provide. Facilitating the setting up of these new services.

• *Promoting new services:* promoting new services by the provision of literature/displays, etc. Liaising with the media and providing information for clients.

• *Overseeing production of client communication materials:* organizing the production and distribution of client communication materials such as newsletters, booster reminders, displays, open day material, newspaper articles, etc.

• *Client surveying:* design of client surveys, overseeing their administration, analysis of and action on the results.

• *Advertising policies and procedures:* production and implementation of advertising policies.

• *Media liaison:* responsibility for liaising/communicating with local and national media, designing practice guidelines for dealing with the media.

• *Public relations:* administering the practice public relations policies and maintaining good public relations at all times.

• *Managing product and services sales strategies:* devising sales strategies and implementing and overseeing new sales initiatives.

This is by no means a fully comprehensive list but gives a flavour of the responsibilities a practice manager may be required to undertake. Obviously no one person can carry out all the duties listed above, but they would be expected take responsibility for them, delegating tasks where appropriate.

REAL-LIFE MANAGERS

We have looked at management roles in veterinary practice and certainly there are an increasing number of managers whose responsibilities fit the above model. However, it is important to realize that the role and responsibilities of managers are still very variable.

A Salary Survey carried out by the VPMA in 2000 also asked managers to list information on type and size of practice, number of staff, their qualifications/experience, time in post, and their job responsibilities. Below are some of the replies.

PROFILE 1

Title: Practice manager
Staff: 10 nurses, 5 receptionists, 6 veterinary surgeons
Type of practice: Equine
Size of practice: 4 sites
Job responsibilities: Asset management, Health and safety, Office management, Marketing, Some financial management
Qualifications/experience: CVPM, CMS, 15 years experience in office administration
Years in the veterinary profession: 8 years

PROFILE 2

Title: Practice manager
Staff: 42 support staff, 11 veterinary surgeons
Type of practice: Small animal, equine and exotics
Size of practice: 4 sites
Job responsibilities: Human resources, Health and safety, Some financial management, Sales and marketing, IT
Qualifications/experience: 15 years experience in customer services outside the veterinary profession
Years in the veterinary profession: 8 years

PROFILE 3

Title: Practice manager
Staff: 4 vets, 4 nurses, 3 support staff
Type of practice: Mixed
Size of practice: 2 sites
Job responsibilities: Bookkeeping, General office management, IT
Qualifications/experience: A levels, previous experience public relations and advertising manager
Years in the veterinary profession: 28

PROFILE 4

Title: Practice manager
Staff: 12 vets, 11 nurses, 20 support staff
Type of practice: Mixed
Size of practice: 4 sites
Job responsibilities: Bookkeeping, Marketing, Personnel, Financial planning
Qualifications/experience: Always worked in the practice
Years in the veterinary profession: 40

PROFILE 5

Title: Practice manager
Staff: 6 vets, 7 nurses, 6 support staff
Type of practice: Mixed
Size of practice: 2 sites
Job responsibilities: Personnel, Financial planning, Bookkeeping, General office management
Qualifications/experience: Administration officer
Years in the veterinary profession: 4

PROFILE 6

Title: Practice manager
Staff: 6 vets, 10 nurses, 6 support staff
Type of practice: Small animal
Size of practice: 4 sites
Job responsibilities: General office management, Personnel, Financial planning, Marketing
Qualifications/experience: NVQ Level 5 in management, training officer in HM Forces (Army)
Years in the veterinary profession: 6 months

The survey illustrates well how varied practice managers' roles, qualifications and experience can be at the present time.

While some individuals carry out a fairly comprehensive management role, others only have limited management responsibilities. We are all fairly clear what would be expected of a receptionist, nurse or veterinary surgeon in practice; this is often not the case with the practice manager.

Qualifications and experience also vary greatly, from the manager who has no formal qualifications, but has worked in the veterinary profession for 40 years, to the public relations and customer services officers and the CVPM holder.

The type and size of practice differ considerably as do the number of personnel the manager is responsible for, with one manager having responsibility for 53 staff and another for 11.

THE CHANGING ROLE OF THE PRACTICE MANAGER

Management in veterinary practice is being seen as a more important function than in the past. This management needs to carried out in a professional manner in order to be effective. Increasingly, many veterinary practices are looking to employ qualified or experienced managers to run their practices. The number of managers holding the CVPM increases each year and the qualification is regarded by the profession as a benchmark of quality in veterinary management.

Business managers from outside the veterinary profession are also being employed in increasing numbers and they bring with them experience from other professions and disciplines.

As practices increase in size, management roles are becoming more specialized and the role of the general manager for these practices may become a thing of the past. The Practice Manager is slowly but surely becoming a 'real' manager as opposed to an assistant or administrator, not involved in decision making or policy formulation.

Management is now being taught as part of the Veterinary Nursing Degree, and more veterinary nurses as well as administrative staff are looking to move into management roles.

With time the practice management function is likely to become more uniform and managers better qualified to manage. The four key areas of change are likely to be:

- better qualified managers
- more defined management role
- more management specialization as practices increase in size
- more responsibility for managers.

CHAPTER CONTENTS

Managing your job 31
What are you supposed to be doing? 31
How well are you doing it? 32
What are you going to do next? 34

Managing your time 34
Personal time management 34
Delegation 39

Yourself 42
Mental and physical well-being 42
Stress 42

5

Managing yourself

Every veterinary practice is unique. Consequently, every practice manager's job description and work pattern will be slightly different. You may be full-time, part-time, an administrator, overall manager, financial manager or stock controller. You may be an employee or a managing partner. But before you can effectively manage any aspect of the practice, you need to make sure you can manage yourself.

This involves managing:

- your job – responsibilities, performance, progression and ambitions
- your time – organization of work priorities, delegation and planning
- yourself – maintaining a stress-free body and mind.

MANAGING YOUR JOB

Job satisfaction does not simply happen. You need to actively work towards a well-defined job role, assess your performance, recognize your ambitions and plan your future progress.

What are you supposed to be doing?

Uncertainty over roles is a common cause of job dissatisfaction. Many first-time employers of practice managers do not have a clear idea of what they want their manager to do, or even what a manager can do. This can lead to real frustrations for both manager and employer later on.

- If you don't know the extent of your responsibility and authority, how can you decide what to do?
- If you don't know what you are supposed to be doing, how can you decide if you are doing it well?

Managing partners need to ensure that the other business partners and employees understand the balance of management and veterinary work undertaken. If this is not made clear, then there is the risk that practice members might think you are not pulling your weight in the practice.

Joining a new practice is a chance to start off with a well-defined role. It is vital to have clear agreement about what the job entails: this should be discussed at your job interview. Don't be afraid to ask your prospective employers what duties and responsibilities they want their new manager to have. If you get the answer, 'Well, you know, just manage the place', then be warned! In this case it might be a good idea to provide a potential job description for the employer to look through. You might find it helpful to use a checklist like the one shown in Figure 5.1, which is based on the management responsibilities listed in Chapter 4, 'What is a veterinary practice manager?'

Misunderstandings over job roles can mean some managers are expected to be responsible for aspects of the practice over which they are given no authority to act. For example, being expected to improve profitability without being allowed to see details of the partnership accounts! Setting out your expectations at interview will highlight any potential problems in this area.

If you are already employed, but feel you have unclear or contradictory job roles, then ask your employer for a meeting to clarify the situation. Chapter 22, 'Who should do the managing?', gives more details about allocating the management functions within a practice, and some pitfalls to avoid. Job descriptions are covered in detail in Chapter 7, 'Managing human resources – recruitment'.

How well are you doing it?

Everybody needs feedback on how they are performing in their job – both from the point of motivation, and addressing mistakes. As practice manager you need to ensure that you are getting accurate, honest feedback on your role in the practice. This can be from two routes:

- assessment by others (practice owners, colleagues and staff)
- self-assessment.

Management task	**Person responsible**		
Human resource management	***Manager***	***Owner***	***Other***
Implementing employment legislation	✓		
Staff recruitment and selection		✓	
Job descriptions	✓		
Contracts of employment			✓ Solicitor
Staff induction	✓		
Appraisals	✓		
Staff training	✓		✓ Head Nurse
Staff motivation and teamwork	✓		✓ Head Nurse
Staff discipline		✓	
Payroll			✓ Bookkeeper
Sickness/holiday monitoring	✓		

Figure 5.1 Extract from a management responsibility checklist.

Before you or anyone else can judge how well you are doing, it is vital to know what you are supposed to be doing, and what goals you are working towards.

Performance assessment by others is generally achieved using some form of appraisal system. Even if there is not a formal practice-wide appraisal system set up, you can develop one for yourself. If there is an appraisal system in the practice, make sure it extends to the management roles as well as the rest of the employees. Appraisal systems are covered in Chapter 10, 'Human resources – training and appraisals'.

Self-assessment of performance is often a continuous subconscious activity, contributing to your feelings of self-worth. 'I feel good because I managed that grievance well,' or 'I really should have been able to reduce the debtors more this month.'

It is important to take the time to do a deliberate, rational self-assessment on a regular basis, however. Only by looking at each aspect of practice management in turn will you really accept all the things that you are doing well, but take for granted.

- What have I done well?
- What have I done badly?
- What have I not done at all?

Then think in more detail about what the reasons are behind your good or poor performance.

- Why did it go well?
- Why did it go badly?
- Why did it not happen?

You need to understand why things go well, so that you can continue to repeat the success. Was it down to good planning, having the right skills, or good teamwork?

It is equally important to pinpoint why things may not have gone so well, in order to rectify the fault. Was it due to inability (training need), lack of time (time management need, inadequate staffing levels), or insufficient authority (review job with employer). Simply sweeping the problem under the carpet will not help you progress.

An example of self-assessment of management tasks is shown in Figure 5.2. Specific inadequacies can be overcome. 'The report was bad because I didn't give myself enough time,'

What went well?	**Why?**	**Action needed/lessons learnt**
Open day	Well planned Staff worked well as a team	
Practice meeting	Good notice of meeting Kept to time Action-orientated discussions	Use these techniques in all future meetings
What went badly?	**Why?**	**Action needed/lessons learnt**
Installation of new phone system		
– More expensive than expected	Poor analysis of costs	Always double check maintenance costs as well as installation
– Substandard service	No background info in company	Follow up more customer references in greater detail
Introduction of appraisal system – behind schedule	Unhappy about own ability to conduct appraisal interviews	Training needed

Figure 5.2 Self-assessment of management tasks.

or 'The waiting room hasn't been decorated because I don't have the authority to spend the money.' Above all, identifying specific reasons for your poor performance are far more positive than sinking into general despair or irritation. 'I'm no good at dealing with the staff, and never will be,' will not help you. Use the outcome of self-assessment to discuss at your appraisal, and to plan future objectives.

What are you going to do next?

Whether you are a new or established practice manager, your job will evolve over time. New challenges and opportunities will arise at the practice, and you will expand your skill and knowledge base. Any future plans the owner has for the practice will have an effect on the management role. Regular reviews of your place in the practice are an essential part of managing your job.

Some ideas and pointers for the future of veterinary practice and its management are discussed in Chapter 21, 'Where do we go now?'

MANAGING YOUR TIME

Poor time management is a major cause of stress for all members of the practice team. Good management of your time is essential for several reasons.

- You have to find the time to carry out all the tasks you need to do to manage the practice.
- Your time at work is a valuable resource, and it is your duty to use it in the most efficient and effective way.
- Good personal time management will allow you to enjoy your work more.
- Unless you have good control of your own time, you cannot hope to persuade other practice members to organize their time.

Telephone calls and meetings are essential communications tools, but both need careful management to ensure they do not become time-wasting sessions. Delegation is a vital part of time management, and is one often poorly used in veterinary surgeries.

Personal time management

'Time management can't work in veterinary practice' is a much-heard lament. Certainly, many standard books or courses on time management seem to refer to more controlled workplaces. In veterinary practice, we like to feel a bit 'special', and tend to assume that other organizations don't have the same level of disruptions. But most businesses will have to deal with very similar problems – demanding clients, missed appointments and staff crises.

The vagaries of veterinary practice that make time management so difficult are the very reasons that we need to manage the controllable parts of our time to the best advantage. Emergencies are much less disruptive if the normal appointment system runs to schedule and has built-in provision for some unexpected arrivals. Management crises are more easily dealt with if the day-to-day administration is under control.

Bear in mind, as we talk of 'time management', that due to the laws of physics we can't actually do anything about the passage of time! What is really meant is 'management of your use of time'.

Myths of time management

In an ideal world, a perfect manager would be able to plan and use their time in such a way that they could do each task in the right order, with the right amount of time, get it finished on time, never rush, and be happy!

This perfect manager does not exist, any more than the ideal world does. Do not set yourself this impossible goal of perfection – it will only lead to feelings of frustration and inadequacy when you fail to achieve it.

Reality will never be perfection, busy times occur, crises happen – but by being aware of time management tools you should be able to sensibly manage the way you use the majority of your time.

Signs of poor time management

The signs of poor time management can often be summarized by the animal model 'headless chicken' syndrome – running around totally unfocussed with no apparent purpose! *Be honest, how often do you find yourself:*

- having to break off one task to do something else more urgent?
- letting yourself be distracted from major tasks?
- spending a day sorting out a filing cabinet when all you wanted was one bit of paper?
- putting off tasks until the last minute?
- trying to accomplish everything at once?
- re-doing jobs which were rushed?
- being interrupted and distracted by other people?
- being unprepared for meetings or appointments?
- doing several things simultaneously?
- having no real idea why you are doing something?
- not knowing what to do first?
- working late or at weekends 'to get on top of things'?

Poor time management is a vicious circle. Items don't get filed because you don't have time to do it. Then it takes much longer to find them again (if you can find them at all). Mistakes get made because you are in too much of a hurry, and then you waste even more time having to re-do them.

Time management is not difficult, but it does require discipline. You need to be constantly aware of what you are doing and why you are doing it.

What are *you doing?*

If you don't know how you are spending your time (apart from 'badly'), it is difficult to know how to use it better. The starting point of time management is to list and analyse how you are currently using your time; and which interruptions and distractions are having the biggest effect on your working day. Exactly how you come up with that list is up to you.

Almost all time management books and courses start with the principle of keeping a time log. This involves writing down each task you do, and how long you spent doing it, over the course of a week. However, use of a time log is one of the main reasons for the 'Time management can't work in veterinary practice' cry. In some practices this is can be a possibility – especially if the manager is lucky enough to have an office and an assistant. The idea is that you keep a notebook with you at all times, and note down the time at which you start each task.

The reality of many practice managers' jobs does make keeping a time log very hard, if not impossible. How do you record folding bills with one hand, signing reports with another, whilst talking to a client on the phone and gesturing to the nurse that you want tea, not coffee?

But you can at least sit down a couple of times a day – at lunchtime and the end of the day – and make a rough guess about what you spent your time on. Use one column to list what you would regard as 'tasks' and another for 'interruptions'. An example is shown in Figure 5.3.

What should *you be doing?*

Often the first attempt to improve time management involves spending a long time making a

Task	Time	Interruptions	Time
Payroll	2 hrs	Unscheduled rep calls	45 min
Stationery order	15 min	Phone calls – unsolicited sales	25 min
Bookkeeping	1.5 hrs	Phone calls – client queries	20 min
Credit control	1 hr	Temporary reception cover	30 min
		Minor staff queries	15 min
Total for day	**4.75 hrs**	**Total for day**	**2.25 hrs**

Figure 5.3 Daily time analysis.

list of everything we are going to do today, and then aiming to cross as many things off as possible to make ourselves feel good. In an extreme case, people add completed tasks to a 'to do' list, simply so the number of ticked-off items looks even longer!

Simple lists like this guard against tasks being forgotten, but do nothing towards making the most use of your time. Often the easiest, least urgent tasks are done first, 'to get them off the list', leaving more critical but time-consuming items undone. There is also no control over what goes on the list in the first place.

True time management involves deciding what you actually need to do, before making the list. If you already have a list, take a quick look at it now. How many of the things on that list do you really have to do? How many of them are going to make any progress at all towards your objectives?

Most 'to do' list tasks can be divided into the following categories:

- Routine tasks – payroll, monthly budget reports
- Goals – e.g. to organize a new telephone system
- New incoming tasks – dealing with post, telephone calls, staff queries.

Routine tasks can be added onto your list at more or less the same time each day, week or month. You tend to know how long they take to do, and simply need an allocation of time. But do question them on a regular basis. Would computerizing the payroll save time? Could somebody else be trained to do the monthly invoicing?

Goals need to be broken down into SMART objectives. These are discussed in more detail in Chapter 7, 'Business planning'. In summary, these are objectives which are Specific, Measurable, Action-oriented, Realistic and Time-based.

Simply putting 'Sort out new computer system' on your to-do list is not going to help you very much. Instead, you might identify the following tasks:

- Specify hardware requirements of printers and monitors by Friday.
- Arrange a meeting with head nurse and senior partner to produce provisional software specification next Monday.
- Send specifications to x, y and z computer companies asking for a quotation to be received by dd/mm/yy date.
- Arrange to visit a, b, c veterinary practice for live demonstration of products by dd/mm/yy date.

Incoming tasks are the dangerous ones. They can leapfrog to the top of your to-do list, in the same way that your 'worst' clients claim more attention than your 'gold star' ones.

All new incoming tasks should be 'vetted':

- Does it need doing at all?
- Can someone else do it instead?
- How important is it?
- How urgent is it?

The difference between importance and urgency is illustrated in Figure 5.4.

Improving your time management

Bad time managers are not necessarily lazy. Often they seem to be very busy, but still never get things done.

Use your time analysis notes, and your incoming task categorization, to identify and eliminate all the Unimportant non-urgent tasks from your day. You should not be doing these at all. Remember to aim for a long-term solution. For instance, don't just ask the receptionist to filter out the junk mail, get her to cancel it at source wherever possible.

Urgent but unimportant tasks are decoys. These demand your attention at once, but are unnecessary – e.g. un-screened telephone calls, minor staff queries. If you don't recognize them for what they are, it is easy to overestimate their importance.

Important urgent tasks are often crises. These have to be dealt with as a priority. If most of your time is taken up with these 'A1' tasks, you are increasing the risk of stress and burnout.

Important non-urgent tasks: most of your genuine management tasks should fall into this

Urgency

Importance

Important urgent – A1	Important non-urgent – A2
Crises Overdue deadlines	Planning
Unimportant urgent – B1	**Unimportant non-urgent – B2**
Incoming phone calls Interruptions by other people	Junk mail Gossiping Internet surfing

Figure 5.4 Importance and urgency of tasks.

category. It is vital to deal with these before they turn into Important urgent ones.

Be realistic about what you can and can't control.

- Deal with Important urgent tasks – you have to!
- Focus on the Important non-urgent ones – do them before they become urgent!
- Control the Unimportant urgent tasks and keep them in their place.
- Eliminate the Unimportant non-urgent ones.

You also need to differentiate between efficient and effective use of time. Being efficient means increasing the number of credit control letters and phone calls you get through in a day. Being effective means spending time setting up a better debt prevention system.

Controlling common time wasters

It is quite easy to eliminate the totally unimportant, non-urgent tasks. It just requires a little discipline not to get involved with them.

The unimportant but urgent ones are more difficult – because they seem urgent. They normally demand answers right now, and because individually they often seem quite trivial, tend to be dealt with there and then, rather than rescheduled. These are things like staff queries, unfocussed meetings and telephone calls.

Staff queries

We all like to be available for our staff, but you can't make the best use of your time if you are constantly interrupted by 'How do you do ...?', 'Can I just ask you ...?', 'What do you want me to do with ...?'.

- ***'How do I?'/'What do I do with?':*** These are the things like 'How do I change the fax roll?'. Often it seems easier to do it yourself, but it will be much more effective use of your time to show them how to do it properly. Make a note of the common queries, and either improve the provision of training in that area, or make more use of delegation.

- ***'Can I have your advice on?':*** Staff will need to discuss some things with you. However, rather than staff expecting to be able to ask for your immediate response at any time, try to set aside a specific time of day that staff can approach you. This may be the time that you find most difficult to concentrate on other matters anyway! Having been approached, you can decide whether to continue the discussion then, or to make a mutually convenient time to follow it up.

- ***'You've got to sort this out':*** There will always be genuine times when they do need your instant help, whether it is a client demanding to see the manager, or some other emergency. Make sure they don't feel unable to call on you in these circumstances.

Meetings

An effective meeting allows you to discuss topics and problems with one or more other people, consider solutions and draw up an action plan. A bad meeting simply takes valuable workers away from their jobs, airs a lot of complaints or 'good ideas' and is totally unproductive and de-motivating as nothing will ever come of it. Meetings as a communications tool are discussed fully in Chapter 9, 'Teamwork and communication'. Remember to bear the following points in mind to make the most effective use of your time in meetings.

- Know why the meeting is being held, and what it is trying to achieve.
- Is a meeting the best way of achieving it?
- Only invite the people who are absolutely necessary.
- Set a timescale and keep to it.
- Keep discussions on track.
- Use written submissions before the meeting to avoid lengthy explanations.
- Always work towards an action plan and follow it up.

A meeting with no action plan and follow-up is nothing but a gesture of good intentions and a waste of time. Worse still, it is de-motivating, as nothing will happen as a result.

Telephone calls

Both incoming and outgoing telephone calls are aspects of your work which can make a huge difference to your time management. Incoming calls take no notice of what you are doing at the time, and expect you to instantly transfer all your attention to them. Outgoing calls can be frustrating if the recipient does not have the correct information with them.

Incoming calls

- Have some means of call screening if possible. Even if you do not have a personal secretary, consider using a caller display monitor.
- Try to develop specific times of day for routine calls. If receptionists know they are to tell sales reps to phone back between 3 and 4 pm, then you won't be disturbed by staff having to constantly check if you are available to take a call.
- Start off by warning the caller how long you have to spend with them. Then it becomes their responsibility to get their point across in the time available.

Outgoing calls

- Make notes before you start on what you want to ask.
- If the person you want isn't available, try to make a specific appointment to call them back.
- Try not to get distracted by small-talk.
- Keep a clock visible – even a stopwatch to highlight how long you have been on the phone.

No time for time management?

More drastic action will be needed if you have reached the 'Stop the world, I want to get off' stage. You must be able to find a breathing space to plan your future strategy.

Time management problems should be dealt with in work time – encroaching into 'home time' will only make matters worse. A common mistake is trying to catch up by doing more of the same – 'If I work all evening and weekend, I'll be able to do time management next week.' You won't – the same poor time management will ensure that all you have achieved by Monday is exhaustion and just as many things still to do. Another mistake is to take a holiday and try to work it all out at home: you may come up with your perfect solution… until you get back to your desk with a week's worth of queries waiting to be dealt with. You will slip back into the old bad habits again very quickly.

You will need to enlist the help of other practice members, employers and colleagues, to help you.

The first reason you need your colleagues' help is that you need an initial short-term **ban on incoming tasks**. Do not accept telephone calls, or deal with interruptions from staff. If you are a managing veterinary surgeon, block out your appointments for a day; if you are a head nurse, take yourself out of the nursing rota. Shut the door if you have your own office, and let everyone know you are not to be disturbed except in case of fire! If you explain to them what you are trying to do, everybody will be on your side. If you don't, they will just think you're being awkward, selfish and grumpy!

Clear your desk. Don't get side-tracked trying to sort it out at this stage – it's too late for that now. Just put everything into a large cardboard box. This is a psychological boost simply not to be staring at a mass of paperwork and post-it notes, not to mention old coffee cups.

Turn your computer screen off – if you don't you'll be tempted to check e-mails or some other documents.

Make a list – use a new pen and clean pad of paper if it makes you feel better! List all the tasks that you feel you 'need' to do. Divide them into the four categories based on Importance and Urgency as described earlier. If possible, ask a trusted colleague to help you with this – a devil's advocate to prompt you every so often, 'What will happen if this does not get done?' 'Why can't someone else do it?'

Forget the unimportant category totally. Or throw that bit of the list into the cardboard box if you have to keep it.

Are any of the tasks absolutely vital (practice cannot function without them) and very urgent (i.e. within 24 hours)? Are you truly the only person who can do them? Just as well you haven't been run over by a bus, then! Get on and do those now, before going any further.

Then go through the rest of the list, and mark beside each item its Urgency (days, weeks, months), Importance (does it have to be done at all?) and ease of delegation (do you have to do it?). Sort the list – starting with the important, urgent items that require personal action, working down to the non-urgent, less important ones which can be delegated. Remove any items that simply don't need doing at all.

If the box of stuff that was originally on your desk is still in the box at the end of the month, then it wasn't important enough for you to need it in that time. There is no need for you to look at it now, just ask someone else to sort through and file or bin the contents.

Keep it up

Let the boss know that the reminder sign above your desk saying 'Why am I doing this?' is not a reflection of the overall job.

Don't get totally rigid about time management. The worst signal you can send out to the rest of the staff and other people is that you don't have time for them. Sooner or later that sort of attitude will backfire on you. 'Well, I would have told you about XYZ, but I know you don't like us to talk to you without an appointment.' The whole point of using time management tools is that you can get through the basics more efficiently. Use the time you have 'saved' to be more available to staff and clients. The important thing is for everybody to know where he or she stands. Pre-time management you might have been available to talk anytime – or you might have bitten someone's head off for no obvious reason (apart from them not being psychic enough to know you had an urgent deadline). Now you can schedule difficult tasks for the time you are most effective (be that morning or afternoon), and let staff know you are available at other times, when you are doing things which can easily be interrupted.

Delegation

Delegation is vital for all members of the practice. Veterinary surgeons need to be able to delegate to nurses; nurses in turn may delegate to other support staff or students. Someone else to do some of your work for you – sounds wonderful, doesn't it? But delegation is not easy; perversely, the more you need to do it the harder it is.

'It's quicker to do it myself' is the excuse most managers use to avoid delegation. This is a very short-sighted view, and the effects of not delegating work can be devastating in the long term for both managers and staff.

Don't confuse delegation with simply allocating a task to someone else. Allocating a task is saying, 'Please water the hanging baskets, they are wilting.' The only feedback someone allocated a task will get is a complaint if it's not done. And they will expect to be told every time you want them to do it again. Delegating a responsibility is saying, 'You are responsible for the appearance of the hanging baskets. This will involve feeding, watering and replacing the plants as necessary. We expect a colourful, healthy display all summer and your budget is £XX'.

Why managers don't like delegating

There are many reasons why people do not like delegating parts of their work responsibilities:

- Time – *'It's quicker to do it myself.'*
- Pessimism – *'They always get it wrong anyway.'*
- Loss of control over the tasks being done.
- Fear of losing their job or status if others can do the work.

The most painless time to delegate is when you don't have to. That is, while you still have time to discuss with the staff member what it is you are making them responsible for, and what authorities and help they will get. Once you realize that you are snowed under with work, you may not have the time and patience to delegate properly, and then the first two excuses become self-fulfilling prophecies.

Some people genuinely find it hard to hand over a task or responsibility to someone else. They tend to make it worse for themselves by staying to watch, and you can almost feel them itching to take over again. If this sounds like you, then break yourself in gently. Start by delegating small tasks (not simply mundane or idiot-proof ones), and force yourself to walk away and do something else.

Remember – the sign of a good manager is that the place does not fall apart as soon as you take a day's holiday. Some managers feel they are not doing their jobs properly unless they do it all themselves, and may view delegation as 'passing the buck'.

Managers might also be prevented from delegating tasks by other factors, such as:

- There simply is not another person there.
- The people you ask say no, because they do not have the time or do not want the responsibility.
- Your superior wants you to take personal responsibility for the task or project.

Problems such as staffing numbers, workload and attitude will need to be tackled at source before any delegation can occur.

Why you should make more use of delegation

Delegation is not a one-way process. It benefits not only you, but also the person being delegated to, and the practice as a whole.

One of the initial reasons to make more use of delegation is to free up more time for you. However, it will not be an instant fix: you will need to 'invest to save'. Taking a little bit of time to effectively delegate a task will free up far more of your time in the long run.

Delegating a task to somebody else is a declaration of trust and confidence in that person. Transferring responsibilities can have a powerful motivating effect on staff, provided that it is done in the right way.

The way in which staff members respond to (and offer) delegation is often a good pointer to promotion to future team leader roles.

Delegation increases and diversifies the skills of the staff members, and ensures that more than one person is able to do each task.

Effective delegation

Firstly you need to decide:

- What are you going to delegate?
- To whom?
- What instruction/tools do they need?
- How much authority are you going to give them?

Don't just delegate the bits you don't like doing – give your co-workers interesting tasks to do as well. If all you ever give them to do is mundane filing or stamp sticking, they'll start to dread the next 'job' you give them. Sometimes it will be unavoidable: someone has to do it, but make sure that sometimes you give something they can be proud of too.

Don't automatically delegate only to your 'next in command'. More junior staff should be given a chance to take on more responsibilities too. However, don't leapfrog any official chains of command; the head nurse won't be very pleased if one of her trainees suddenly disappears off doing something for you. Involve any heads of department in the selection of staff to be delegated to. But don't delegate the delegating – it can turn into Chinese whispers if you ask the head receptionist to ask the Saturday receptionist to do such and such.

The person you select needs to be given the tools to do the job. This might be access to information, time in which to do the job, money or materials. Failing to do this will completely de-motivate the employee, as they will be unable to do what has been asked of them. If you want a nurse to run clinics, you must find her a room to do it in, and allow her to take time out from her normal nursing rota.

Explain to them what it is you want them to achieve, and make sure they understand it.

Give them sufficient instruction to be able to do the job, but leave room for some initiative on their part too. Remember, part of the reason for delegating is to stretch and develop the staff. The balance point will depend upon the staff member you have selected. Someone who has shown initiative in the past will need fewer detailed instructions than a junior staff member being given their first assignment.

Make sure they have sufficient authority to do the job. If they will need to order supplies, make sure the supplier will accept an order from them. If they need access to computer information, make sure they know any necessary passwords. You may need to set an upper limit on authority: 'Sort out the repairs to xx, but let me know if it is going to cost over £yyyy.'

Don't just abandon them! But also don't just stand over them while they do it. They need to know you are interested in how things are going, but that you will not intervene unless they ask you to (or things are going really badly!). Give them feedback and subtle help as required.

Let them know when they have done a good job. And let everybody else know too.

If delegation goes wrong

Although you have given someone else the responsibility for organizing, carrying out and completing the task, and also the right to be recognized for a job well done, the ultimate responsibility still remains with you.

Minor problems might arise, for example if the staff member is constantly asking questions about the tasks given. This might be because you gave them insufficient information, or that the person lacks the confidence to deal with the task. Some people are simply insecure – if there is someone to double-check with, they will; if not, they get on with it.

If something goes disastrously wrong, you can't simply turn round and blame the employee: 'Well, it's not my fault, I told X to do it.'

You need to ask yourself:

- Did I pick the right person?
- Did I explain things well enough?
- Did I give them all the information they needed?
- Did I make it clear they could ask for help?
- Did I give enough supervision?

Even if it turns out that the employee totally ignored some of your basic instructions, do not make a public scapegoat of them. Other staff will not want to take on future responsibilities if they think they will be publicly shamed if things go wrong.

However, you can't just pretend a mistake didn't happen. You need to talk it through with the employee, but in a way that allows you both to learn. Was there something that cropped up unexpectedly? Or had you missed something out? How should the staff member react next time they have a similar situation?

Finally, don't forget there will be many times you need to have something really boring and simple done. Don't think you have to go through a whole delegation procedure just to get your booster reminders stamped. Just tell someone to do it. Nicely, of course!

YOURSELF

The management of your job, and your time, will be much easier if you are in control of your 'self'. Both physical and mental fitness are essential if you are to cope with the varied aspects of practice and home life.

Your attitude of mind makes all the difference between regarding a difficult day at work as simply being 'a bad day' or 'the end of the world'. If you are physically healthy then you will recover more easily from a hard day.

Any imbalance in your 'self' will leave you much more susceptible to problems such as stress or depression.

Mental and physical well-being

Although often regarded as two separate aspects of yourself, your mental and physical fitness are interdependent.

Just as mental stresses will have physical effects (racing pulse, sweating, shaking), so physical neglect will reflect on your mental abilities. You will not be effective if you only had a few hours sleep, and you are bound to be crabby if you've downed 6 cups of black coffee by lunchtime.

The physical aspect is often the one that gets neglected once you start trying to sort out other things. In an attempt to work that bit harder, faster and get that last thing done which will suddenly make everything better, the things that suffer are exercise, eating and sleeping.

Physical exercise is going to help you sleep better, and aid relaxation. And you can't count running around the surgery trying to find someone to take a phone call as exercise.

If you spend a lot of your day at the computer, remember to give your eyes a break every so often. Ideally this needs to be something that gives the eye muscles a change – don't just swap looking at a screen for looking at a magazine the same distance away. Look out of the window, concentrate on something moving or watch the traffic go by.

Take some time out to think about how you function. Don't get obsessed by navel-gazing, or giving yourself a self-destructive character assassination. Do spend a little time once in a while simply jotting down a few strengths and weaknesses – there are bound to be parts of the job which come naturally or which you enjoy more than others. You wouldn't be human if you didn't have a few faults: is it a tendency to be impatient, to be a workaholic and expect the same of others, or that you over-react to interruptions? Unfortunately it often takes a crisis or cross words from an upset member of staff before these are recognized.

As with anything else, if you recognize your strengths, you can make best use of them. If you recognize your weaknesses, you can either try to overcome them, or at least be honest and accept them; tell the staff, 'OK, I know I'm crabby until after my second cup of tea in the morning – can you leave any difficult problems until after then!'

Everybody has more effective times of day, depending on their personal biorhythms – learn to work with them, not against them. Schedule tricky work for when you are most effective, more routine chores for the lower parts of the day.

Stress

Stress is the buzzword of modern society. Everybody is talking about it, writing about it, having e-mail chat sessions about it. People are getting stressed because they think they have stress, and almost feel guilty if they don't have it – are they not working hard enough?

Work-related stress must be taken seriously. The employer has a legal duty to ensure that their employees are not made ill as a result of their work – and that includes stress-related illness. These aspects of stress are covered in Chapter 18, 'Health and Safety'.

What is stress?

Stress is a demand on the body's physical or mental resources. When faced with a source of stress, the body's alarm system takes over. Hormonal and neural signals prepare the body for a 'fight or flight response'. This aspect of stress is totally normal and very useful. It is the way you are able to run that bit faster to get out of the way of a dangerous situation.

Some stress is good, giving that extra 'high' that you need to get through the day. This is the stress that makes you try that extra bit harder to complete the difficult task. It may be the buzz of finishing a tricky operation, or that 'It's been a busy day but we've done OK' feeling. A low level of stress is needed to maintain performance; in a zero stress situation, apathy often rules.

But some stress is counterproductive – either because the stress response is inappropriate, or because there is simply too much of it. There are two reasons why the stress response causes a problem in life, i.e. what we regard as 'stress':

1. The 'fight or flight' response is not the most socially acceptable way of dealing with modern problems. Hitting the cause of your stress (boss or computer screen) is rarely permitted, and neither is running away. We are therefore having to 'bottle up' our stress response, leading to continued stress symptoms of increased heart rate, dry mouth and nervous tension.
2. On-going exposure to stressors results in eventual exhaustion.

Causes of stress

There are standard lists of well-known stressors, such as moving house, getting divorced, or death of close relatives. These are undoubtedly stressful circumstances, however well the individuals concerned appear to handle them. But it should be remembered that different situations are stressful to different people.

Sometimes people may appear to be worked up about quite trivial matters. This is often due to the cumulative effect of stressors. The 'final straw' that causes someone to blow their top is often quite mundane, such as a jammed paper feed in a printer. Stresses at home will combine with work stressors.

External causes of stress are more easily understood by friends and colleagues. 'I'm not surprised he's stressed, having to deal with all that paperwork.' But much stress is generated internally, as a result of personal expectations or low self-esteem. This can be much harder to accept personally, and for others to take in. 'I don't know why she's so wound up about that report, it looks good enough to me.'

Common external causes of stress within veterinary practice are:

- dealing with clients – their demands and expectations
- treating patients – animals may be uncooperative, or have difficult conditions to cure
- the 'care versus profit' dilemma
- emergencies and out-of-hours work
- managing staff
- running a business
- responsibility without authority
- lack of clear targets and goals
- increased information. In its way, 'ignorance was bliss'. Whilst striving for excellence is good, the increased communication about what is clinically and administratively possible is causing stress in those whose ideals are above their abilities.

Internal stressors include things such as:

- feeling out of control
- peer pressure
- high personal expectations
- low self-esteem
- inefficient working patterns.

Signs of stress

Different people have different reactions to the stress they do receive. However, the classic responses include physical, mental and behavioural signs such as:

- muscle tension
- sleeplessness

- apprehension
- cold sweats
- racing heart
- mood swings
- depression
- loss of concentration
- excess consumption of drugs such as coffee, chocolate, alcohol, legal and illegal medications
- Under- or over-eating.

Stress is contagious. If one member of the practice is snappy, apathetic or suffering from mood swings, then it will start to upset other staff. If stress leads to absence from work, then the staff left to cover become more at risk from stress themselves.

Dealing with stress

Dealing with a stress problem requires several approaches.

- Remove the underlying cause.
- Control the symptoms.
- Improve your resistance to stress.

In theory, you can remove the cause of stress, and all will be well with the world. But reality is not like that, and the practice reorganization/partnership break-up/difficult staff member cannot be removed 'just like that'. You will need to be able to continue functioning in the face of stress for long enough to be able to do something more permanent about it.

Remember that stress is cumulative, and if you can remove some of the minor stressful factors from your life, then those remaining will be easier to cope with. So change what can be changed – if a dodgy piece of equipment needs fixing, then fix it rather than curse every time it doesn't work! If the morning rush hour gets your blood boiling before you even get to work, then try leaving earlier when it isn't so busy, or use alternative transport.

It is important to understand whether the causes of your stress are external or internal. Major stress relief tactics such as changing jobs will only work if the main stressor was directly related to that job, for example poor staff rotas leading to excessive weekend and night work. If your major stressor is your own inability to accept the occasional mistake, then changing jobs, moving house or swapping partners will not help you!

Controlling the symptoms of stress, and improving the body's resistance to it, often go hand in hand. The main ways of doing this are:

- nutrition
- relaxation
- exercise.

You are what you eat, and caffeine and chocolate will rapidly enhance your stress reactions, adding to feelings of jitteriness and preventing sleep. Replacing stimulants with calming herbal drinks will help combat stress. Eating proper meals instead of snacking on 'junk' food will help you cope better with the day's demands. Foods high in sugar will give a quick lift, but this is rapidly followed by a 'down', as the body reacts to the blood sugar levels. Food additives are a common cause for concern nowadays, and are implicated in many health problems.

Distraction, by watching TV or reading a book, will give short-term relief from stress by taking your mind off your difficulties. But really this simply puts off the problems until you are forced to face them again. True relaxation actually affects the physiological mechanisms of the body, acting as an antidote to the stress reaction. It lowers respiration and heart rates, and unwinds muscle tension. There are many classes offering relaxation techniques such as yoga and breathing exercises. Many of these exercises can be practised at work – at lunch or coffee time. You might initially feel a twit doing deep breathing in the staff room – but a lot less of a twit than losing your cool with someone.

Not only does physical exercise improve your fitness, get you out of the house and aid general health, it also helps to use up all those surplus 'fight or flight' hormones flying round the body. You can't hit the boss, but you could play squash. You can't run away from the tax inspection, but you can use those primed muscles to jog round the block at lunchtime instead.

There is a wide range of self-help books about combating stress, which cover the subject in much more detail. A professional stress counsellor will be able to give you a more personal approach to dealing with your stresses. The wide range of alternative and conventional medical solutions to stress can be overwhelming, and the recommendation of a counsellor or friend will be of great help in finding the best way for you.

The veterinary profession recognizes the serious problems caused by stress. Two support organizations exist within the profession. The Veterinary Helpline offers sympathetic discussion, information and practical advice on emotional, addictive and financial problems. The Veterinary Surgeons Health Support Programme was established to help combat problems of alcohol and drug abuse.

CHAPTER CONTENTS

Where are we now? 47
The audit 48
The SWOT analysis 51

Where do we want to go? 52
The business plan 53

6 Business planning

We have looked at the role of today's practice manager and the areas of management they may be responsible for. A practice manager or a veterinary surgeon wishing to undertake the management of his or her practice is faced with innumerable management tasks. Knowing how and where to start the management process can be a nightmare. There are however two very simple questions which all managers need to ask:

1. Where are we now?
2. Where do we want to go?

Whether you are taking on a new management role or reviewing your present role, these two questions must be considered and answered before any kind of management strategies can be effectively implemented. If you don't know where you are, you will have great problems finding the right road to continue your journey. If you don't know where you want to go, how will you ever manage to get there?

It's the same with management. You need to be very clear what the present situation is, what management policies and procedures are in place and how management is presently carried out. You also need a management/business plan to help you decide where you want to go so that you know what you are aiming for and how you can achieve those aims.

WHERE ARE WE NOW?

In order to find out where you are, you should start by carrying out a practice audit.

The audit

The audit is an inspection or examination of the practice and its management. It is also an information-gathering exercise which will enable you to assess and prioritize your management tasks.

The audit should carefully examine the following areas of the practice:

- premises
- services
- clinical standards
- staffing
- marketing and sales
- PR and communications
- internal management systems
- client base
- future plans.

You will need the help of your staff to carry out many parts of the audit; they are nearer to the ground on day to day matters than the manager and are a source of much detailed information. A number of brainstorming sessions will identify many strengths and weaknesses in the different areas you examine, as well as providing you with material for your future wish-list of where you want to go.

Premises

Make a careful inspection of the premises and answer the following questions (you will find many more as you tour the practice):

- Is the fabric of the building, internal and external, in good condition? If not, list what needs to be repaired.
- Is the signage good, or could it be improved?
- Is the car park lit at night?
- Are the premises clean inside and out, not forgetting the car park? Do you have enough space, do you have a litter bin and a dog loo, for example?
- What refurbishment is required in public and staff areas?

Services

Look at the services the practice provides and does not provide (you will think of many more than are listed below):

- Do you provide a full range of operations or do you refer? Are you happy with this or should the practice be carrying out more specialist operations?
- How many consultations does the practice carry out in an average week, could there be more, how long are they, is this the right length, is the length varied?
- Do you hold nurses' clinics, puppy parties, etc.?
- Do you refer or act as a referral centre for other practices?
- Do you have a website?
- Do you have a veterinary surgeon specializing in exotics or specific species?
- Do you have pet healthcare supplies, and where is the nearest pet shop?
- Do you have a practice ambulance used to collect and return animals?
- What sort of client reminder service do you have for boosters and worming, etc.?
- Do you hold farmers' meetings to promote new services and improved animal care and management?
- Do you have large animal health programmes?

Clinical standards

What are the clinical standards of the practice (the non-veterinary manager will require input from vets and nurses to complete this area of the audit):

- What particular clinical/surgical skills do the veterinary surgeons and nurses possess?
- Do you need to recruit for other skills?
- What CPD is undertaken to improve skills?
- Do any of the veterinary surgeons have a certificate, or are they presently studying for one?
- What is the practice drug policy, what choice do veterinary surgeons have, are the most modern /effective drugs being used?
- What surgical equipment is there, does it need upgrading, what extra equipment is needed?

Staffing

Your staff are your greatest expense and your greatest resource, so assess them carefully:

- What are your staff ratios, and are they adequate?
- How good is teamwork?
- Do you carry out appraisals, and are they effective/successful?
- What is the standard of client care skills?
- What staff training/CPD is provided, is there a budget, is there a training plan, is training recorded?
- What recruitment and selection procedures are in place?
- Do all staff have job descriptions and are they up to date?
- Do all staff have access to, and do they follow, practice policies and procedures?
- Are there any problems with staff – difficult staff members, etc., and what needs to be done?

Marketing and sales

The way a practice markets and sells its services can greatly affect its success and help it to ward off competitors. Ask the following questions:

- What is the practice image?
- What marketing methods/initiatives are in place?
- What packages, discounts, etc., are offered to large and small animal clients?
- What literature and IT is used for marketing?
- What is the standard of client care?
- What marketing skills do staff possess, do they need further training?

Public relations and communication

PR is taking on an increasingly important role in veterinary practice relationships with clients. The following are relevant questions:

- Is there a client newsletter, and how is it distributed?
- Is there a farmers' newsletter?
- Is there a practice brochure?
- Is there a practice website?
- What relationship does the practice have with the local media, does the practice use the media to the full?
- Does the practice have open days, client evenings and events?
- Does the practice sponsor local events?
- Does the practice have a presence at local agricultural shows?
- Does the practice liaise with local animal charities and animal rescue organizations to help raise awareness and encourage rehoming of animals?

Internal systems

Look at the following internal systems: IT; health and safety; stock control; cash flow; account management; insurance management; fees and mark-ups.

IT

- What is the standard of software, and does it need to be upgraded?
- How is the database used, and what general, management and financial information can be extracted?
- Is the hardware adequate, or do you need more?
- Is the computer used for stock control, or could it be used?
- Do you have a website?
- What word processing facilities are there?
- What is the standard of printers and scanners?

Health and safety

- Have you a named health and safety officer?
- Is all health and safety up to date, or what still needs to be done?
- Have all the risk assessments been carried out?
- Has COSHH been carried out?
- Do you regularly review health and safety procedures?
- Do you provide staff health and safety training?

Stock control

- How is stock control organized, is it manual or computerized, could/should it be improved?

- What stock levels do you have, are they enough, are they too much?
- Are you receiving the best wholesaler and drug company discounts, and how do you know?

Cash flow

- Do you monitor cash flow?
- Is cash flow under control?
- Do you need a better system?

Account management

- Who manages client accounts and debt control?
- How big is your debtors' list, and is this acceptable?
- What debt control policy/procedures do you have?

Insurance management

- Are you getting the best deals on all practice insurances?
- Should you be looking at other insurance companies?

Fees and mark-ups

- What are your fee levels and when were they last increased?
- How do they compare with other local practices?
- Should fees be increased?
- Are the operation fees enough, and are time and materials being adequately charged for?
- What is your drug mark-up, and is it enough?
- Do you monitor drug price changes and alter fees on a regular basis?
- Do you have dispensing charges?
- Do you charge for nurses' time when they are called out?

Clients

You need to know about your clients in order to plan future client services and targeting.

- Who are your clients?
- How many large animal, equine and small animal clients do you have?
- How many active clients do you have?
- How many bonded clients do you have?
- Where do your clients live, what are the demographics of your area?
- How many pets are registered?
- What are the herd and flock sizes you provide veterinary care for?
- What is the split between species, and is it changing?
- Is your client database detailed enough?
- Do you regularly survey clients to find out their needs and opinions?
- Do you have a client care policy/strategy?
- Do veterinary surgeons make regular client care visits to farming clients?

Future plans

It is important to bear in mind any future plans there may be for the practice, as they will influence any decisions made on the audit. For example, if the practice is to expand or move premises in the next year there is little point in enlarging the car park or carrying out long-term refurbishment.

- Is expansion planned?
- Are new premises planned?
- Are new services planned?
- Will staff levels change?
- Will there be a change in partnership?

This is by no means a comprehensive audit list but it does give an idea of the areas managers should look at when trying to assess in management terms the existing practice position.

The type of audit you carry out and the areas you look at will naturally depend on the type of practice, the services the practice provides, the number of sites, and so on, but the process of auditing will be the same.

You are highly likely to end up with an enormous and daunting 'wish-list' of things to do and change, and of course because of financial and time constraints there is no realistic way you can achieve all this immediately. However, the next step is to prioritize your wish-list, assess what is the most and least important, most and least expensive, most and least time-consuming

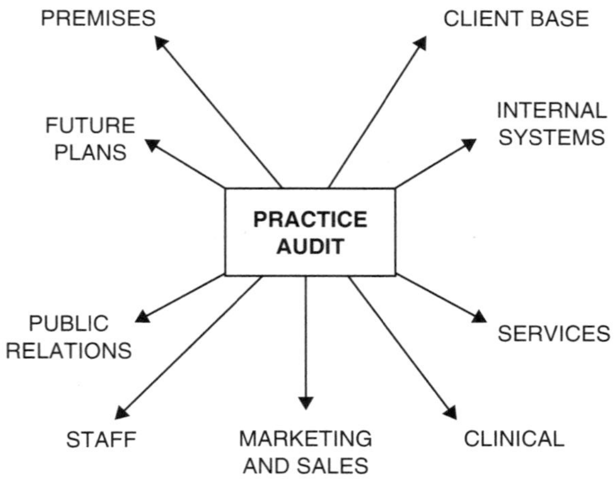

Figure 6.1 The practice audit.

and then weigh up the order of tasks to be undertaken. This is the beginning of your management plan. The audit is summarized in Figure 6.1.

By carrying out the audit you are well on the way to establishing a very clear idea of 'where the practice is', and what needs to be achieved. The rest of the journey will be taken up with identifying the practice strengths, weaknesses, opportunities and threats. This second part of the journey is best undertaken by carrying out a SWOT analysis.

The SWOT analysis

The SWOT analysis is a simple technique which identifies the practice's **S**trengths, **W**eaknesses, **O**pportunities, and **T**hreats.

Each of these areas should be considered in turn so that an overall picture can be built up of:

- the positive aspects of the practice, what it does well and what factors give it strength
- the gaps in the practice functioning and the factors which cause weakness
- the areas where the practice can expand, develop and improve by taking advantage of existing opportunities
- the negative aspects and internal and external factors which pose a threat.

One of the best ways of carrying out a SWOT analysis is to hold a number of brainstorming sessions with practice staff. It may be better to do this in groups rather than have a full practice meeting, especially if the practice is very large and/or has a number of sites.

The SWOT analysis should be considered in all areas of the practice. Box 6.1 suggests just some of the areas to look at.

You are likely to be aware of most of the strengths, weaknesses, opportunities and threats, but by setting them out in a formal way you can see the practice situation as a whole as well as

Box 6.1 SWOT analysis: some areas for inclusion

Premises Location Appearance Car parking Opening hours	**Services** Staff skills Clinical skills Equipment Clinics Specialisms Diversification	**Clients** Client base Bonded clients Client care Pet population Herd and flock numbers Clinical skills
Finance Economic climate Agricultural climate Fees Future capital investment Mortgage Interest rates	**Sales and Marketing**	**PR skills**
IT provision	**Competition**	**Legislation**
Partnership structure	**Management systems**	

possible connections between some of the audit results and the SWOT analysis.

The SWOT analysis completes the picture of 'where you are', enabling you to start looking forwards to where you are going.

Box 6.2 shows an example of a SWOT analysis for a mixed practice on the outskirts of a small market town in a predominantly rural area.

WHERE DO WE WANT TO GO?

Having established just exactly 'where you are' and looked at the practice strengths, weaknesses, opportunities and threats it is then time to decide where you actually want to go on your journey.

As a Practice Manager you may well have lots of bright ideas for progressing the practice, making money, developing services, improving staff training, attracting new clients, etc. However, moving the practice forward has to be a joint exercise involving all practice members. Everyone in the practice will have ideas and views on how they see the practice moving forwards and you need to tap into these before any real planning starts.

Box 6.2 Sample SWOT analysis

STRENGTHS

Location
- greenfield site on edge of town within walking distance
- large car park
- easy access
- attractive surroundings

Staffing
- well trained staff
- trainee and qualified nurses
- good teamwork
- dedicated staff
- vets, good clinical skills, 1 with certificate, 2 doing certificates

PR
- good PR
- good relationship with local paper

Clients
- 25% bonded
- good reports from surveys on client care
- clients in medium/high economic bracket

Services
- nurses' clinics
- consultations 8.30 am–7.30 pm Mon–Fri, 8.30 am–4.00 pm Sat, 10.00 am–2.00 pm Sun
- operations carried out each day
- referral clinic for dermatology and acupuncture

Partnership
- strong 4-vet partnership

Stock control
- computerized stock control
- 3 weeks stock held
- drug discounts monitored

WEAKNESSES

Marketing
- No marketing plan
- Staff not well trained in this area
- Poor veterinary support

IT
- no dedicated person to act as 'trouble shooter'
- poor back-up from computer company
- data retrieval system needs improving

Planning
- no written business plan

Finance
- large mortgage
- poor debt control

OPPORTUNITIES
- New housing estate being built on the edge of town
- Branch surgery has chance to move to larger premises and expand
- Newest vet is interested in developing an exotics clinic
- Practice nurse has expressed desire to work with local schools encouraging children to be aware of pet healthcare
- Neighbouring practice is selling its L/A side of the practice, giving this practice first refusal
- Practice has land on which it can build
- Conference centre on first floor which can be used for external meetings/functions and training

THREATS
- A corporate practice surgery has opened in the town
- New pharmacy regulations may affect drug sales and there is a large agricultural merchant in the town interested in expanding their business
- Farming economy is depressed, after effects of Foot and Mouth Disease
- Reduction in pet population
- Rising cost of implementing Health and Safety legislation
- Economic situation – possibility of another recession looming

A partners' brainstorming meeting is the most important starting place at which the manager can present the current practice situation, the audit results, and the SWOT analysis and ask the question, 'Where do you want to go from here?' It is vital to have all the partners' views on how the practice should develop. It is their business which is to be changed and their money at stake, and they must be in agreement on future plans.

Continue to consult staff, and ask for ideas from employees:

- How can the practice improve its services?
- What new services could be provided?
- What new products would clients buy?
- How can client care be improved?
- What training is needed?
- Do rotas need updating?
- Are staffing levels adequate?

The list could be endless, so it may be advisable to identify the 5 or 6 most common suggestions to attack/take on board first.

It is now that the planning proper can begin. Ideally a planning team should be established to devise, develop and drive the practice plan. The team may simply consist of the practice principal/partners and practice manager, or preferably may also include nursing and reception representatives. It is important to look at the overall aim of the practice; does it have a mission/vision statement, or more simply a catchphrase on the logo such as 'Caring for your Pets' or 'Because we Care', etc.? Constantly keep this overall aim in mind so that it can be used to guide you through the planning process.

The business plan

It is easy to have a wish-list of areas you want improving or developing in the practice, but wishes can only be realized by careful planning. Planning is about establishing and achieving overall aims, particular objectives and specific targets.

Aims

Aims are general overall statements of where you want to go or what you want to be, such as *'We aim to provide the highest quality of care for all our clients and their animals.'*

Objectives

Objectives are the statements showing how overall aims will be achieved, for example,
'We will provide the highest quality care for all our clients and their animals by:

1. *Having well trained and qualified staff*
2. *Providing the highest quality clinical care*
3. *Providing an efficient appointment system*
4. *Using modern, up-to-date equipment',*

and so on.

Targets

Targets are the specific ways in which the objectives are achieved. For example, if we look at objective 2:
To achieve the highest quality of clinical care the following targets will be reached:

1. *We will have a veterinary surgeon with a radiography certificate by ...*
2. *We will have 4 qualified nurses by ...*
3. *We will establish an acupuncture clinic by ...*
4. *We will purchase a new dental machine by ...*

Having decided upon a number of clear objectives for the future, the next step is to design the detailed business plan which will enable you to reach these desired objectives.

The business plan should contain:

- The overall practice vision – the philosophy of the practice and where it is heading in the future
- The objectives – the ways in which the practice vision will be reached. This can be divided into different areas, e.g. finance, staffing, client care, marketing
- Targets – specific tasks and targets required to attain objectives and the time scale within which these targets must be completed
- Action required – clear statements on how the targets will be achieved and who will be involved in carrying out the actions

- Time scale – it is vital to set a time scale for the targets; there must be completion dates to aim for. However, these are not set in stone and when the business plan is reviewed dates may be altered if appropriate.
- Budgetary implications – no plan is complete without careful consideration of costs and a careful assessment must be made of the expenditure required to implement the plan as well as any revenue implications
- Review date – the business plan must be reviewed on a regular basis, which may be yearly or as frequently as every 3 months depending upon circumstances.

All business plans must be 'SMART':

- **S**pecific
- **M**easurable
- **A**ction-orientated
- **R**ealistic
- **T**imed.

Specific

You must be very clear what you are trying to achieve. State specifically what the objectives and targets will be without ambiguity. Allocate tasks to specific people/departments with specific resources.

Measurable

All targets must be measurable. If your target is to increase the number of dental operations you must state what that increase is to be, for example five more dentals per week or 10% more dentals per month. If you cannot measure the targets you will not know if you have achieved them.

Action-orientated

The plan must be realizable by being based on specific actions, so to increase the number of dental ops will require actions such as dental care promotions, targeting older pets, examining all pets' teeth at consultations, etc.

Realistic

Your plans must be realistic and achievable. It is no good setting a target of increasing dental operations by 80% over the next 2 months and then failing to reach the target when a target of 5% over 3 months could have been achieved. Unrealistic targets can be very de-motivating. If realistic targets are reached, you can always set a new higher target when you revisit the business plan.

Timed

Timed actions are one of the keys to success of all business plans. All actions/targets must be timed. Increase dental operations by 5% means nothing unless you say by when, and requiring a veterinary surgeon to get a certificate in radiography could take many years if you don't specify an achieve-by date.

Business plans may be set for 1 year, 3 years, 5 years etc. so that you have short-term and long-term objectives catered for. Alternatively you may have a single business plan which you revisit on a very regular basis such as every 3 months, to assess what has been achieved, how the plan needs to be modified and what needs to be added.

Figure 6.2 shows an excerpt from a detailed business plan with the first set of targets completed for the first objective in the client care and marketing area.

The plan sets out specific targets, for example to produce a client newsletter four times a year. This target is clearly measurable and the actions needed to achieve it are listed, such as 'Appoint an editor, decide on content.' It is a realistic target as publication four times a year is achievable and the actions required have been timed, such as 'Appoint an editor by the end of January.'

By use of a carefully considered and constructed business plan you will have identified exactly where you are going and how you are going to get there. The one thing to remember of course is that as soon as you do get there, you will be making plans to go even further. The essence of a good business plan is that it is on-going: planning never stops.

Area	Objective	Targets	Actions required	Person responsible	Timescale	Costs	Revenue	Review
Client care and marketing	1. To promote practice services to existing clients and attract new clients	1. Produce a client newsletter 4 times a year	1. Appoint editor	– practice manager	– by end Jan	– staff time	More products and services sold to clients	
			2. Decide on content	– editor and practice manager	– by mid Feb	– staff time		
			3. Liaise with printer	– editor	– by end Feb	– staff time	Possible new client income	
			4. Produce proof copy	– editor	– by end March	– staff time		
			5. First copy of newsletter to clients	– editor	– by 1st April			April
		2. Develop a website						
		3. Have a regular veterinary column in the local paper						
		4. Hold an open day						
	2. To have promotions and displays in the waiting room							
Staff training								

Figure 6.2 Excerpt from business plan.

CHAPTER CONTENTS

Why are staff important? 57
Staff costs 57

What do you want from your staff? 58
Qualities 58
Skills 59

What do your staff want from you? 59

Recruitment 61
1. The job description 61
2. Candidate personal/skills profile 62
3. Advertising 63
4. Interviewing 64
5. Candidate acceptance 67
The contract of employment 67

Discipline 68
Misconduct 68
Gross misconduct 68
The disciplinary interview 68

7

Managing human resources – the importance of staff, recruitment and discipline

Staff are the greatest resource of a veterinary practice and they are also one of the practice's greatest expenses. For these two reasons alone it is vital that this human resource is well managed.

WHY ARE STAFF IMPORTANT?

Every member of the practice team plays an important part in the functioning of the practice, whether they be experienced vets, veterinary nurses, trainees, receptionists, administrative staff or animal care assistants.

Staff costs

Staff are expensive to 'run and maintain'. Consider an expensive piece of equipment which the practice might buy for £15,000. This equipment will be insured, used carefully, well maintained and treated with respect for the work it can do. It may last for ten years in the practice before it is replaced with a more modern machine, and will most likely have earned its keep, as well as being written off against tax well before its useful life is at an end. £15,000 is a significant investment but consider the investment in a member of staff whom you employ for ten years:

- Salary
- National insurance
- Staff benefits – e.g. healthcare, disability insurance
- Uniforms

- Sickness pay and cover
- Accommodation
- Car or mileage allowance
- Training
- Recruiting costs
- Practice social events.

This would probably add up to more than ten pieces of the expensive equipment above. The practice is making a very large financial investment in every member of its staff, and it makes sense to manage and care for those staff in the best way possible so that they, like the piece of equipment, give a good return on the investment made in them.

It should never be forgotten that staff are the practice's only source of income. Primarily this is income generated by the veterinary surgeons, but increasingly nurses and receptionists are developing an earning capacity by running healthcare clinics and promoting product and service sales.

Of course staff are not only important from a financial point of view. Staff can make or break a practice; they are the ambassadors for the practice both inside the building and outside in the community. They are your shop window; clients see nurses and receptionists long before they penetrate the inner sanctum of the consulting room, and the treatment they receive influences this perception of how good the practice may or may not be. The veterinary surgeons in the practice must also provide excellent client care skills, as well as the clinical skills to treat the owner's animals if the demanding and discriminating owner is to remain with the practice.

Staff management takes up a high proportion of a manager's time and is often the most difficult (as well as the most rewarding) aspect of managing the practice. A good people manager requires experience, communication skills, sensitivity and perhaps most of all, patience. Well-managed staff can improve practice productivity, attract and bond clients and increase profits, while badly-managed staff can lose the practice clients, money and even its livelihood.

WHAT DO YOU WANT FROM YOUR STAFF?

On the surface this may seem a simple question, but in reality we ask a very great deal of our veterinary staff, probably a lot more than is asked from staff in comparable small businesses.

Below are just some of the qualities and skills we expect from veterinary staff.

Qualities

- *Commitment:* we automatically expect our staff to be totally committed to the veterinary practice in the same way that the partners/owners are committed. We expect them to work long hours, stay late and nurse the very sick animals in the small hours of the morning. We may well pay our staff to do this, but money does not always compensate for time away from home and family and is not necessarily related to an employee's degree of commitment.

- *Hard work:* the hard work seems to go without saying. Working in a veterinary practice is not a soft option and it is remarkable how hard most veterinary staff willingly work.

- *Confidentiality:* confidentiality is vital to the work of a veterinary practice. We expect total confidentiality from our staff at all times.

- *Loyalty:* we expect our staff to be loyal to the practice, never to criticize any aspect of the practice or its work to others outside the practice whatever they may actually think.

- *Stability:* a good practice will invest time and money in training staff. This is a long-term investment, and most practices will expect staff to stay with the practice for a number of years.

- *Care:* almost without exception it is the care provided by the practice staff which leaves the lasting impression in a client's mind. No amount of excellent clinical skills can compensate the client for a perceived lack of care or understanding of them or their animal.

• *Flexibility:* the nature of veterinary work requires staff to be flexible in their working hours. The rigid 'nine to five' employee is not for the veterinary practice team.

• *Cheerfulness:* we ask our staff to be cheerful in all circumstances but especially when dealing with clients. A pleasant smile and greeting from the receptionist or nurse creates such a good impression of the practice and makes the client feel welcome.

• *Teamwork:* this is one of the keys to a successful practice. Each member of staff must be able to work as a good team member, providing help and support to other team members as well as fulfilling their particular role in the team.

Skills

• *Expertise in their chosen area:* this is the obvious requirement for all staff employed by the practice. The veterinary surgeons must have good clinical skills in order to deal with the animal, and just as important, good people and communication skills to deal with an increasingly demanding clientele. Nurses are now expected to take on more and more demanding nursing and clinical roles, and reception work involves a high degree of computer work, communication skills and organization.

• *Sales skills:* today's veterinary practices have a greater dependency on the sale of products and services, and sales is now an integral part of the staff role within the practice.

• *Marketing skills:* as competition between practices increases so the quality of the practice marketing skills becomes more important. All staff should be involved in the marketing of practice services, be it by the production of displays, special offers, development of new services or the simple procedure of informing clients of the services and benefits the practice has available.

• *People skills:* the veterinary profession is all about people as well as their animals. It is vital that staff can relate to and communicate well with all types of client. After all it may be the dog who is ill, but it is the owner who will have the information required to help the diagnosis and it is important that the veterinary surgeon and nursing staff can obtain this easily from the client. Veterinary staff must also be able to relate well to each other to enable the smooth running of the practice. Poor communication can be one of the greatest stumbling blocks to the efficient running of a practice.

• *Computer skills:* a very high proportion of practices are now computerized, not only in terms of client records but also websites, e-mail facilities and word processing, and employees must increasingly be computer literate.

• *Teaching skills:* most veterinary staff need to be able to explain veterinary procedures, give advice on preventative healthcare treatments and on the administration of medicines. In particular the veterinary surgeon should be able to explain a diagnosis in simple layman's terms to clients who generally speaking have a limited knowledge of veterinary science. The practice requires staff who can provide all this information to the client in a clear, concise and understandable way.

• *Debt collection:* this is one of the least pleasant aspects of working in a veterinary practice, but is a very necessary skill which all staff, but especially receptionists, should possess.

WHAT DO YOUR STAFF WANT FROM YOU?

We may well have a long list of what we require from our employees but we should never forget the hopes and aspirations as well as the basic needs and requirements they themselves will have.

If each party can fulfil the other's needs we have the perfect combination of employee and employer. In reality there is of course always a certain degree of compromise.

Most staff are looking for some or most of the following requirements from their veterinary employer:

• ***Respect:*** for many staff this is one of their most important requirements. Staff have the right to be treated with consideration and respect for themselves and their abilities, whether they be an experienced veterinary surgeon or a part-time receptionist.

• ***Money:*** this is a basic need and comfort factor. A fair day's pay for a fair day's work is what most employees are looking for. Until fairly recently it was always the case that 'everyone wanted to work in a veterinary practice' and would do so for almost any salary. In many cases wages were low and numbers of applicants for jobs were high. Employment legislation and the emergence of an increasing number of qualified VNs is changing this, but the message is that staff should be paid fairly for what they do if they are to feel they have the respect of the practice and not feel that they are being exploited.

• ***Security:*** job security is less of an issue today now that legislation safeguards employees after 12 months employment, but it is nevertheless one of the basic needs of most staff.

• ***Interest/stimulation:*** to obtain the best from staff they need to have a keen interest and be stimulated by what they do. Even in a veterinary practice there are the mundane jobs, and these should be interspersed with more stimulating work procedures to maintain staff interest.

• ***Promotion/progression:*** not all staff wish to progress through the practice or be promoted to head receptionist/nurse, etc., but for those who do it is important to discuss roads to promotion and responsibility so that they have something to aim for and goals to reach.

• ***Good working conditions:*** this should really go without saying; all staff should expect and have a right to good working conditions, in terms of working time, health and safety and environmental conditions.

• ***Challenges:*** most staff enjoy a challenge and the satisfaction of achieving a set goal. It is by challenges that staff progress and take on more responsibility.

• ***Responsibility:*** many staff will say they want more responsibility, and this has to go not just with accountability but also with coaching for the responsibility. A good manager will delegate responsibilities to those staff willing and able to take them on, and provide help and support while the employee learns and masters the new role.

• ***Training/skill development:*** training is an essential part of developing staff and improving the practice services. Many more staff expect on-going training at work, and staff training and development programmes are becoming common in many practices.

• ***Thanks and praise:*** this is the simplest item of all to provide for your staff but is often the

Box 7.1 Expectations

STAFF EXPECT FROM THE PRACTICE ↓	THE PRACTICE EXPECTS FROM THE STAFF ↓
RESPECT	EXPERTISE
MONEY	COMMITMENT
SECURITY	HARD WORK
PRAISE	CONFIDENTIALITY
TRAINING	LOYALTY
RESPONSIBILITY	CARE
CHALLENGES	LONG SERVICE
PROGRESSION	GOOD COMMUNICATION
GOOD WORKING CONDITIONS	FLEXIBILITY
PROMOTION	CHEERFULNESS
STIMULATION	

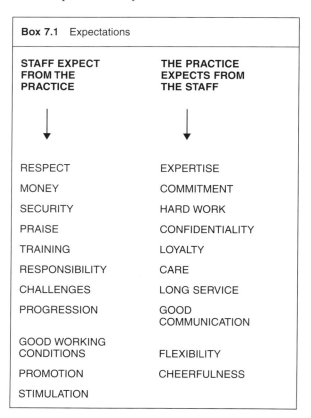

most overlooked. A word of praise or an occasional thank you when deserved can often be more motivating to an employee than a pay rise. Saying thank you costs nothing but produces great rewards for the employer.

RECRUITMENT

Recruiting new staff is one of the most important procedures in the management of a veterinary practice. Staff are your most important resource and their recruitment requires time, effort and financial resources for success.

The real cost of recruitment is very high when you consider the different areas involved in employing one new member of staff. Recruitment costs are made up from the following areas:

- Time – this is an expensive recruitment item and usually not costed in the recruitment budget
- Advertising – it is not cheap to advertise for staff and a small boxed advert in a publication such as the Veterinary Record can cost £200 per week
- Interviews – these are not only time-consuming but can be expensive if candidates' costs are reimbursed
- Administration – there are the costs of stationery, and postage (all applications should be replied to), and the administration time
- Clothing and equipment – new employees will require new uniforms and equipment
- Induction and training – the new employee will not necessarily be able to start the job without training, and induction training can take time
- Probationary appraisals – appraisals during the probationary period help to assess the new employee's progress but do cost money in terms of employee and appraiser's interview time and administrative work
- Dismissal – sadly sometimes the wrong candidate is chosen and has to be dismissed. This is the most expensive part of recruitment, as the whole process has to start all over again.

Bearing in mind how much effort and money goes into selecting a new member of staff, it is important to plan and execute the recruitment process. Recruitment can be broken down into the following procedures:

1. Job description
2. Candidate personal/skills profile
3. Advertising
4. Interviewing
5. Candidate choice and acceptance.

1. The job description

It is important that you have a very clear idea of the job you are offering so that you can select the best person for the post. The best way of doing this is to have a detailed job description. In the recruitment and selection process, job descriptions have four main uses.

Firstly they provide the information needed in determining the selection criteria and producing the personal and skills profile of the potential employee. It is at this stage that the job – if it is not a new post – can be reviewed and changed to suit present and future needs of the practice. Secondly job descriptions inform applicants of the nature of the job (the job description can be sent to the candidate with the application form). Thirdly they avoid misunderstandings about the job at the interview, both on the part of the candidate and the employer, and lastly they ensure that the newly-appointed staff understand the primary purpose and principal functions of the job and its place in the structure of the organization.

Job descriptions are essential documents which clarify the role of the employee and set the boundaries of the job. They are also invaluable for the good management of appraisals, training and discipline. Employee appraisal and training are discussed in Chapter 10, 'Human resources – training and appraisals'.

The ideal person to write a job description is the person who is actually doing the job, in collaboration with the practice manager or person responsible for personnel. As jobs change and new job descriptions are required the employee whose job it is should always be consulted in the writing of the new job description. The situation is obviously different if a new job is being created, but staff who will be working with the new appointee are likely to be very helpful in the formulation of some of the aspects of the new role.

The job description should contain the areas of information listed here.

Job title

Consider the job title carefully and use words that are descriptive of the job. If the job has changed since the last appointment it may be necessary to change its title. Many employees place a high importance on job title, and potential applicants may be influenced by the style and status the title reflects.

Major purpose of job

This sets the scene for the more detailed description later. This statement should make clear the main purpose of the job and the principal activities.

Location

It is important to include the location/s, as the practice may have a number of sites where the employee may be asked to work.

Hours of work

Make this very clear, state if overtime and holiday/sickness cover are required.

Lines of authority

The employee must understand to whom they are directly responsible and should report, and which members of staff (if any) are directly responsible to them. It is important that reporting lines and lines of authority are clear so that no misunderstandings arise and positions within the organization are not undermined.

Main duties

List here the main duties the post involves. There may be unspecified duties: do not forget to include 'Any other relevant duties which may be required'. This allows flexibility for the employer to request other reasonable additional work which may arise but is not listed on the job description. If the duties begin to alter significantly, a new job description may need to be supplied.

Knowledge and skills required

This is a statement of skills required to fulfil the role. It can be useful to refer to during appraisals or when discussing the need for further training.

Training

Make clear what training will be provided and what is required to be undertaken as part of the job.

An example of a head receptionist's job description is shown in Figure 7.1, and that of a veterinary nurse in Figure 7.2. Figures 7.1 and 7.2 can be found at the end of the chapter.

2. Candidate personal/skills profile

It is important to have a very clear idea of the skills and personal qualities you require from a new employee before attempting to select candidates for interview. A personal/skills profile enables you to set out those qualities and skills in a logical manner and is of great use not only when comparing applications but also when assessing candidates at interview. Did they match up to the qualities you specified? Did they have the skills required?

A profile form provides a guide to the kind of qualities and skills you may require from a new employee. An example of this is shown in Figure 7.3 at the end of the chapter.

The profile can be divided into 2 sections: personal qualities and skills required.

Personal qualities

• ***Appearance:*** do you want someone who looks smart and tidy? Does it matter how clearly they speak? If they are dealing with clients, what sort of manner should they have?

• ***Personality:*** who will they be working with, and how will you avoid employing someone who does not get on with the other staff? If they are working with clients, what sort of personality will be required?

• ***Flexibility:*** do you want overtime to be done? Do you want weekend work carried out? Do you want someone who can cover for sickness, etc.?

• ***Travelling time:*** how far away from work is it acceptable for them to live?

• ***Driving licence:*** do you want them to be able to drive? If so, they need a current UK driving licence.

• ***Date available to start work:*** how soon do you want them to start and how long would you wait?

• ***Health and fitness:*** will they be required to lift and carry?

Skills

• ***Education:*** what qualifications would you like them to have?

• ***Work experience:*** do they need to have had previous experience, and if so, what kind?

• ***Computer skills:*** what computer skills do they require?

• ***Specialist skills:*** are there any special skills required to carry out this job?

• ***Communication skills:*** does the job require good communication skills? Is teamwork involved?

• ***People skills:*** will they be working with clients? How will they need to relate to the rest of the staff?

• ***Special work interests:*** does the job require them to have a particular interest in, or develop certain aspects of it?

The profile is by no means comprehensive, as the qualities and skills are of course entirely dependent on the job in question and each manager will create their own profile. It does however serve as a starting point for thinking about what you require from your new employee.

Beside each quality or skill, list what you require from your employee. The completed profile will provide you with a very comprehensive picture of the kind of person you are looking for. It is unlikely that you will find someone who fits the profile perfectly, but at least you have an ideal in mind.

3. Advertising

There are three main questions to ask when placing adverts for new employees in veterinary and other publications:

- What is it going to say?
- Where will it be put?
- How long will it be put there?

What should the advert say?

The advert requires a number of essential ingredients in order to attract a potential applicant's interest.

An attractive logo of practice name is eye-catching and the job title should be obvious to see. A little information about the practice, the work it does, number of vets and support staff and its location should be included. The main body of the advert should describe the job, detail the sort of person who is required and list any other benefits the job may provide, such as accommodation, pension, etc.

Some practices simply ask for a Curriculum Vitae, while others send each enquirer an application form. A full job description should be sent to each enquirer with the application form so that they can make a considered decision whether or not this is a job they would like

Practice logo/name Job title What the practice does About the job (duties, hours, etc.) The person required The benefits Contact name and details Application/CV ***Closing date***

Figure 7.4 Advertising a job.

(this saves their time and the practice time). An example of the contents required in an advert are shown in Figure 7.4.

Where will you advertise?

Most veterinary and veterinary nursing and practice manager jobs are advertised in the Veterinary Record. Veterinary nursing jobs also appear in the nursing journals and publications such as *Veterinary Times*, and practice manager jobs often appear in local regional newspapers. Support staff and trainee veterinary nursing jobs are usually advertised in the local press.

How long will you advertise?

The answer is really for as long as it takes. Many publications offer deals for multiple weeks advertising (4 for the price of 3). One advert for one week may however be sufficient if the employment market is overflowing with the sort of employee you are looking for. In reality you will probably have to advertise professional posts for a number of weeks to ensure maximum exposure of the advert, but it is money well spent if you attract the right person for the job.

If you look in the classified section of the veterinary press you will see hundreds of different types of advert. Some are bold while others look quite insignificant. It is likely that most will do the job they set out to. However, if there is a shortage of the type of candidate you are looking for an eye-catching, well set out, informative advertisement will attract more attention and therefore hopefully more candidates to choose from.

It should not be forgotten that many vacancies are filled not by formal advertising, but by word of mouth; this is particularly common for practice manager posts. It is certainly worth using any contacts in the veterinary world who may know of potential applicants before advertising some posts. But care should be taken that by doing this, you are not restricting choice and taking the most convenient, though not necessarily the most successful or effective, route to recruitment.

4. Interviewing

Selecting for interview

The selection process for interviewing is important, and time should be spent assessing the applications and measuring them against the personal profile and skills you have set.

Decide how many candidates you wish to interview. Normally six would be ideal; any more and the time element becomes a problem, any less and you will find adequate comparison of candidates difficult.

Use the following selection criteria to choose the candidates: personal profile, letter of application, CV and application form, and recommendations.

Personal profile

Consider how well the candidate matches the requirements of the personal profile you drew up.

Letter of application

Consider the way the letter is set out, its neatness (the handwriting if it is hand written), and the grammar, as well as the content and reasons given for wanting the job.

CV and application form

Study this carefully, look for gaps in employment, check that experience is relevant, and look for indications given of future ambitions. Look at hobbies, interests, etc., and whether the candidate sounds like the sort of person who would fit in with existing staff or into the locality.

Recommendations

Take into account any recommendations that may have been given: these can be worth their weight in gold.

Now divide the applications into 3 groups: A. Yes – interview; B. Possible – only interview after group A interview; C. No – do not interview.

All staff who are going to be on the interview panel should carry out the above procedure. If you end up with more than six applications in the A group, go through it again to select the best six. If you do not manage to find six suitable applications for group A, consider carefully before you move any of group B into group A.

When you have selected those candidates for interview, send the offer of interview letter. This should contain a job description including salary range – if one has not already been sent with an application form – a practice brochure, map and details of time and place and what to do when they arrive.

The interview

Ask yourself the following questions:

1. Who is going to interview the candidates?
2. Where are they going to be interviewed?
3. When are they going to be interviewed?
4. What questions do you want to ask?
5. How long will the interview be?
6. Who will show the candidates around the practice?
7. How will you analyse the interview?
8. Will you have second interviews?
9. What records will you keep?

Ideally, candidates should be interviewed by their immediate superior and the practice manager or managing partner. It is unwise to have too many people interviewing as this can be intimidating and disorganized, but for the more responsible jobs, such as heads of departments and veterinary surgeons, a third interviewer may be required. So for example if interviewing a nurse the ideal interviewing panel would be the practice manager and the head nurse. For a head nurse, the panel might be a senior partner, a partner responsible for small animal surgery and the practice manager.

Interviews should take place in a quiet room away from the hustle and bustle of the practice and where there will be no interruptions.

Timetable interviews so that all the interviewers are free. Try to carry them out over a short period of time, one or two days, so that all the candidates are fresh in the interviewers' memory, and don't schedule the interview for the candidate who lives 200 miles away for 9.00 a.m.!

The interview questions should be designed to obtain information in the following areas:

- work experience and technical/clinical abilities
- teamwork
- client care
- computer skills
- personality
- practicalities.

Examples of interview questions are given in Figure 7.5 at the end of the chapter.

The length of the interview is a matter of practice choice, but time constraints inevitably restrict the length to one or two hours at the most.

The candidate should be shown around the practice, ideally before they are interviewed, so that the interview is in a better context and they can ask questions about what they have seen. It is often a good idea to ask one of the candidate's potential colleagues to give the practice tour. The candidate will be able to identify with this member of staff and the member of staff can assess how the candidate might fit in with other members of the team. Remember that you are also trying to sell the job to the candidate. So make sure you sell the benefits of working with the practice. It would be sad if the best candidate turned down the job because they had not been given the right impression of the practice.

In some cases there will be second interviews, either to introduce the short-listed candidates to other members of staff or to enable a final decision to be made. You will need to consider the interview process again, and plan how it will be carried out by the same method as before.

Very careful records should be kept of the interview. These should include:

- the original personal/skills profile
- the questions asked
- the candidate assessment form
- any other relevant material.

The record of the successful candidate will be of use during employee appraisals. But the records of all interviewees should be kept for at least 6 months in case you should be unfortunate enough that a candidate questions your decision, suggests some form of discrimination and asks for reasons why they were not offered the post.

The structure of the interview

There is a logical order to an interview, which if followed enables a smooth progress from greeting to farewell:

- Welcome the candidate, this is polite and indicates friendliness.
- Introduce the candidate to the interviewers and explain their role in the practice.
- Invite the candidate to sit down. Indicate where they should sit and do not place them in front of a row of interviewers. Have the seating arrangements as informal and comfortable as possible.
- Put the candidate at their ease; this helps to break the ice and makes the candidate a little more comfortable. Ask them what their journey was like or if they know the area, etc.
- Explain the interview procedure. Make sure the candidate understands how the interview will be conducted and how long it will be.
- Let the candidate introduce themselves; this also helps to relax the candidate. Ask them to talk about themselves, where they live, their family, and their career to date.
- Now ask the interview questions as arranged beforehand with colleagues, but always be prepared to alter or abandon questions if necessary, especially if a 'new line of enquiry' arises.
- Always give the candidate time for questions at the end of the interview.
- Ensure you have references. If the candidate did not supply references when they applied for the post, ask for them now if you think you may consider offering the candidate the post. Make sure you have full contact details. It is important to have a very clear idea of what you want to know about a candidate before taking up any references. Consider the job requirements and also their performance at interview, and decide what you need to know from the candidate's referee. Note any doubts you have or inconsistencies displayed by the candidate, and make sure you follow them up with the referee. Taking up references on the phone is a good method of checking on a candidate's suitability for the post. You can generally interpret more from a telephone conversation than a letter, and you have the added opportunity to ask further questions if required.
- Explain to the candidate what will happen next. Tell them when a decision will be made and how the job offer will be made (by letter, telephone, etc.), if there are second interviews and how to claim expenses – if this is the practice policy.
- Thank the candidate for coming. Maintain the politeness and friendliness to the closing of the interview. Leave the candidate with a good impression of the practice.

Candidate assessment

Once the interviews are completed, a decision has to be made. It is very useful to complete a Candidate Assessment Form for each interviewee – as shown in Figure 7.6 at the end of the chapter. The assessment form relates to the person/skills profile drawn up for the ideal candidate, and allows the interviewer to rate the candidate and comment on their skills and qualities. At the end of all the interviews these assessments can be compared in order to help choose the right person for the job. There are three golden rules when making this important decision:

- *Rule number 1* Be as absolutely sure as you can that this is the right person for the job, and if in doubt do not appoint.

- *Rule number 2* Do not take second best, however tempting this may be; re-advertise. The right person is out there somewhere.
- *Rule number 3* Listen to your staff; they are the ones who have to work with the new employee. If they don't think they can do this, do not make them try and probably fail.

5. Candidate acceptance

Reply to ALL the letters of application; this is only polite, and if not done can leave a very bad image of the practice. A standard letter can be used, as the reply is simply a formality.

For those applicants who were interviewed a more personalized letter is preferable, especially if the candidate was very good at the interview.

The letter offering the job to the lucky candidate should include the following information:

- the formal offer of the job
- contract of employment
- the start date
- a statement regarding any existing holidays the person may be taking
- uniform/dress details
- reporting for work details – where and to whom
- a contact name for information before employment starts
- a request for confirmation of acceptance of the post.

There is only one final step to take, and that is to inform employees of the appointment. This may be done by the usual communication channels such as the staff newsletter or even a memo. Brief details of the new employee should be given, as well as the date they will be starting.

There are always mistakes made when recruiting staff. No interview system is infallible, and most veterinary practices will have tales of the recruiting mistakes they made. However, by following a planned and considered selection process your chances of recruiting the best person for the job, rather than the 'Employee from Hell', are very much increased.

The contract of employment

A contract of employment is an agreement between two parties, enforceable by law. It is a contract of service and comes into being when an employee agrees to work for an employer in return for pay. The contract of employment comes into effect as soon as a job has been offered and accepted. Initially the contract is simply the terms of employment discussed at the interview, or written in the letter offering the job. The terms of the contract are the rights and obligations which bind the parties to the contract.

All employees who are employed for more than one month must receive a written contract of employment. The contract must be given to the employee within two months of their starting work. Ideally the contract should be given to the employee the day they start work. The contract of employment (whether oral or written) is legally binding and cannot be altered without the employee's consent, except under particular circumstances. An employer may wish to vary the terms of the contract because of changed economic circumstances, or due to a reorganization of the business. Areas of change may be, for example, pay rates, hours worked, duties or place of work. An employee may wish to vary the contract to increase their pay or working conditions.

An existing contract of employment can be varied only with the agreement of both parties. Any employer wishing to alter an employee's contract should first seek legal advice.

The contract of employment should contain the following information:

- name of employer
- name of employee
- job title
- place of work
- date when employment began
- details of pay and benefits
- payment details (monthly, weekly, hourly)
- pension scheme
- holiday entitlement
- sickness rules
- disciplinary rules
- grievance procedure and who grievances should be reported to

- length of notice to be given (by employee and employer).

Two copies of the contract should be signed by both the employee and employer, and a copy kept by each.

It is advisable to seek legal help and advice when initially drawing up contracts to ensure there are no loopholes or ambiguities.

Throughout the whole recruitment process the manager must be aware of the danger of discrimination against the candidates. Discrimination is dealt with in Chapter 8, 'Principles of Employment Law'.

DISCIPLINE

The objectives of disciplinary procedures are to maintain the standards of the organization. Every practice should have its own disciplinary policy, which may be contained in the practice or staff manual. The disciplinary policy should be given to all new members of staff when they commence employment. The main areas for disciplinary proceedings are attendance, job capabilities, health and safety, behaviour and honesty.

Misconduct

Misconduct is normally accepted to be poor attendance, poor work standards, breach of the practice health and safety regulations, breach of practice and client confidentiality, refusal or failure to carry out instructions, or unacceptable behaviour. Such misconduct will attract the following types of disciplinary procedure: oral warning, two levels of written warnings, and dismissal, as set out in Box 7.2.

Oral warning

The oral warning might be given for unacceptable standards such as continual mistakes in sending out practice accounts.

Written warning

The written warning is for a more serious offence, such as dispensing the wrong medicine to a client, or for continuation of an original offence, such as still making mistakes in sending out the practice accounts.

Final written warning

The final written warning is for continued failure to improve after the written warning, or for serious misconduct such as being rude to a client.

Dismissal

Dismissal would be for still further failure to improve after the final written warning, or for gross misconduct.

Gross misconduct

Gross misconduct would normally be considered to arise in case of theft, falsification of records, fraud, assault, malicious damage, the use of drugs or alcohol on the premises, or serious negligence, and would incur immediate dismissal.

The disciplinary interview

Before going ahead with a disciplinary interview, gather the facts promptly, take statements from individuals concerned, and record everything in writing. Be clear about the complaint and whether or not you actually need to take disciplinary action rather than simply talking to the employee on a less formal basis, providing counselling or more help and training. If you do decide to go ahead with the proceedings, ensure that the individual is aware:

- of the nature of the complaint
- that the interview is a disciplinary one
- of the time and location of the interview
- that they have the right to be accompanied at the interview.

Always arrange for a second member of the management team or member of staff to be present at the interview, even if the employee has decided to be accompanied.

The disciplinary interview should be conducted along the following lines:

- Introduce the people present.
- State the purpose of the interview.
- State the nature of the complaint.
- Show the supporting evidence.
- Allow the individual to state their case, and consider and question any explanations they put forward.
- If new facts emerge, decide if further investigation is required and adjourn the interview to investigate if necessary.
- Always call for an adjournment before reaching any decision.
- Come to a clear view of the facts.
- Decide on balance of probability which version of the facts is correct, if they are disputed.
- Decide on the penalty based on the gravity of the breach of discipline, previous disciplinary proceedings in similar cases, and the person's disciplinary record and general record.
- Reconvene the interview.
- Inform the individual of the decision and their right to appeal.
- Explain what actions are needed for them to improve their performance or behaviour, and what the time-scale is for the improvement.
- Record all the interview proceedings.
- Confirm disciplinary action in writing to the individual, unless it is an oral warning.

Monitor the individual's progress/performance and discuss it with them on a regular basis, providing help and advice where and if necessary.

It is important to remember that an employee's disciplinary record must be 'spent' after a fixed period of time (normally decided by the practice and usually 6–12 months in length). After this time, assuming that the employee has acted positively on the disciplinary requirements of the interview or oral warning, their disciplinary record can no longer be taken into account should they be asked to attend a future disciplinary hearing, even if they are for the same offence as before.

If the employee appeals against the disciplinary decision an appeal interview must be held and should be conducted along the same lines as the original disciplinary interview. If new facts emerge, do not be afraid to overturn the previous decision.

Every practice will have their own notion of what they regard as a disciplinary offence, and so must act in accordance with their disciplinary policies. However, it is essential to seek legal advice before any disciplinary proceedings are undertaken and many organizations such as the Federation of Small Businesses (FSB), the Veterinary Practice Management Association (VPMA), and the British Veterinary Association (BVA) provide free legal advice lines for their members.

Box 7.2 Misconduct and management response

MISCONDUCT	GROSS MISCONDUCT
↓	↓
ORAL WARNING	IMMEDIATE DISMISSAL WITHOUT NOTICE OR PAY IN LIEU OF NOTICE
↓	
WRITTEN WARNING	
↓	
FINAL WRITTEN WARNING	
↓	
DISMISSAL	

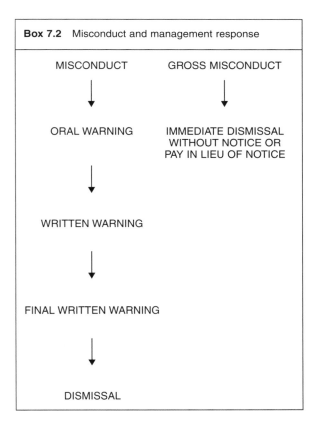

VETERINARY PRACTICE NAME/LOGO

JOB DESCRIPTION

TITLE

Head Receptionist

MAJOR PURPOSE OF JOB

To organize and co-ordinate the Practice Reception facilities and staff in order to provide a friendly, efficient and effective reception service to our clients

LOCATION OF JOB

This job is based at the main surgery but there may be occasions when duties at our two branch surgeries will be required

HOURS OF WORK

- 8.30 am–4.30 pm Monday–Friday
- 8.30 am–1.00 pm 1 Saturday in every 4
- Overtime will be required

LINES OF AUTHORITY

- Responsible to the Practice Manager
- Responsible for all reception staff in the main surgery

MAIN DUTIES

- To organize reception rotas, including holiday and sickness cover
- To organize and maintain effective debt control
- To send monthly client accounts
- To oversee reception staff
- To produce waiting room displays
- Reception staff discipline
- Reception staff training
- To maintain computerized client records
- To attend monthly heads of departments meetings
- To attend weekly meeting with Practice Manager
- To organize and chair monthly reception meetings
- To undertake general reception duties
- Any other relevant duties which may be required

KNOWLEDGE AND SKILLS REQUIRED

- A sound knowledge of Practice policies and protocols
- Good client care skills
- Good staff management skills
- Competence in the use of the practice computer and word processing systems
- Up-to-date knowledge of practice services and products
- Sound knowledge of common veterinary terms
- Familiarity with commonly used veterinary drugs
- Working knowledge of common veterinary treatments and operations
- Sound clinical knowledge of areas relevant to reception services

TRAINING

- Attendance at relevant in-house training sessions
- Attendance at appropriate external training courses which will enhance skills and personal development

Figure 7.1 Sample job description: head receptionist.

VETERINARY PRACTICE NAME/LOGO

JOB DESCRIPTION

TITLE

Veterinary nurse

MAJOR PURPOSE OF JOB

To act as a veterinary nurse in the practice nursing services team, which supplies surgical skills and animal care to the veterinary team as well as providing excellent client care

LOCATION OF JOB

This job is based at the main surgery

HOURS OF WORK

- 8.30 am–4.30 pm or 10.00 am–6.00 pm Monday–Friday
- 1 night duty per week and 1 weekend duty in every 5 weeks

LINES OF AUTHORITY

Responsible to the Head Nurse

MAIN DUTIES

- To provide surgical nursing support to the veterinary team
- To provide animal nursing for hospitalized animals
- To act as consulting room nurse when required
- To dispense animal medicines
- To maintain practice hygiene standards
- To sterilize surgical equipment
- To assist in X-raying animals
- To provide pre- and post-operative animal care

KNOWLEDGE AND SKILLS REQUIRED

- A sound knowledge of Practice policies and protocols
- Qualified Veterinary Nursing skills
- Good client care skills
- Competency in the use of the practice computer and word processing systems
- Up-to-date knowledge of practice services and products

TRAINING

- Attendance at relevant in-house training sessions
- Attendance at appropriate external training courses which will enhance skills and personal development

Figure 7.2 Sample job description: veterinary nurse.

JOB TITLE	
PERSONAL PROFILE	
SMARTNESS SPEECH BEARING MANNER	
PERSONALITY	
FLEXIBILITY	
TRAVELLING TIME FROM HOME	
DRIVING LICENCE	
DATE AVAILABLE TO START WORK	
HEALTH AND FITNESS	
SKILLS PROFILE	
EDUCATIONAL STANDARD Also include here numeracy and written skills	
WORK EXPERIENCE	
COMPUTER SKILLS	
SPECIALIST SKILLS	
COMMUNICATION SKILLS	
PEOPLE SKILLS	
SPECIAL WORK INTERESTS	

Figure 7.3 Personal skills profile.

This is just a small selection of general questions which could be used when interviewing veterinary, nursing and support staff. Clinical questions obviously depend on the practice concerned.

- What attracted you to apply for this post?
- How does this job fit in with your long-term career objectives?
- We are looking to develop nursing clinics for our clients; how would you approach setting up a weight clinic in the practice?
- Work in a veterinary practice is not always 9–5. How flexible can you be with your working hours?
- How easy will it be for you to provide the cover we will require when other staff are away on holiday or ill?
- What computer skills and experience do you have?
- What qualities do you possess that make you a good vet/receptionist/nurse?
- Why do you think it is important for clients to insure their pets?
- What do you see as the main aims of a veterinary practice today?
- Veterinary practices provide more services and sell more products than they used to. What sales and marketing skills do you have and how would you feel about promoting new products and services?
- What experience have you of dealing with difficult or awkward clients?
- What would you do if you are on your own in the waiting room, you are dealing with a client at the reception desk and the phone rings?
- What do you see as your main strengths both at and outside work?
- We are able to provide increasingly more sophisticated treatment for pets but at a financial cost to the client. Where do we draw the line?
- How would you like to develop your interest in surgery?
- What other interests or specialities do you have?
- What is the secret of good teamwork?
- What do you see as the role of veterinary support staff?
- How do you think any changes in the right to prescribe will affect the veterinary profession?
- How do you see the veterinary profession in 10 years' time?

Figure 7.5 Interview questions: examples.

POST...

NAME...

DATE...

RATING: 1 = POOR 2 = AVERAGE 3 = GOOD 4 = VERY GOOD

ASSESSMENT	**SCORE 1–4**	**COMMENTS**
PERSONAL QUALITIES		
SMARTNESS		
SPEECH		
BEARING		
MANNER		
PERSONALITY		
HEALTH		
FLEXIBILITY		
ABILITY TO FIT IN WITH STAFF		
CLIENT CARE SKILLS		
DEPENDABILITY		
ASSERTIVENESS		
TEAM MEMBER QUALITIES		
COMMUNICATION SKILLS		
SKILLS/EXPERIENCE		
EDUCATION		
RELEVANT EXPERIENCE		
COMPUTER SKILLS		
NUMERACY		
RECEPTION SKILLS If applicable		
NURSING SKILLS If applicable		
CLINICAL SKILLS If applicable		
OTHER SKILLS		

TOTAL SCORE [ ]

RECOMMENDATION...

....

Figure 7.6 Candidate assessment form.

CHAPTER CONTENTS

Discrimination 75
Sex discrimination 75
Race discrimination 76
Disability discrimination 76
Age discrimination 76
Equal pay 76

Maternity rights 76

Rights for working parents 77

The right to time off for family emergencies 77

Part-time work 77

Human Rights 77

National minimum wage 77

Working time regulations 78

Redundancy 78

Dismissal 78
Minimum period of notice 79

8

Principles of employment law

Employment law is an enormous and ever-increasing area which managers must be aware of. This chapter is intended to make the reader aware of some of the more important pieces of employment legislation which will affect the running of the veterinary practice. Managers should always seek legal advice before taking any actions which may relate to, or affect, employees' rights under the law. Legal advice may be obtained from the free veterinary helplines mentioned in Chapter 7, *'Managing human resources – the importance of staff, recruitment and discipline'*. Information on current employment legislation can also be obtained from the Department of Trade and Industry (DTI) website, www.dti.gov.uk and the ACAS website, www.acas.org.uk.

DISCRIMINATION

Discrimination means treating someone less favourably, at present, because of their sex, race or disability.

Sex discrimination

Under the Sex Discrimination Act 1975 (as amended), employers should not discriminate on grounds of sex, marital status, or because someone intends to undergo, or has undergone, gender reassignment. Sexual discrimination also applies to recruitment and training. The advertisement, interview, terms and conditions of employment, training opportunities, promotion, retirement and dismissal must all be free of any discrimination. Sexual harassment may also come under the discrimination umbrella. If an employer fails to deal with sexual harassment in the workplace, they may be guilty of discriminating against the employee.

Race discrimination

The Race Discrimination Act 1976 makes it unlawful for employers to discriminate on grounds of race, colour, nationality (including citizenship), or ethnic or national origins.

Disability discrimination

The Disability Discrimination Act 1995 makes it unlawful for an employer with fifteen or more employees to discriminate against current or prospective employees who have or have had a disability. Discrimination occurs when due to the employee's disability an employer treats them less favourably than they would treat other employees and cannot justify the different treatment. The different treatment cannot be justified if by making a 'reasonable adjustment' the employer could remove the reason for the discriminatory treatment. A 'reasonable adjustment' is any actions the employer could reasonably take to prevent putting the disabled person at a disadvantage compared with a non-disabled person. Any employer who employs 20 or more employees has a statutory obligation to employ a quota of disabled employees. Currently that quota is 3%. If the employer is unable to recruit the required quota they may apply for a permit to allow the employment of non-disabled persons for that quota.

Age discrimination

Discrimination on the grounds of age will become unlawful by 2006.

Equal pay

The Equal Pay Act 1970 makes it unlawful for employers to discriminate between men and women regarding payment for 'like work'. Men and women must be given equal treatment in terms and conditions if they are employed on 'like work' or work found to be of equal value. Equal pay is not restricted to remuneration alone, but includes most terms in an employment contract. Terms covering special treatment because of pregnancy or childbirth are not covered. Individuals may complain to an employment tribunal under the Equal Pay Act 1970 up to six months after leaving the employment. They may claim arrears of remuneration for a period of up to two years before the date of their tribunal application.

MATERNITY RIGHTS

The EU Pregnant Workers Directive sets out the following maternity rights:

- 14 weeks continuous leave before or after childbirth
- paid time off for antenatal examinations
- no dismissal during the period of pregnancy and maternity leave
- contractual rights preserved during maternity leave, e.g. company car, holiday entitlement but not remuneration
- pay at a rate of not less than the appropriate sick pay during the maternity period.

Maternity leave may commence at any time the female employee wishes after the eleventh week before the expected week of childbirth. Statutory Maternity Pay (SMP) is paid by the employer for a maximum period of 18 weeks provided the employee has been employed for 26 weeks ending with the fifteenth week of confinement.

The mother may return to work at any time before the end of the 29 weeks starting at the week of birth. She must notify her employer in writing 21 days in advance of the intended date of return.

When the employee returns to work she must be reinstated in the same kind of employment as she had previously on terms and conditions no less favourable than before.

RIGHTS FOR WORKING PARENTS

The Employment Bill 2001 contains far-reaching proposals regarding the rights for working parents and their employers. The main proposals which may well come into force during 2003 are:

- 6 months paid and 6 months unpaid maternity leave for working mothers.
- 2 weeks paid paternity leave for fathers following the birth or adoption of a child, to be taken during the first 8 weeks of the child's life. This Statutory Paternity Pay (SPP) will be set at £100 per week.
- SMP increased from £62 to £100 per week.
- The SMP payment to be increased from 18 to 26 weeks.

THE RIGHT TO TIME OFF FOR FAMILY EMERGENCIES

In many cases employees now have the right to take time off work to deal with an emergency involving someone who depends on them. A husband, wife or partner, child or parent, or someone living with the employee as part of their family can all be considered as depending on them. Others who rely solely on the employee for help in an emergency may also qualify.

An emergency is considered to be when someone who depends on the employee:

- is ill and needs their help
- is involved in an accident or assaulted
- needs them to arrange their longer-term care
- needs them to deal with an unexpected disruption or breakdown in care, such as a childminder or nurse failing to turn up
- goes into labour.

The employee can also take time off if the dependent dies and the employee needs to make funeral arrangements or attend the funeral.

The employee must tell their employer as soon as possible why they need to be away from work and how long they expect to be off. The time the employee can take will be as long as is required to deal with the emergency. For example, if a child falls ill the employee may take time off to take the child to a doctor and arrange for their care. The employee must make other arrangements for the child's long-term care.

There is no legal obligation for the employer to pay the employee when they take time off for family emergencies.

PART-TIME WORK

The Part-time Workers Regulations 2000 ensure that part-time workers are not treated less favourably than comparable full-timers in their terms and conditions. This means that part-time workers are entitled to:

- the same hourly rate of pay
- the same access to company pension schemes
- the same entitlements to annual leave and maternity/parental leave on a pro rata basis
- the same entitlement to contractual sick pay
- no less favourable treatment in access to training.

HUMAN RIGHTS

The Human Rights Act came into force on 2 October 2000 and incorporates into UK law certain rights and freedoms set out in the European Convention on Human Rights.

Some of the main points in the act are:

- the right to a fair trial
- the prohibition of slavery or forced labour
- the right to privacy
- the right to freedom of thought, conscience and religion
- the right to freedom of expression
- the right to freedom of association, including joining a trade union
- the prohibition of discrimination.

This piece of legislation may well be used by employees claiming against their employer for discrimination.

NATIONAL MINIMUM WAGE

All full-time and part-time employees in the United Kingdom have the legal right to a minimum level of pay.

On October 1st 2001 the minimum hourly rate for employees aged 22 years and above became £4.10. The minimum hourly rate (development rate) for employees aged 18–21 years inclusive became £3.50. The development rate can also apply to workers aged 22 years and above during their first six months in a new job with a new employer and who are receiving accredited training.

From 1st October 2002 the minimum hourly rate for employees aged 22 years and above will be £4.20 and the minimum hourly rate for employees aged 18–21 years inclusive will be £3.60.

WORKING TIME REGULATIONS

The Working Time Regulations 1998 implement the European Working Time Directive and parts of the Young Workers Directive, which relate to workers of 18 years and over.

The basic rights and protections for employees are:

- a limit of an average of 48 hours a week which an employee can be required to work (though workers can choose to do more if they want to)
- a limit of an average of 8 hours work in 24 which night workers can be required to work
- a right for night workers to receive free health assessments
- a right to 11 hours rest each day
- a right to a day off each week
- a right to an in-work rest break if the working day is longer than 6 hours
- a right to four weeks paid leave per year.

Some employment areas such as transport and fishing are excluded from the Working Time Regulations. Veterinary practice is not one of these areas. Present thinking is that time spent by home-based veterinary surgeons and nurses on call, at the disposal of their employer but not carrying out any duties, does not count as working time under the Working Time Regulations. This would not be the case if the employee is required to be on call at premises other than their own home.

REDUNDANCY

The Redundancy Payments Act 1965 allows for employees to receive redundancy payment if they have at least two years' continuous service since the age of 18. Only employees working under contract can receive redundancy payments. Redundancy must be caused by the employer's need to reduce their workforce, and the disappearance of the employee's job.

The amount of redundancy pay is related to the employee's age and length of service and ranges from half a week's pay to one and a half week's pay for every year of continuous service. There is a maximum payment for twenty years' employment.

If a business changes ownership the employee's contract of employment is automatically transferred to the new employer and the employee is not entitled to any redundancy payment due to the change of ownership. Subsequently any redundancies will be subject to all the normal regulations.

If an employee is given notice of redundancy they may leave early by arrangement with their employer and still qualify for payment. However, for redundancy payment to come into operation, the minimum period of notice which the employer has to give must have started by the time the employee gives their notice.

DISMISSAL

Legislation lists five specific types of reasons which can justify dismissal:

- Conduct – normally for disciplinary reasons
- Capability – when the employee is unable to satisfactorily do the job through lack of ability, qualifications or health
- Redundancy
- Statutory requirement – when for example an employee who is required to drive has lost their licence and there is no other suitable job available

- Other substantial reasons – for example in certain cases where an employee is taken on, on a temporary basis, to replace a worker suspended for medical reasons who is then reinstated.

For an employer to dismiss an employee fairly, they must have a valid reason for the dismissal and act reasonably in treating that reason as sufficient for dismissal. When an employee has reason to resign because of certain conduct by the employer, this is considered 'constructive dismissal' and may amount to unfair dismissal.

If an employee is unfairly dismissed or resigns due to 'constructive dismissal' they are entitled to claim reinstatement and/or compensation through an employment tribunal. Awards are based on actual loss of earnings and benefits, plus compensation. Before any employee is dismissed, legal advice should be sought.

Minimum period of notice

Employees are entitled to a minimum of one week's notice once they have had four week's continuous employment. Entitlement increases to one week's notice for every year of service, up to a maximum of twelve weeks, after the employee has worked for the business for two years.

Payment in lieu of notice may be offered to an employee as long as the payment covers the period of notice.

CHAPTER CONTENTS

Teamwork 81
The team mix 82
What makes a successful team? 84
Team leadership 84
Team motivation 84
The advantages of teamwork 85
Why do teams fail? 85
The difficult team member 85

Communication 85
Who should be told? 86
When should they be told? 86
What should they be told? 86
Where should they be told? 86
Who should be in control of communications? 90

Managing change 90
Barriers to change 90
The steps to achieving change 91
Changing of the culture – looking to new ways of working 91

9

Human resources – teamwork, communication and managing change

A great deal is talked about developing and encouraging teamwork in veterinary practice. In essence the whole practice is the team. For many years there has been very good teamwork, particularly in smaller practices where communication has been relatively easy and employee numbers small. As practices have grown in size and communications have become more difficult, the emphasis on developing teamwork has increased.

Good teamwork and communication are essential ingredients in all practices. We are living in a changing veterinary world, and managing the changes requires highly-developed teamwork and communication systems.

TEAMWORK

Teamwork can be summed up by the 5 Cs:

- Co-operation
- Combination
- Commitment
- Contribution
- Communication.

Teamwork is the co-operation and communication between a group of committed individuals who combine and contribute their talents, experience and personal qualities. Put more simply, it is success through people.

We can all work very productively and efficiently on our own and achieve great things, but the advantage of teamwork is that productivity is increased, quality is often improved and the members of the team together encourage greater motivation and commitment among individuals, as shown in Figure 9. 1.

The advantage of a team is that:

Together Everyone Achieves More

The veterinary practice is one big team of people working together for a common objective. However, in the larger practices within this big team are smaller teams which have to liaise and co-operate if the 'team' as a whole is to function efficiently. There will be nursing teams, reception teams and administration teams as well as the veterinary team and the management team. Some employees may well be in more than one team, for example the head nurse who as well as being in the nursing team is likely to play a part in the management team. This is illustrated in Figure 9.2.

The team mix

Teams benefit from the differences rather than the similarities between people, and the strengths of one member of the team will often

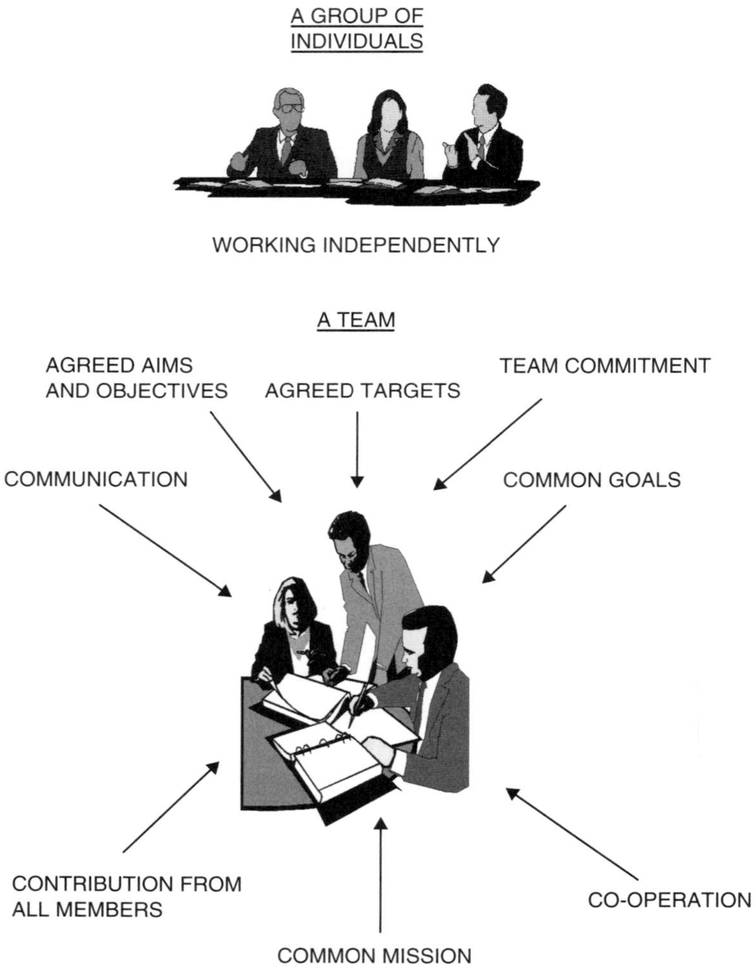

Figure 9.1 Independence vs teamwork.

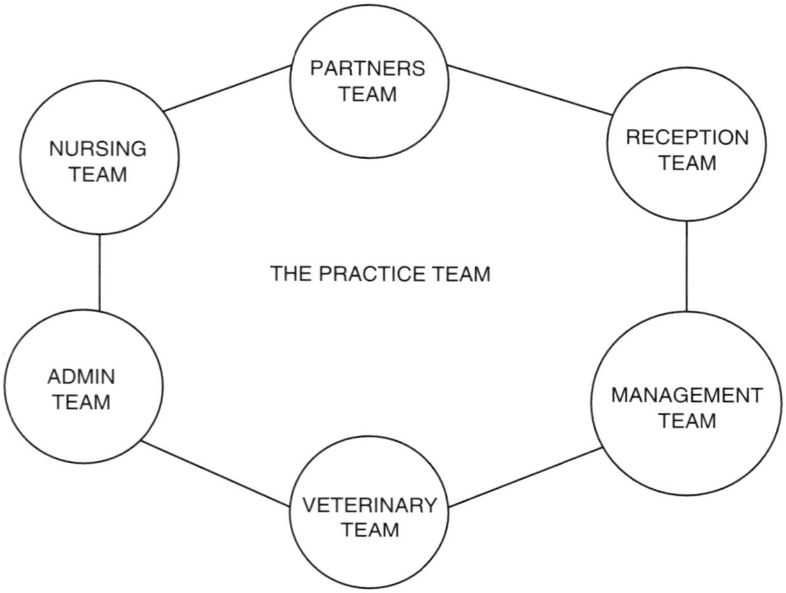

Figure 9.2 The practice team.

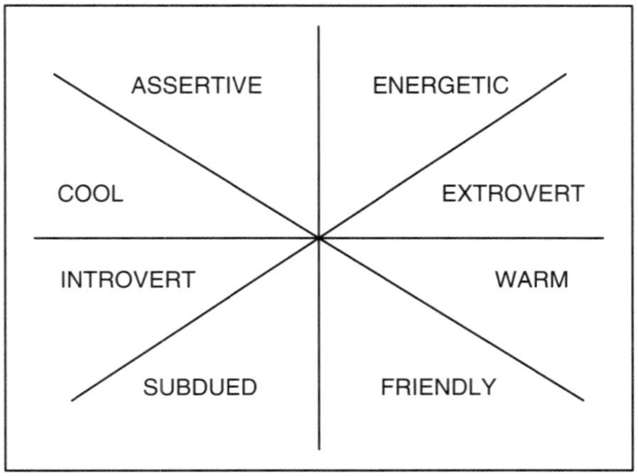

Figure 9.3 The team mix.

compensate for the weaknesses of another. Teams also benefit from having a mix of people with different personalities and skills.

As individuals we are all different. We may be extrovert or introvert, energetic or subdued, cool or warm towards others, assertive or retiring. Working on our own these characteristics may influence our output considerably, sometimes for the better and sometimes for the worse. In a team situation the ideal is to have a mix of all these characteristics so that a balanced view is produced of the work being carried out. This is shown in Figure 9.3.

Generally we exhibit five main types of behaviour in a work situation:

1. The Co-ordinator – the potential team leader, who makes sure objectives are clear and everyone is committed to the work programme, the new idea or the problem encountered.
2. The Challenger – who questions deficiencies and presses for improvements and results.
3. The Doer – who simply gets on with the task in hand.
4. The Thinker – who carefully considers all ideas and options.
5. The Supporter – who eases tensions, maintains harmony and working relationships.

If we have this mix in our team we are creating a balanced working situation where input from the different behavioural types produces an ideal working group.

What makes a successful team?

A successful team is usually small. In a veterinary practice groups of 6–8 would be ideal. The team must have strong leadership from within, and each member must adhere to the 5 Cs (commitment, communication, contribution, co-operation and combination). The individuals within the team should know themselves, their strengths and weaknesses, and know the other members and their abilities. Listening to team members, sharing ideas, successes and failures, all contributes to team strength. The team individuals should be able to jointly analyse problems and review and modify procedures. Above all, team members should be flexible, friendly towards others and not compete.

A successful team must have:

- a purpose
- good relationships
- good communication
- all the members performing well
- confidence in each other
- appreciation of each other
- the willingness to support each other.

As well as good leadership the successful team must be well trained, coached and appraised, and if this is provided, motivation and commitment are far more easily achieved.

Team leadership

The influence and usefulness of team leaders comes not from any hierarchical supervision but from their ability to lead from the front and train and coach their team members. Team leaders need to be able to co-ordinate the team skills and dovetail the strengths and weaknesses of individuals in the team. Perhaps their most important skill is their ability to facilitate the process of change. The team leader must by necessity be a highly-motivated member of the team who can instil this same motivation into their colleagues. Team leaders are often chosen by the manager, but increasingly they are chosen by the teams themselves, and in some cases the role of leader is taken on by different members of the team for set periods of time. There are some teams which operate without a leader at all, each member of the team taking responsibility for different aspects of team organization. In this situation there is a definite need for on-going training for team members to help them manage working as a group and making joint decisions.

Team motivation

Team motivation is vital for successful teamwork. Motivation is achieved by:

- The leader – without motivation from a team leader the members of the team will struggle to achieve motivation.
- Other members of the team – motivation is infectious, those who are seen to be motivated instil motivation into others.
- Having goals – the team must have agreed, achievable goals to aim for and to be motivated by when they are reached.
- Rewards – the rewards may be simply reaching goals or targets, or being thanked. Some rewards may of course be financial, such as bonus schemes.
- Personal development – this is a great motivator for many employees; it may be the gaining of a VN qualification or simply the attendance at a day's course relevant to the employee's role in the practice.
- Appraisals – a successful and productive appraisal which results in the further development of the team member can be one of the best ways to maintain motivation (appraisal is dealt with in Chapter 10, 'Human resources training and appraisals').
- Ownership of roles – ownership and empowerment are great motivators. Being given real responsibility for tasks can improve personal performance and motivation. It may be, for example, giving a nurse personal responsibility for a nurses' clinic or behavioural consultations, or putting one of the receptionists in charge of client accounts or pet insurance.
- Teamwork – teamwork itself motivates individuals by the variety of tasks they perform, the autonomy they are given and the identity

they feel as 'part of the team'. The social contact they have with other team members, as well as the responsibilities and opportunities for learning and development, are also good motivators. Box 9.1 illustrates the reciprocal nature of motivation.

The advantages of teamwork

Teams improve work productivity because everyone is working together to achieve common goals and outcomes. They also improve the quality of the work. Ownership of a task ensures a pride in a 'job well done' and a greater commitment to quality. Perhaps most important of all, teamwork improves staff motivation and commitment.

Why do teams fail?

Teams fail for a variety of reasons, principally:

- The team members do not know the practice goals
- The individual members do not understand their roles within the team
- The goals set are unrealistic
- There is poor training
- There is poor communication within the team
- There is poor communication between the team, other teams and the practice
- There is poor delegation within the team
- The team is made up of the wrong people.

Box 9.1 The reciprocal nature of motivation

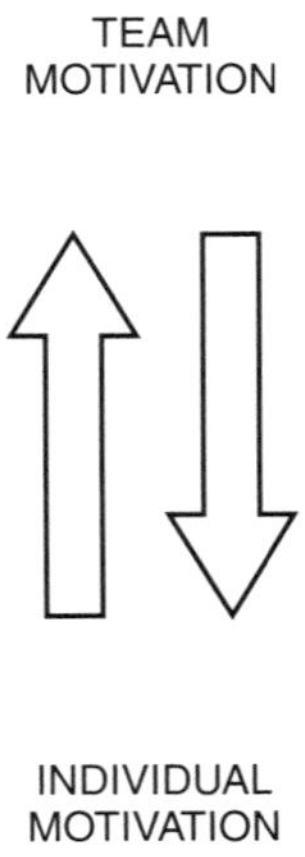

Any one of these reasons can cause a team to fail, but usually team failure is due to a combination of reasons and top of the list is often communication.

The difficult team member

The concept of teamwork is of course excellent, but establishing teams from a limited number of existing individuals can be very difficult. This is often the case in a veterinary practice. We do not always have the luxury of choosing the right mix of individuals and we often inherit existing groups of people whom we have to form into teams. We have to work with the material we have, and try to impart as many of the principles of good teamwork as we can.

We all have had experience of the difficult team member. These people can be a nightmare. The standard solution to difficult team members (if we cannot integrate them into their existing team) is to move them to another team and give them a different role. This is all very well in a large organization but virtually impossible in a veterinary practice. Perhaps the best answer to such a problem is to remove these individuals from the team and give them ownership of specific responsibilities. It is better to make use of their talents in this way than have constant friction in an otherwise efficient and happy team. We have to accept that some people are simply not team players and are better left as solo performers.

COMMUNICATION

The key to good teamwork, and a successful practice, is communication. Communication is important so that all the practice members:

- always understand the practice aims and objectives
- are kept up to date with new services, procedures, policies, plans, etc.

- can work as a team with common objectives
- can maintain good relations
- do not jump to incorrect conclusions through having inadequate information.

Always consider the 5 Ws of communication:

1. **W**ho should be told?
2. **W**hen should they be told?
3. **W**hat should they be told?
4. **W**here should they be told?
5. **W**ho should be in control of communication?

Who should be told?

Unless information is confidential, the best policy is to tell everyone. Then no one is left out, no one's feelings are hurt and there is no excuse for not having the correct information.

When should they be told?

Most information should be communicated as quickly as possible; second-hand information is usually wrong. However, there are obviously some things which are less important and can be communicated in, say, a staff newsletter.

What should they be told?

Generally it is best to tell everyone as much as possible. There will of course be some confidential information for the eyes of the partners and manager. But with this exception, it is better to give too much information than not enough. However, do not fall into the trap of drowning staff in irrelevant information. Clinical facts may not be relevant to administrators and the new photocopier maintenance contract may not be of interest to anyone except the practice manager!

Where should they be told?

There are a number of different internal communication methods. Each has its place within the organization and will be effective if used in the correct circumstances.

- *Internal memos:* if used occasionally for important or immediate information these can be very effective, but generally speaking the fewer pieces of paper that are floating around the surgery the better. The number of memos that are produced is inversely proportional to the likelihood of their being read!

- *Notice boards:* notice boards are useful but do need to be kept tidy and carry up-to-date information. They are better used for specific purposes such as health and safety, where new information can be posted for all staff to see immediately.

- *Staff newsletters:* staff newsletters are a very good way of communicating with staff. They can be used to provide information on management, clinical and social issues. The newsletter should be produced on a regular basis, and if much of its input is from staff it will tend to have a greater impact. Staff ownership of the newsletter can be very effective both in its production and contents, so that the publication acts not just as a means of communicating information from the management, but also as a way of bonding staff through a common effort.

- *Internal e-mail:* in large organizations or split practices and premises this is an increasingly useful way to communicate with staff.

- *One to one:* one to one communication is happening among staff all the time. It may also be necessary for the manager or head of department to have one to one meetings with particular members of staff regarding problems, discipline, etc.

- *Informal communication:* this is an excellent way of maintaining communication lines and may be through the staff BBQ, night out bowling or simply a group of receptionists or nurses going out for a meal. This is a slightly different form of communication where staff get to know each other outside work. This improved knowledge of each other helps tremendously in day-to-day working situations.

• *Appraisals:* appraisals are an excellent way of communicating with staff on a personal basis, and are dealt with in Chapter 11, 'Client care'.

• *Team briefings:* communication within a good team should be happening all the time but it is also helpful to hold reasonably regular team briefings when the whole team meets to discuss the current projects, issues of the moment or potential problems.

• *Meetings:* good internal communication in veterinary practice is essential and meetings are one of the ways to achieve this. The meetings must however be efficient and effective. Poorly organized meetings waste time and de-motivate staff, as well as costing money in lost time.

Effective meetings should:

- be short – a maximum of 1 hour
- start and end on time
- have an agenda for all those participating
- have minutes taken and distributed
- have action points produced by name and date
- be controlled by a chairman
- be small – but keep all relevant personnel informed via minutes, etc.
- have facts and figures and handouts available
- involve all members of the meeting
- stick to the subject
- give adequate notice of being held.

Meetings are a very valuable means of communication but it is important to hold the right number. Some managers can become rather over-enthusiastic about the number they hold. The reaction of 'Not another meeting!' by staff is to be avoided at all costs. The number of meetings held depends entirely on the structure of the practice and the issues to be discussed. Informal meetings are of course happening all the time, information is being passed on to appropriate members of staff and problems are being sorted out. This is how it should be in a good practice, but there is also the need for more formalized, structured meetings to discuss specific items.

It can be very helpful to draw up a plan of the necessary meetings the manager should organize and/or attend. The meeting planner shown in Figure 9.4 lists the meeting structure in

MEETING	FREQUENCY	STAFF ATTENDING	DATE	TIME
ALL STAFF	2 times per year	All staff		
PARTNERS				
PRACTICE MANAGER AND MANAGING PARTNER				
PRACTICE MANAGER AND INDIVIDUAL HEADS OF DEPARTMENTS				
RECEPTIONISTS				
NURSES				
SECTION/ DEPARTMENTAL HEADS				
SECTION/ DEPARTMENT				
CLINICAL				

Figure 9.4 Practice meeting planner.

a fairly large practice which is departmentalized, and should be used as an illustration of how to set about planning the meetings that your practice needs. They are likely to be quite different from those illustrated, but the principle of planning and organizing the meetings remains the same. The planner allows the manager to see the structure of practice meetings and set times and dates for them so that they can be integrated into the working of the practice.

Staff meetings

These should normally be held only once or twice a year unless they are needed for very special reasons. Full staff meetings are difficult to hold, as there never seems to be a time when all staff are available. It is likely that they will have to be held in the evening, and the provision of refreshments is often usual. Many practices will pay staff overtime for attending staff meetings out of hours, or give time off in lieu. Probably more than any other meeting this is the one which should be kept to time, as it is out of working hours and staff may well have other home commitments.

Partners' meetings

Monthly partners' meetings are essential for the efficient running of a practice. The practice manager should attend these meetings to report on financial and other relevant practice matters. It is at these meetings that practice policy is discussed and new plans and strategies approved.

Practice manager and managing partner meetings

The practice manager requires support and input from the partners, and in the case of larger practices there is likely to be one partner who has the remit for overseeing the practice management. It is always difficult to plan meetings during the veterinary working day, but it is important that these meetings are not missed or regarded as less important than routine clinical work by the vet. (Without good management there may not be the clinical work to do.) The meetings need not be very long, say a maximum of half an hour, but it is here that the manager can discuss any problems or issues where he or she requires help, advice or approval.

Practice manager and individual heads of department meetings

If the practice has separate departments for nursing, reception, administration, etc. the manager should meet on a regular basis with the heads of those departments to discuss staff and organizational matters. This enables the manager to keep abreast of what is going on in each department and provides back-up and advice for the head of department.

Receptionists' meetings

It is important that all receptionists have time at least once a month to discuss administrative and client matters as a group. This meeting is difficult to achieve as many receptionists work shifts, so getting them all together at the same time can be a problem. This may be the only occasion that some receptionists see each other. It is important to try and hold these meetings and distribute minutes and action points to those who miss the meeting.

Nurses' meetings

These are the same as the receptionists' meetings and provide valuable input time for discussion of nursing/clinical issues.

Heads of department meetings

In a departmentalized practice heads of departments need to communicate on a regular basis in order to avoid crossed wires and misunderstandings between the different disciplines. This is a time to iron out problems and discuss any difficulties one department may be causing another without realizing.

Departmental meetings

A number of times a year it is useful to have full departmental meetings where the workings of the department can be discussed and changes and improvements planned. The practice manager should attend these meetings.

Clinical meetings

Veterinary surgeons need to talk to each other on a regular basis about case studies, drugs, clinical procedures and so on. If possible a weekly meeting before morning surgery starts is ideal. There are an increasing number of practices which set time aside for such meetings, perhaps starting the day 30 minutes later in order to hold them. It is considered time well spent.

Meeting structure

A badly held meeting is worse than having no meeting at all. The structure of the meeting is important if productive discussion is to be achieved and results obtained. Meetings should follow a set format and always have an agenda, even if it is only a meeting between two people such as the practice manager and a head of department. A typical agenda is shown in Figure 9.5. Someone should be designated to take the minutes of the meeting and set the action points. This is a task which requires practice, and for those assigned the task some training should be provided. The set format and paperwork allow records to be kept, actions set to be checked and any disputed points to be verified. It can be surprising how often referrals back are made to discussions and decisions

1.00 pm Wednesday 28th June 2002

Practice meeting room

AGENDA

1. Welcome
2. Apologies for absence
3. Minutes of the meeting on 20th May 2002
4. Action points from meeting on 20th May 2002
5. Items for discussion
    1.
    2.
    3.
    4.
    5.
6. Any other business
7. Date of next meeting
8. Close of meeting

Figure 9.5 Departmental meeting.

made at meetings. The example of a meeting agenda sets out the format of a typical meeting.

The procedure of the meeting should be as follows:

- *Welcome* – it may seem unimportant but it is a courtesy to welcome the members of the meeting and thank them for attending.

- *Apologies for absence* – simply note the people who could not attend the meeting. Sometimes someone will be unable to attend but has registered their feeling/opinion on certain matters to be discussed at the meeting.

- *Minutes of the last meeting and matters arising* – read through the minutes of the last meeting and discuss any matters arising. In many cases these matters will be included in items for discussion during the meeting.

- *Action points and review* – action points from the previous meeting should be read through and reported on. This may be the incentive for staff to complete the actions they committed to at the last meeting.

- *Specific items for discussion* – this is the main business of the meeting and where most of the time will be spent. Items for discussion will be listed on the agenda and discussed in order. Do not have too many items for discussion, as you will be tempted to rush each item in order to get through them all. It is better to have another meeting at a different time if there are too many items for discussion in one meeting.

- *Any other business* – this is the time for any items not included in the agenda to be discussed. Usually they are matters which have arisen since the agenda was produced or they are small items which did not really warrant being included as a specific item for discussion on the agenda.

- *Date of the next meeting* – always set the date of the next meeting before closing the meeting. This ensures everyone knows the date and removes the hassle of checking later with everyone what would be an appropriate date.

- *Close the meeting* – officially close the meeting. Once the meeting is closed there can be no more discussion.

Who should be in control of communications?

In most cases responsibility for good internal and external communications rests with the manager. The manager should have a tight hold on the internal communications network and be in a position to assess how well it is operating and to make any necessary changes to ensure continuous and efficient communication among all staff. This responsibility does not preclude the delegation of tasks such as the production of the staff newsletter, organization of social events and some of the meetings, but the manager should always be fully aware of how effective these communication methods are and how they are being carried out.

MANAGING CHANGE

We are living in a rapidly changing world, and coping with and managing change is not easy. The manager must not only cope with change in the veterinary practice but also provide a smooth passage for the veterinary staff exposed to the changes. Managing change successfully is all about taking people with you as you move from the current steady state, through the pain of change, into the hopefully planned but unknown territory.

There are two types of change, incremental change and major change. Incremental change is the slower but constant change we all experience, the 10% increase or decrease in staff, the extension to the premises, the gradual development of new services, etc. Major change is the 25% redundancy, the move to a new building, the restructuring of employee roles.

Barriers to change

There are a number of barriers to change:

1. *The culture of the practice:* all practices have established policies and protocols. This is the

way they work, and change must take existing ways and methods into account if it is to be successful. The 'we've always done it like this' attitude can be a great barrier to any form of change, if the development does not allow a smooth integration of new and old methods, with the final outcome being the embracing of a new system.

2. ***Employee attitude:*** change is frightening and threatening to many people. Naturally one feels safer with the 'devil one knows'. It is the manager's role to portray the change as exciting and beneficial to the employees.

3. ***Lack of management strategies:*** change which is badly planned is going to be even more threatening to practice staff. Good strategic planning is essential. Aims, objectives and targets must be set, and a timescale decided upon.

4. ***Poor communication:*** if staff are not kept informed of plans they will assume the worst and be far more resistant to accepting the changes. Communication at all stages all the time is essential.

5. ***Insufficient skills:*** it is no good trying to manage any change if the skills required are absent. If a practice wishes to set up nursing clinics, they must have the skilled nurses available to run them. If a new computer system is to be installed, all staff must be trained to use it.

The steps to achieving change

Ability to change

First and most important of all, analyse the practice's ability to change. Are there the resources and opportunities to make the changes, is the likelihood of success good, will the results be worthwhile, and is the time right? Relate the ability to change to building a new veterinary practice:

- Can you afford it?
- Is there land to build on?
- Will you get planning permission?
- Is the location good?
- Will the new building satisfy your needs for more money, more space and the ability to develop services?
- Should you do it now or next year, what are present bank interest rates, what are your competitors doing?

Tailoring the change

Tailor changes to fit in with the people in the practice and the practice culture. You will still be working with the same people and the culture of the practice will not alter overnight, so changes must embrace existing situations in the practice.

Planning the change

This is the key to managing change. Plan the process at every stage. Have objectives and timed targets, continually monitor and review your plans, and don't be afraid to alter them if necessary.

Communicating the change

Make sure you communicate the plans to everyone at all stages. Keep all staff informed. No information means mis-information, rumours and gossip, the very things which will work against successful change and staff co-operation.

Team management

Create a management team to implement the plans. If possible draw the team from all sections of the practice; this will provide expertise and input from all areas, creating a balanced view of intended changes and their implications for the practice. Making a success of change requires shared vision – among all staff – and understanding of the changes by everyone.

Changing of the culture – looking to new ways of working

- *Communication* – with everyone all the time

- *Experienced help and counselling* – for those who have difficulty coping with change
- *Strong leadership* – to guide the practice through the change
- *Stakes in the change* – all staff must see what's in it for them
- *Benefits for all* – the change must be beneficial for all, not only in financial terms but also in job satisfaction and working conditions.

Change is with us and it will always be here. There are two ways of dealing with it: reactively – by responding only when one has to and when it is often too late, and pro-actively – by planning for change and trying to keep, if not one step ahead, then at least in the vanguard of change. Always remember that 'if you do what you have always done, you will get what you have always got.' The good manager wants more than this.

CHAPTER CONTENTS

Training 93
Induction training 94
Initial job skills training 96
On-going training and development 97
Obstacles to training 97
Developing a training programme 98

Appraisals 102
Who should be appraised? 102
Who appraises? 102
How often should appraisals take place? 103
The five golden rules of appraisal 103
The paperwork 104
The appraisal process 104
The appraisal interview 104

10

Human resources – training and appraisals

TRAINING

It is not so long ago that staff training simply meant sending your vets on a clinical update course to carry out a new procedure, your nurses to college to gain their VN qualification, or training support staff in-house to carry out their specific roles in the practice. For some practices it did and does still end there, the staff having been 'trained' and the commitment to training now at an end.

Today staff training is starting to be viewed from a different perspective, being seen as vital to the successful functioning of any veterinary business however small or large. Training requires a commitment by the practice and the training manager, to the development and sustaining of a training programme which will enhance staff skills. All training must be quality training and result in the improvement of staff skills or services to the client, and of processes and procedures within the practice. Training is also about the progression of staff roles and responsibilities, and of the continued development of the staff and the practice, as outlined in Figure 10.1.

The main advantages of training are:

- the improvement of the practice, departmental and individual performance
- the achievement of new business objectives through better-trained staff
- the production and maintenance of job satisfaction
- the achievement of improved staff motivation and commitment

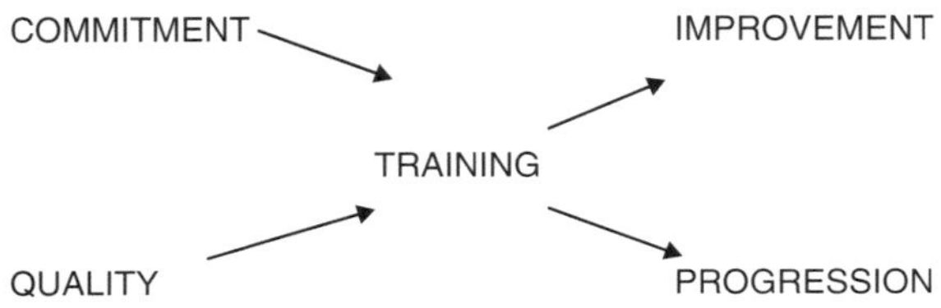

Figure 10.1 Central nature of training.

- the increase in practice income through greater efficiency and effectiveness
- the provision of a quality service to clients.

Implementing a staff training and development programme in your practice is time-consuming and requires the commitment of all members of the practice, but in particular that of the training organizer who is likely to be the practice manager.

The training process can be divided into three stages:

1. Induction training
2. Initial job skills training
3. On-going training and development.

The most important thing to remember is that training never ends. However long an employee has been with the practice, there is always more to learn and new skills to develop, because the work of the practice and client needs are always changing.

Induction training

The new employee on their first day at work is going to ask, 'Where am I?', 'Who is everyone?' and 'What am I expected to do?' Your new employee can be left to find out the answers to these questions themselves, or you can help them by providing the answers during the first stage of their training – induction. Induction is about all the steps an employer can take to ensure that new employees settle into their jobs quickly, happily and effectively.

The first day at work

Before any new employee begins work, all staff should be made aware of their appointment and when they will start working for the practice. In particular the people the new employee will first meet should be briefed on the date and time of their arrival.

A reporting time (such as 9.00 am) and place (for example reception) should be set for the new recruit. They should be welcomed by reception staff and met promptly by the manager or person delegated to begin the induction process.

One of the first formalities should be the completion of any necessary paperwork. It is useful to have a checklist of documents required both by the practice and the employee, as shown in Figure 10.2.

The employee should be given their full job description and contract of employment and the practice or staff manual if there is one. If the practice does not have a staff manual the employee should be provided with such basic information as; fire and first aid procedures, the health and safety policy and the practice disciplinary policy. On that first day it is also very helpful for the employee to be provided with a staff list, organization chart and if the practice is large, a floor plan. Uniform, protective clothing, locker keys, etc. should also be handed out at this stage. You will require from the new employee their P45 and details of a bank account into which their salary will be paid, as well as details of next of kin, doctor's telephone number, etc. The manager should spend some time with the employee at this stage explaining the fundamental procedures and systems of the practice, i.e. the basic housekeeping.

Once all these practical details are out of the way the rest of Day One induction training can proceed. Figure 10.3 gives an example of a Day One induction programme for a new receptionist and provides a basic guide to how any programme needs to be tailored to the new employee and their role in the practice.

The new employee should be introduced to the practice staff, and given a tour of the practice. It is a very good idea to allocate a member of staff to the new employee, to be the starter's 'friend'. They will give the starter the lowdown on things such as tea and coffee arrangements, staff rooms, cloakrooms, the do's and don'ts of

ITEM	SIGNATURE	DATE
JOB DESCRIPTION		
CONTRACT OF EMPLOYMENT		
P45		
SALARY PAYMENT DETAILS		
NEXT OF KIN		
DOCTOR'S TELEPHONE NUMBER		
ORGANIZATION CHART		
ROTA		
STAFF LIST		
PRACTICE FLOOR PLAN		
PRACTICE/STAFF MANUAL		
First aid regulations		
Fire regulations		
Health and safety regulations		
Disciplinary regulations		
Health and Safety Policy		
UNIFORM / PROTECTIVE CLOTHING		
LOCKER KEYS		
CAR DOCUMENTATION		
TRAINING PROGRAMME		

Figure 10.2 New employee documentation checklist.

TIME	ACTIVITY	PERSONNEL INVOLVED
9.00	Meeting practice manager and paperwork	Practice manager
10.30	Coffee with head receptionist, discuss rota, etc.	Head receptionist
11.00	Health and safety briefing	Health and safety officer
12.30	Lunch	Allocated 'friend'
1.30	Observation in reception area	Receptionists on duty
3.00	Tea and overview of reception activities	Head receptionist
4.30	Debriefing with practice manager to discuss the day and any queries	Practice manager

Figure 10.3 Day One induction timetable.

the practice, etc. The rest of the day should be spent getting to know the practice and the particular area where they will be working. Under no circumstances should the new recruit be asked to work on the first day, as this is their day of observation and making themselves familiar with the practice surroundings. At the end of the day it can be very helpful to have a de-briefing meeting with the practice manager or head of department, just to iron out any queries or problems which may have arisen. The practice manager should also discuss with the new employee the induction training programme which has been designed for them, explain how it will operate, and how it will be assessed.

Induction training programme

Induction training programmes may last one or two days or up to two weeks, depending on how they have been designed and what is appropriate for the practice and the new employee.

OBSERVATION	TRAINEE	TRAINER	COMMENTS	DATE
CAT SPAY				
BITCH SPAY				
CAT CASTRATE				
DOG CASTRATE				
LUMP REMOVAL				
ANAESTHETIC ADMINISTRATION				
RECOVERY				
DISPENSARY				
LABORATORY				
CONSULTING ROOM				
NURSES' CLINICS SUTURE REMOVAL CLIP CLAWS WEIGHT OLDER PET DENTAL				
PUPPY PARTY				
EUTHANASIA				
ETC.				

Figure 10.4 Induction training observation checklist.

The aim of the induction programme is to familiarize the new employee with all the work of the practice and enable them to place it in context with their own specific job. The longer induction programmes will combine observation of other areas in the practice with practical work in the employee's specific area, so that they are learning their own job as well as observing those of others.

Figure 10.4 illustrates an observation checklist for a new receptionist. It is important that both the trainee and trainer sign the checklist to ensure that the observation has taken place and that the trainer is happy that the trainee understands both the process and what they have observed.

Initial job skills training

Job training involves three kinds of training:

1. theory
2. observation
3. practice.

All three kinds of training will be used to teach employees new skills, but it is important to understand that people have different learning styles. When designing a new employee's training this must be borne in mind.

There are four main learning styles:

1. *Activist* – those who want to 'have a go' and have 'hands on experience' right from the start. These people will benefit from a very practical training programme.
2. *Theorist* – those who want to learn about a new skill first. These people will benefit from theory and observation training before putting their knowledge into practice.
3. *Reflector* – those who are cautious and methodical. An observation-based programme will benefit these people.
4. *Pragmatist* – these are the planners who learn, design and then test out their skills. These people will learn best from a theory-based training programme.

Specific job training should be carefully planned with the skills required and the individual in mind. The training programme should have scheduled time set aside for training the employee and for the employee to carry out

Name.. Job Title...

SKILLS REQUIRED	SKILLS ACQUIRED	TRAINEE SIGNATURE	COMMENTS	TRAINER SIGNATURE	COMMENTS	DATE

Figure 10.5 Training competence checklist.

personal study. There should be dedicated trainers committed to the programme, and a timetable should be set for reaching training targets. A training competence checklist will help to assess the progress of the training. It should list the skill areas required by the trainee, and be completed by both trainee and trainer as the training progresses, as shown in Figure 10.5.

On-going training and development

On-going training and development is for all staff for all their working life. Training never ends; there are always new services to provide, products and equipment to use, processes to learn about and skills to develop. Ideally practices should aim to develop a training culture in which all staff are aware that training is one of the normal activities of the practice.

Developing a training programme is time-consuming but rewarding, not just to the employees who are learning but to the manager who sees the fruits of their labour and to the practice owners who see increased productivity and enthusiasm.

Obstacles to training

As with most other activities that involve change there are obstacles to overcome before plans can go ahead. The main obstacles to staff training are staff attitude, money, time and resources.

Staff attitude

This is possibly the most difficult obstacle to overcome. Some staff will see more training as a threat; they will worry that they cannot learn what is expected of them and will resist at every opportunity. Avoiding this scenario requires careful staff consultation at all stages of the training planning. Involve the staff and ask them for ideas, help and opinions on what is required. It is important that they have ownership of their own training and that they have participated and agreed in its design. Show them the benefits of more training and personal development, not just to the practice but to themselves.

Money

You can only train within your budget, so do not be over-ambitious. It is better to do a little well than too much poorly. Concentrate on the most important areas that require training, and develop long-term training plans.

Time

Time is always a problem for veterinary practices and it is important to be realistic about how much time staff will have for training. Do not place them under pressure to carry out training or they will resist it.

Resources

Apart from the obvious resource of money, other resources such as training space, internal trainers, expertise, training equipment and availability of local courses can all be obstacles. They need to be considered at the outset of the training programme development.

Developing a training programme

First establish the aims of the programme, i.e. what are you trying to do, what do you want the training to achieve?

You may, for example, be trying to achieve some of the following:

- enable all members of staff to carry out their respective roles more responsibly, effectively and efficiently
- improve staff performance
- enable staff to attain job satisfaction
- develop new skills
- develop new services
- promote teamwork
- motivate staff.

In whatever area you are looking to train, first establish the overall aims of the practice, and then work towards more specific aims. For example, if you are considering the training needs of reception staff, look at:

1. Aims and objectives of the practice
2. Aims and objectives of reception
3. What staff skills are needed to achieve these aims and objectives.

In this way you can establish the core skills and knowledge required by the reception staff.

One of the core skills identified in reception would be booking appointments. The knowledge required to book appointments would be:

- consultation times
- operating times
- booking procedures
- telephone skills
- communication.

Look at all the core skills and all the knowledge required, assess the standard of knowledge which already exists among the reception staff, look at any new knowledge required, say, for developing new services or procedures, and identify the overall training needs.

Identifying training needs

There are a variety of ways to identify training needs:

- ***Brainstorming*** – this involves gathering together all the staff for whom training is to be designed and giving everyone an opportunity to make suggestions on the training needed.

- ***Questionnaires*** – send questionnaire to all staff asking them to identify areas where they consider they require training.

- ***Interviews*** – interview staff individually to discuss their training needs.

- ***Observation*** – the manager's own observation, or that of the heads of departments, team leaders, etc. are valuable in assessing the training requirements of staff.

- ***Appraisals*** – if the practice carries out annual appraisals, training and development needs will be discussed at these meetings.

Designing the training programme

Having established the core skills all staff require and the need for specific training among staff, it is time to consider who will undertake the training, the method of delivery, when training will be carried out, how long it will take, and how much it will cost.

The programme should be designed to satisfy both the short-term and long-term outcomes which the practice requires of the training. In the case of product familiarity, Figure 10.6 shows an example training programme where in this case short-term training might be a better knowledge

Core skill	Training required	Method of delivery	Trainer	Training time	Venue	Complete by	Cost	Employees to be trained	Training outcomes
New product familiarity	Knowledge of all new products Use of products	Talks Leaflets	Drug reps Vets	Lunchtime 1–2 pm	Seminar room	On-going	Food for lunch	All nurses and receptionists	Short term – better knowledge of products Long term – more product sales

Figure 10.6 Practice training plan.

of new products while long-term training might be training for increased product sales.

One of the best ways to design the programme is to draw up a training plan for each section of practice staff and make training decisions in the areas suggested in Figure 10.6.

Core skill. Identify the core skills which staff must possess.

Training required. Identify the training required by staff to fulfil the core skill needs.

Method of delivery. How will the training be carried out? Consider staff learning abilities, the practical considerations of staff being away from work, numbers of staff to be trained, the most effective way of training, and the cost. In some cases a lunch-time talk by a drug rep or leaflets on new products may make up the training while in other instances an external two-day course may be required.

Who will train? In some cases training will be carried out in-house by vets or nurses, but there will be some training which requires outside trainers, external courses or distance/internet/CD Rom/training.

When will training take place? In an ideal world training should always take place in working hours, but in the real world of veterinary practice this can often be difficult. Whenever possible, training should be carried out during working hours and lunchtime. If there is lunchtime training, provide food and give a short rest break before training starts. Distance/private learning is becoming increasingly popular and there are now a variety of training CD Roms and internet packages. However, this type of learning does not suit everyone and the manager should be careful to ensure how well the employee will manage with this type of training.

Where will training take place? If the practice has a dedicated training/meeting room, much of the staff training can take place there. If this is not the case, external courses may be a better option, as well as home study using IT-based courses.

When should training be completed? There must be a target for the completion of specific courses. Inevitably these targets will sometimes have to be changed but it is very important that there are targets to aim for. Some training, such as new product awareness, will of course be on-going and it may be that there are set times when this training always takes place.

How much will it cost? Training can be expensive, not only in the cost of the course but also the staff time, cover time and travelling time. All these costs must be considered when estimating the full price of the training and be within the budget set for staff training.

Who is to be trained? Some training will be for all staff, but some will only be for specific members of the practice. It is important to identify who is trained in what, so that the full training plan can be completed.

What training outcomes do you want? This may seem obvious but it is easy to rush into staff training and not look carefully enough at what the end result of training needs to be. It is only by knowing what outcomes you wanted that you will be able to assess if the training has been successful.

Individual training plans

It is very helpful for each member of staff to be given their own training programme, as this gives them a clear idea of what training there will be, how it will be organized and what is expected of them at the end of the training. It is also extremely useful during an appraisal to have the training programme to refer to and discuss. The individual training plan can be a replica of the master practice plan in format but designed specifically for the individual's own training needs.

Monitoring training

It is only by carefully monitoring staff training that you can measure its success. There are many ways to monitor, but perhaps appraisal interviews are one of the best. Here the manager has a chance to talk to each employee, discuss training and development, and look at the best way that individual training needs are being satisfied. Evaluation forms are also a good way of monitoring training. At the end of any training period the employee should be asked to complete an evaluation form which asks some or all of the following questions:

- What did you expect to learn from the course?
- How did the course meet up to your expectations?
- If it did not meet your expectations, how could it be improved?
- How has the course helped you to carry out your job better?

Staff CPD record cards are a good way not only of recording training but also measuring its success. An example of such a record card is shown in Figure 10.7.

Although the record card is primarily for the employee's use and benefit, it is another piece of documentation which should be brought to the appraisal interview to be discussed. The record should include home study, courses, and in-house training, etc. The employee, as well as the manager, can see at a glance how much training has been received during the year. Other monitoring methods include feedback from trainers, supervisors and of course clients (especially if the practice has client focus groups). The manager is also going to receive feedback from departmental heads and staff supervisors on how successful courses have been in improving individual performance.

Evaluating training

You can evaluate training both quantitatively and qualitatively.

Quantitative evaluation. This method of evaluation involves looking at what the training has cost and comparing it with increased productivity rates and/or improved profits. Measuring such productivity rates or profits is not easy, as there will always be other factors involved, but general trends can often be seen which can be attributed to specific actions such as training. It is also worthwhile looking at the attendance rates on the courses. Did all the required staff attend, and if not, why not? Did you spend money on an internal course which was poorly attended because of work commitments? How could this be improved in the future?

Qualitative evaluation. We are looking here at opinions and views expressed by individuals in the practice. Hearsay evidence is always a little suspect, but if a significant number of similar comments are received it is reasonable to attribute some weight to them. Feedback can also be measured using specific client surveys.

TRAINING RECORD

NAME.. JOB TITLE.......................................

TRAINING RECORD FROM 1st JANUARY 200.... TO 31st DECEMBER 200....

DATE OF TRAINING	**TITLE OF COURSE**	**INTERNAL OR EXTERNAL TRAINING** **If external state where course was held**	**LENGTH OF COURSE**	**COMMENTS ON COURSE**

Figure 10.7 Staff training record.

Reviewing training

Review training on a very regular basis, asking yourself the following questions:

- Have individual, departmental and practice training objectives been achieved?
- Is more training needed?
- Is less training needed?
- Is different training needed?
- Has training kept within budget?
- Are the methods of measuring training adequate?

- Are resources sufficient?
- Are training times appropriate?
- Did all the staff have a reasonable access to training?

Never be afraid to change any of the training programme if it will benefit the staff or the practice. Any programme must be flexible, staff change and the skills required change, as do the methods of training, and it is important to achieve the best mix. If this means altering the training programme, then do so.

Below are some of the do's and don'ts of staff training.

Do:

- be clear what the practice objectives are
- be clear what the training objectives are
- consult staff at all stages
- allocate realistic funds
- monitor
- evaluate
- review.

Do not:

- be afraid of change if the plan is not working
- think training is ever finished
- give up when the going gets tough
- expect to achieve miracles overnight.

APPRAISALS

Small businesses such as veterinary practices can benefit greatly from operating an appraisal system. In some ways the appraisal task is made easier because managers and supervisors will know their staff well. Appraisals can help improve employees' job performance by identifying strengths and weaknesses. They also determine how the strengths can be best developed and utilized and the weaknesses overcome.

The performance appraisal is a very effective means of ensuring that managers and their staff meet regularly to discuss past and present performance issues, and to agree what future action is appropriate on both sides. Appraisals should always be positive, they should also be continuous, and once begun they should be carried out on a regular basis, usually annually. The appraisal should assess an employee's performance, look at past achievements and agree objectives for the future. It should build on the employee's strengths and help resolve any weaknesses. Successful appraisals will increase individual and thereby practice productivity and performance, and help develop an individual's potential. A well-organized appraisal system will increase staff motivation and commitment, but a poorly-managed appraisal is worse than no appraisal.

One very important point to make is that appraisals should never be linked to pay. The appraisal is used as a tool for developing a staff member's skills and abilities. It should be constructive, positive, and encouraging to the employee. Linking pay to the outcome of the appraisal will alter the whole ambience of the interview and remove its relaxed atmosphere.

Who should be appraised?

The answer to this is everyone, including the partners and owners of the practice. For a practice appraisal system to be successful, everyone in the practice must be involved and appraised. This avoids the them-and-us scenario where junior staff are appraised by seniors who themselves are not appraised.

Who appraises?

In most organizations employees are appraised by their immediate managers, based on the assumption that those who delegate the work and monitor performance are best placed to appraise performance. In veterinary practice appraisals are best carried out by an employee's immediate senior. In the case of a small practice this may mean that most of the appraisals are carried out by one person, i.e. the manager or senior partner. In larger practices head nurses and head receptionists would appraise their staff, and in turn be appraised by the practice manager. Figure 10.8 shows a typical appraisal hierarchy.

In the case of partners' appraisal it is probably best if possible for each partner to be appraised

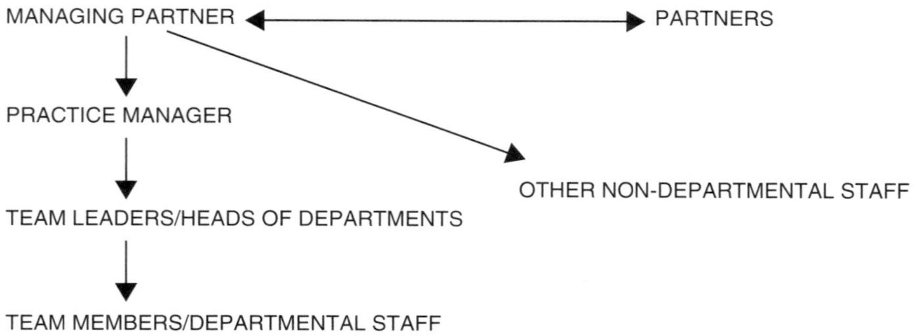

Figure 10.8 Who appraises whom?

by two others. For example: Partner A is appraised by partners B and C; partner B is appraised by C and D; C is appraised by D and A; D is appraised by A and B.

As an alternative to this form of partnership appraisal, in the case of a single owner appraisal from below should be considered, perhaps by a senior administrative assistant or practice manager if there is one. This type of appraisal must be carefully carried out and look at staff support and leadership skills, communication and approachability as some of the important areas for appraisal.

How often should appraisals take place?

Appraisal should be a continuous process, and realistically an annual appraisal is what most practices should be able to achieve. Between the annual appraisal a six-month mini-appraisal can be organized to assess how the individual's training and development is progressing. There are a number of instances where appraisals will need to be more frequent, in particular the appraisals for new employees. To assess how well a new employee is managing, a one, three and six month probationary appraisal can be carried out. These appraisals do not need to be very long or sophisticated but they do provide a set time when the employee and manager can formally get together to discuss any problems, and plan the employee's progress and training needs. They also provide the employee with a guide to how they are doing, and allow any problems or potential problems to be addressed quickly.

The five golden rules of appraisal

Before any appraisal scheme is embarked upon there are five golden rules to follow:

1. ***Gain the commitment of the owners/partners:*** the appraisal scheme will be viewed with mistrust and apprehension by some members of staff so it is important that the partners are seen to be not only backing the scheme but actively taking part in it, by themselves being appraised. The practice will need to spend time and money setting up the scheme and training appraisers, and this must have the backing of the partners.

2. ***Consult and inform staff:*** the appraisal scheme will not succeed if the staff do not give their support. From the very start when the scheme is just being considered, consult staff and provide information to help them understand how the scheme will work and the benefits there will be for them. Listen to their worries and spend as much time as is necessary ironing out difficulties.

3. ***Train the appraisers:*** good appraisals require skilled appraisers. This is not a role that anyone can just take on without some form of training. Training may take the form of an external course, the reading of appraisal articles and booklets, or being trained internally.

4. ***Keep it simple:*** keep the scheme as simple and as straightforward as possible. A complicated scheme takes more time, involves more work, is less acceptable to staff and unlikely to provide any better results than a simple one.

5. ***Establish a system for monitoring:*** it is important to know if the scheme is working well or needs modification. A system should be set up to gather the views of both appraisers and appraisees about how the scheme operates, what problems they have encountered, and how improvements could be made. Monitoring may be as simple as a questionnaire for staff to complete or a more formal regular meeting of appraisers to discuss the scheme.

The paperwork

It is essential to have written records of appraisals to enable both manager and employee to look back at previous appraisals and decisions made as well as providing evidence of on-going agreed training. The documentation provides the history of the employee's development in the practice; it can be used to assess their suitability for promotion, as well as in the worst scenario assess the need for any disciplinary procedure.

The essential paperwork is listed below.

• ***The job description:*** the job description should feature at the beginning of the appraisal form. The employee's performance will be based on how well they are carrying out their job description.

• ***The job profile:*** the job profile allows the employer to highlight the skills and qualities the employee requires to carry out the job description and should be used as a guide when completing the employee's appraisal form. An example of a job profile is shown in Figure 10.9 at the end of the chapter.

• ***The self-appraisal form:*** this form is for the employee to complete before the appraisal interview, and asks questions about their achievements, difficulties, skills and training. The completed form is handed to the appraiser a few days before the appraisal so that they can study it and prepare comments. An example of a job appraisal form is shown in Figure 10.10 at the end of the chapter.

• ***The performance appraisal form:*** this is the form for the appraiser to complete; it is used to assess the performance of the employee over the previous 12 months. There are many ways of assessing performance. Performance scoring is the system used for the appraisal form shown in Figure 10.11 at the end of the chapter. It is important to also make written comments on performance so that the score and comment can be used together to interpret the appraisal. The appraisal form should be passed to the employee a few days before the appraisal so that they can study it and prepare comments.

• ***The training action plan:*** the training action plan is drawn up as a result of the appraisal interview and sets out the training agreed for the employee for the next 12 months. The type of training and courses are listed, and target dates set for the completion of the training. The action plan should be discussed at intervals throughout the year to ensure the training is progressing, and it should be brought to the next year's appraisal for discussion.

The appraisal process

The appraisal process should be carried out in a similar fashion to the flow chart in Figure 10.12.

The appraisal interview

Employees must be given adequate notice of appraisal interviews, and time to complete their self-assessment forms and to study the performance appraisal form completed by their appraiser.

At least one hour should be set aside for the appraisal interview, it should be held somewhere quiet, and under no circumstances should it be disturbed. Seating arrangements should be comfortable and the appraiser should aim to create a relaxed atmosphere; after all this is a constructive discussion on the employee's training, development and progress, not the 'third degree'.

The appraiser should explain the purpose and scope of the interview and ensure that there is a constructive and positive discussion. The employee's job should be discussed in terms of its objectives and demands, and the comments made by the employee and appraiser on the appraisal forms discussed. Future objectives should be discussed and agreed, and the means to achieve them (more training, education, etc.) agreed. It is very important that the appraiser does not promise help or training which cannot be delivered; there should be no rash promises, and realistic goals should be agreed. At the end of the appraisal the appraiser should summarize the discussion and the plans or training agreed.

After the interview the appraiser should summarize in writing the main points of the discussion and the actions agreed, and provide a copy for the employee.

The manager should follow up the interview to ensure that the objectives agreed are being achieved and any training is being carried out; this is where a mini or six-month appraisal can be very helpful.

Appraisals are very useful management tools. They can improve communications and the quality of working life for employees and make them feel more valued by the organization. However, the introduction of a formal appraisal system does not mean that the manager's responsibility for monitoring performance on a daily basis has been removed. The manager should always be aware of their staff's productivity, performance and associated problems, and be able to act quickly to resolve any difficulties or give praise for a job well done.

Below are some of the main points to remember when setting up an appraisal scheme:

- Appraisals need commitment from both staff and owners/partners.
- Keep staff informed and ask for their comments and opinions.
- Staff responsible for appraisals should receive adequate training.
- Appraise everyone in the practice.
- Keep paperwork to a minimum.
- Spend enough time to carry out a thorough appraisal interview.
- Do not promise what you cannot deliver.
- Keep written records.
- Continue to appraise on a regular basis.
- Monitor the appraisal scheme and review if necessary.
- Do not link pay to appraisals.

SKILLS	VERY IMPORTANT	IMPORTANT	NOT IMPORTANT
INTERPERSONAL SKILLS			
Counselling			
Mentoring			
Training			
Communication			
Empathy			
Etc.			
LEADERSHIP			
Motivating others			
Initiative			
Decision making			
Team building			
Etc.			
MANAGEMENT SKILLS			
Planning			
Time management			
Financial decision-making			
Personnel management			
Etc.			
TECHNICAL SKILLS			
Surgical			
Medical			
Nursing			
Health and safety			
Etc.			

Figure 10.9 Job profile, head nurse.

NAME.. JOB TITLE..

DATE..

Please answer the following questions. They are intended to help you and your appraiser achieve the best from your performance appraisal interview, so please answer as honestly and in as much detail as you can.

1. What have you achieved over and above the minimum requirements of your job description in the last 12 months?

   List any difficulties you have in carrying out your work.

2. Please give reasons for your answers. What parts of your job do you:-

   (a) Do best

   (b) Do less well

   (c) Have difficulty with

   (d) Fail to enjoy

3. Have you any skills, or knowledge, not fully utilized in your job? If so, what are they and how could they be used?

4. What support do you feel you receive from your immediate manager, head of department or supervisor?

5. What support do you receive from the members of staff you work with?

6. What additional training have you received in the last 12 months – please enclose your CPD Record Card. Please comment on the training.

7. What training do you think would help you to do your job better?

8. How do you see your job and role in the practice developing over the next 12 months?

9. Are there any constraints on you, which will prevent or impede your ability to develop your job and role in the practice? If your answer is yes, please explain.

10. What work goals/ambitions do you have for the next 12 months?

11. What personal goals/ambitions do you have for the next 12 months?

12. Please list any other comments, questions or suggestions here which you would like to discuss at the appraisal interview.

Figure 10.10 Employee self-appraisal form.

NAME....................................... JOB TITLE................................

APPRAISER.............................. DATE.......................................

KEY: 1 = room for improvement
2 = satisfactory
3 = good
4 = excellent
5 = exceeds expectations

PERFORMANCE	SCORE	COMMENTS
QUALITY OF WORK The extent to which the person's work is accurate, thorough and neat.		
FLEXIBILITY How adaptable the person can be in changed situations		
JOB KNOWLEDGE The extent to which the person possesses the practical/technical knowledge to carry out the job		
PRODUCTIVITY The extent to which the person produces a significant volume of work efficiently in a specific period of time		
RELATIONSHIPS The extent to which the person is willing and demonstrates an ability to co-operate, work and communicate with colleagues, supervisors and clients		
COMMUNICATION ABILITIES The extent to which the person is able to communicate with colleagues and clients		

Figure 10.11 Annual performance appraisal.

PERFORMANCE	SCORE	COMMENTS
ATTITUDE The person's attitude to their job, colleagues, clients and the practice in general		
INITIATIVE The extent to which the person seeks out new assignments and assumes additional duties when necessary		
ATTENDANCE AND PUNCTUALITY		
LEADERSHIP SKILLS The extent to which the person leads and encourages others		
DEPENDABILITY The extent to which the person can be relied upon regarding task completion and follow-up		

APPRAISER'S COMMENTS

Signed... Date........................

APPRAISEE'S COMMENTS

Signed... Date........................

Figure 10.11 (Continued)

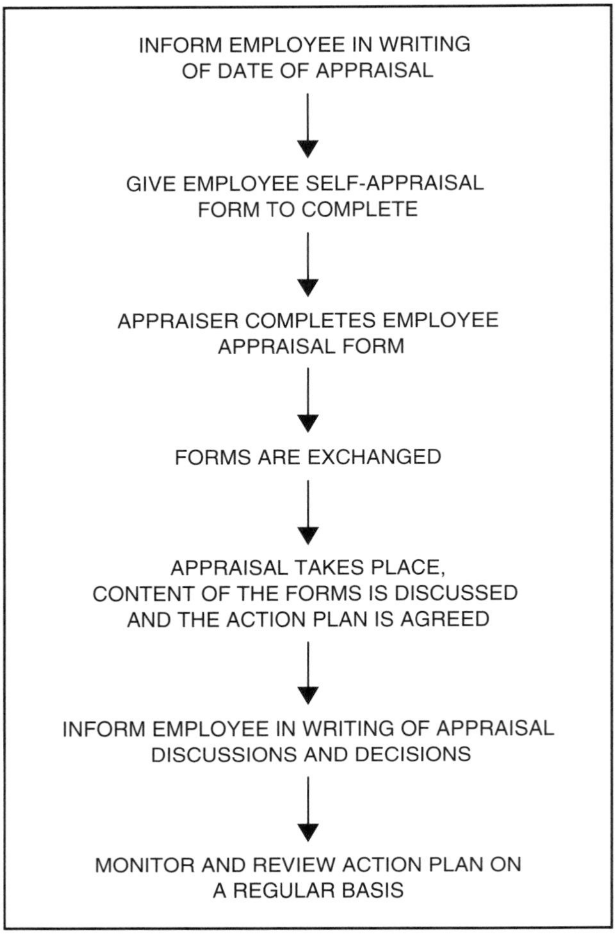

Figure 10.12 The appraisal process.

CHAPTER CONTENTS

What does the client want? 111
The results of good client care 112
The results of bad client care 112

How to provide good client care 112
Client care standards 112

Measuring and maintaining client care 114
Client feedback 114
Staff feedback 116

Dealing with client complaints 116

Dealing with difficult clients 117

Excellence in customer service 118

11

Client care

Most clients judge their veterinary practice not on the clinical treatment their animal receives, but on the client care the practice and its staff deliver. It is difficult for the non-professional to assess the quality of clinical care, but they can and do evaluate the client care they receive and equate its standard to that of the clinical treatment.

Providing good client care is the responsibility of all members of the practice, but it is the manager who has the responsibility to ensure that the standards are set, followed and maintained.

WHAT DOES THE CLIENT WANT?

All client care must be geared to what the client actually wants and not what you as the practice think they want or need. The best way to discover what the client wants is to ask them. This can be done by the use of client surveys or client focus groups. It should be an on-going process, as client requirements will change and what is considered good client care today might be seen as unexceptional in a year's time. Client expectations are continually increasing, and in an environment that is becoming ever more competitive the practice must constantly endeavour to meet and exceed those expectations.

Client requirements will vary from practice to practice but there are a number of common requirements that all clients need over and above good veterinary care for their animal:

- a welcoming and caring atmosphere
- friendly staff

- helpful staff
- convenience
- individual attention
- clean and pleasant surroundings
- respect for the client's time
- time for the client
- advice
- the client and their pet being made to feel cared for.

The results of good client care

A practice which provides good client care is much more likely to retain and bond clients. Those bonded clients will tend to visit the practice more to follow up on pet healthcare advice. Client loyalty is important when client numbers are diminishing, and it is also your loyal/bonded clients who are the best ambassadors for your practice. It is they who will tell their friends and neighbours how caring and helpful the practice is and recommend you to potential new clients as well as to those who are dissatisfied with their present veterinary practice. Happy clients produce happy staff. Fewer complaints and a caring, pleasant atmosphere are in themselves very motivating for staff, and the client care mentality is self-perpetuating.

The results of bad client care

Very simply, fewer clients. This is especially likely if there are competitors close by. Dissatisfied clients will very quickly pass on their feelings of dissatisfaction to their friends and neighbours. Always remember that one dissatisfied client will tell ten others, while one happy client will only tell four others.

HOW TO PROVIDE GOOD CLIENT CARE

The practice should have a policy towards client care which all staff are fully aware of. It may be a simple as 'The practice will provide excellence in client care at all times', but it does need to be stated and written down for all to see in the practice manual, staff manual, practice brochure, etc.

In order to achieve the highest possible level of client care, standards have to be set governing staff actions and behaviour as well as practice routines. These standards should be translated into practice standards/protocols which must be known, agreed and adhered to by all staff.

Client care standards

Standards should be agreed by the owners/partners and manager of the practice and produced in a written form for all staff. It is no good producing a fanciful wish-list of client care standards which cannot be achieved. If there is only one receptionist on duty in the reception it is unreasonable to have as a standard, 'the telephone must always be answered after three rings and clients must never be put on hold'. Standards must be realistic, and workable at the busiest of times.

Standards should be set for all areas of client care. This is illustrated in Figure 11.1.

Below are just some of the sort of questions you should be asking about client care in the practice in order to establish the standards you want to provide.

The building

- Is the practice easy to find?
- Is the signage clear and easy to see?
- Is the building well maintained?
- Is there sufficient car parking?
- Is the car park well lit at night?
- Is the car park clean?
- Is there a dog loo?

The reception area

- Is it clean?
- Does it smell?
- Is it tidy?
- Are there good, useful, informative displays?
- Is the seating adequate and comfortable?
- Is there a children's area or a box of toys, etc.?
- Are there separate cat and dog areas?
- Is there somewhere to tie the owner's dog while they pay the bill?

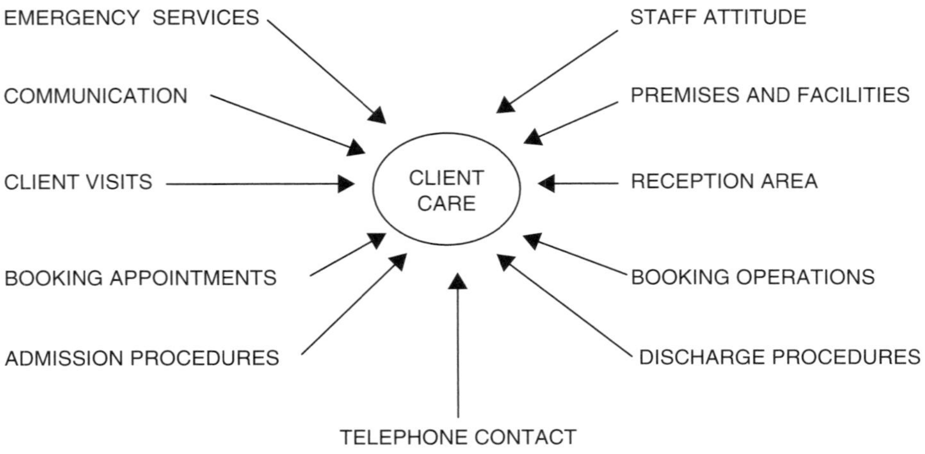

Figure 11.1 Areas of client care.

- Are there plants and flowers, and do they look healthy?
- Is it made easy for the client to pay their bill?

The staff

- Are they smart?
- Have they name badges?
- Are they friendly and caring?
- Do they smile?
- Do they acknowledge clients as soon as they enter the building?
- Do they use both the client's and the animal's name?
- Are they helpful?
- Are they polite?
- Are they sympathetic?
- Are they informative and knowledgeable?

Telephone contact

- How quickly is the telephone answered?
- What is the greeting?
- Are clients put on hold?
- How are bookings and appointments handled?
- How is information given over the telephone?

Booking appointments and operations

- What is the policy on booking appointments and operations?
- Do clients usually get the appointments they want?
- Is enough information taken and given over the telephone?

Admissions and discharges

- Are clients given adequate pre-op instructions?
- Are clients given pre-op appointment times?
- Is there a designated nurse to admit animals?
- Are the clients telephoned when the operation is over?
- Does the nurse who admitted the animals also discharge them?
- Are clients given adequate post-op instructions?
- Are clients given enough time with the vet/nurse for adequate explanation of post-op care, etc.?
- Are the clients telephoned the next day to check how their pet is?

Small animal and large animal visits

- How long does it take the vet to reach the farm after a farmer has called, and does the receptionist contact the farmer if the vet is going to be later than the time given?
- Do veterinary surgeons make regular monthly visits to farming clients?

- How easy is it for a small animal client to have a house visit?

Emergency services

- Are these carried out by the practice or by another veterinary service, and if so, how well does this work?
- What system is used to answer emergency calls?
- How quickly does the veterinary surgeon reach the client after an emergency call?

Client communication

- Is there a client newsletter?
- Are there farmers' newsletters?
- Are there client meetings?
- Are there farmers' meetings?
- Are clients surveyed for their opinions and needs?
- Is there a practice website?
- Are there displays in the reception area for client information?
- Does the practice have open days?
- Does the practice send booster reminders?
- Does the practice send herd and flock health reminders?

Debt control

- Do clients understand the practice debt control policy?
- How are clients asked for money?
- Is pet insurance promoted by staff?
- Do all staff believe that the practice gives value for money?
- Are there as many ways as possible to pay bills – cheque, credit/debit card, etc?
- Does the practice offer an instalment plan?
- Are estimates given?
- Are bills thoroughly explained to clients?
- Are large animal accounts detailed enough?

All these areas and many more specific to your own practice need to be addressed when considering the client care standards you wish to achieve, and always aim to exceed the client's expectations.

MEASURING AND MAINTAINING CLIENT CARE

It is fine to have client care standards, but they are useless if that care is not monitored and measured on a regular basis. The two main ways of measuring standards are:

a) Looking at client feedback, i.e. complaints and compliments, surveys and focus groups.
b) Looking at staff feedback, i.e. staff observation and questioning of care standards and their suggestions for improvements.

Client feedback

All client complaints should be recorded; these may be by letter, telephone call, face to face or even second hand, though care should be taken when assessing this type of complaint. Different members of staff will be receiving these complaints, and a complaints recording system should be set up. This can be a simple form on which every complaint is recorded with the date of the complaint, details of the client, the nature of the complaint, how it was received (telephone, letter, etc.), who received it and the action taken. The complaints should be regularly monitored by the practice manager, and in this way the deficiencies in client care can be identified and dealt with.

Complaints are good news inasmuch as they allow you to put right problem areas. Most clients who complain simply want their complaint sorted out and are not contemplating leaving the practice; sadly it is the clients who do not complain but simply take their business elsewhere who are the bad news for the practice. However, a complaints form can still be quite de-motivating both for the manager and the staff. It is often a good idea to have running in tandem with the complaints form a client thank you or compliments form, just to prove that it is not only complaints that the practice receives or that the manager/owner is recording. The form can be set out in the same way as the complaints form but record all the thank you letters and cards, telephone messages, etc. that the practice receives.

Client surveys and the use of focus groups can be helpful when trying to measure the effectiveness of the practice's client care. Surveys should be carefully designed to find out exactly what you need to know about your clients' care. It may be that you simply want to know how well staff answer the telephone and book appointments, or perhaps how long clients wait for their appointments. Whatever the area, ask specific questions which will provide you with the information you require, such as:

- How long are you happy to wait if your appointment time is delayed?
- How important is it to you to see the same veterinary surgeon each time you come to the surgery?
- If you are put on hold when telephoning the surgery, how long is it acceptable to be kept holding on?

Focus groups made up from your top 20% clients will help you establish the needs of those clients who use you most. A focus group might consist of six to eight client members which meets on a regular basis to discuss particular practice issues which require client input. Clients from your top 20% should be invited to be members of the group for set periods of time, say 12–18 months. Changing the composition of the group brings in new ideas and opinions, and helps to achieve a representative sample of your top clients whose opinion is the most important to you. Groups should meet at a time convenient to the clients. This is likely to be in the evening, and light refreshments should be provided.

Client surveys can be very informative for analysing present client care and for planning new services. They should be carefully tailored to the needs of the practice and the information you require.

There are a number of different types of client survey, each having its own advantages and disadvantages.

Handout questionnaires: these are the questionnaires handed to clients in reception, to be completed at the time and handed back to the receptionist. These surveys are immediate, but not all clients will have either the time to fill in the survey before being called into the consultation or the inclination to complete it afterwards.

Telephone questionnaires: this is in effect cold call interviewing of clients. Although direct and immediate, such surveys may be seen by some clients as an intrusion and there is the danger of questions being answered without thought, just to get the telephone call over with as soon as possible.

Face to face questionnaires: this system employs the personal approach with someone (not from the practice) interviewing clients in the waiting room. Time is a constraint here just as with the handout questionnaires, but the personal approach can often provide more revealing information.

Whatever form of survey you use, it will be time-consuming and expensive. It is therefore very important to plan the survey carefully and ask the right questions. Be very clear what the aim of the survey is: know what it is you are trying to discover. It may, for example, be to assess the quality of client care in the practice, or perhaps more specifically to investigate the effectiveness of the appointments system. Plan the survey by asking yourself some of the following questions:

- What information do you want? – *Always be as specific as possible.*
- How many questions will be asked? – *Do not ask too many, preferably no more than 10.*
- What questions will be asked? – *Questions should be unambiguous, and easy to answer. Consider whether you want simple yes or no answers or comments and opinions.*
- What sort of questionnaire will it be? – *Handout, telephone or one to one.*
- How many clients will be surveyed? – *A minimum of 100 is usually needed.*
- When will the survey be carried out? – *Pick times when you will interview a fair representation of your clientele.*
- How will you involve staff? – *All staff need to be aware of the survey, understand why it is being done, and be given the results.*
- How will you analyse the results? – *Simple yes/no answers can be analysed on a percentage rating. Comments need to be noted and grouped; this is a much more difficult task.*

- What will be done with the results? – *You need to follow up the results of the survey with actions, or the time will have been wasted.*

Client survey questions are not easy to design. For example, if you are considering setting up a nurses' weight clinic, a first question such as 'Would you like us to provide a weight clinic?' is a poor one. 'Are you concerned about your pet's weight and nutrition?' is a much better one. It will discover how important the client feels their pet's weight and feeding is, and how likely it would be that they would attend a clinic. If you are considering extending opening hours, do not ask, 'Would you be interested in the practice opening until 8 pm?' Ask, 'What is the easiest time for you to come to the practice?' The client is almost certainly going to say yes to the first question, while it may be that they would actually consider opening until 7 pm convenient for their needs.

It is wise to carry out a pre-survey test on a small number of clients, or even your staff, to test the suitability of the questions. Any problems can be ironed out at this stage and avoid wasted time later.

The way you conduct the survey will depend much on your circumstances, the time you wish to spend, and the budget you have allowed. Consider the different ways the survey may be carried out, look at the advantages and disadvantages of each, and decide what is most appropriate for you. Most importantly remember that the results are only as good as the thought and planning that has gone into the initial stages of the project.

Staff feedback

All staff should be asked to assess client care standards on a regular basis. This can be done through client care meetings and by the use of client care forms which staff can complete. The forms should be designed to address aspects of client care in the practice about which you want information. They may vary accordingly, but essentially they should be asking staff their opinion on specific aspects of care, how they would rate them – say on a scale of 1–5 – and any comments they may have for improvements, as shown in Figure 11.2. Examples of questions might be:

1. How quickly is the telephone answered?
2. How often are clients seen on time?
3. How often do clients complain about their bills?
4. How often are you unable to make an appointment for a client the day they want it?
5. How well does the booster reminder system work?
6. Do clients always manage to see the vet of their choice?

Your staff will often be the most aware of weaknesses in client care and they will all have their own ideas of how matters could be improved, so listen to them. Give your staff the opportunity to make suggestions for improved client care on an on-going basis. This may be done at staff/departmental meetings as well as more formally by the use of a client care suggestions form.

Having monitored and measured the standard of client care the practice is providing, any suggestions for improvements or identified weaknesses should be discussed and acted upon as soon as is reasonably possible. It is far worse to ask clients and staff for opinions and then not respond to their comments, than it is to have never asked in the first place.

DEALING WITH CLIENT COMPLAINTS

Every practice needs to have a policy on how they deal with client complaints. This gives the nurse or receptionist at the receiving end of the complaint rules and guidelines to follow, and provides them with a greater confidence in coping with the client. Staff should understand when a complaint needs to be passed on to someone of higher authority and who that should be. In many cases it is the practice manager's role to deal with more complex or difficult complaints and non-clinical complaints. Even they will at times need to refer clients to owners or partners if problems cannot be resolved or the manager has not the authority to act upon or resolve the complaint.

CLIENT CARE AREA	PRESENT CARE Assess on scale of 1–5 where 1 is poor and 5 is excellent	IMPROVEMENTS REQUIRED
PREMISES		
RECEPTION		
STAFF ATTITUDE		
TELEPHONE CONTACT		
BOOKING OPERATIONS AND APPOINTMENTS		
COMMUNICATION		
ADMISSIONS		
DISCHARGES		
INFORMATION PROVISION		
ETC.		

Figure 11.2 Staff/practice assessment of client care.

Complaints which are justified need to be dealt with quickly and efficiently. If the client is right in their complaint then it should be made easy for them to complain. This defuses the situation and enables the receptionist to move on to solving the client's problem. It is important that the client receives an apology and is asked how the practice can make up for the mistake. They should always be thanked for their comments and the practice should try to exceed that client's expectations by perhaps sending them a voucher for discount off their next booster or pet food as an apology. If you deal successfully with this group of clients you probably will have bonded them for life to the practice. It's worth noting that 70% of clients with grievances will stay with the practice if efforts are made to remedy the complaint, and that 95% will stay if the complaint is rectified on the spot. So take advantage of client complaints and learn from them, as these complainers may well highlight areas of your service which need improving.

DEALING WITH DIFFICULT CLIENTS

We all have 'difficult' clients in our practices but it is a fact that many clients are perceived as difficult when in fact it is often the staff themselves who have created the myth.

It is very easy to make assumptions about clients because they have been 'difficult' on a previous visit, because they 'look' difficult or because their personality clashes with our own. Staff perceptions can often turn a perfectly mild and ordinary client into a difficult one, which then means they are treated as such, and may well quite justifiably become difficult.

Staff attitude can also affect the attitude of the client. An unsmiling, uninterested receptionist or nurse will hardly be likely to endear themselves to a client, and this means that often quite small difficulties will be made into large ones because the client perceives an unhelpful, unsympathetic member of staff.

Reception staff should also be trained to understand and sympathize with the client's 'hidden agenda', as illustrated in Figure 11.3.

We usually only see the tip of the iceberg when it comes to client feelings, emotions and problems. The receptionist sees a particular behaviour and response from the client without understanding all the other emotions, attitudes, feelings and problems that are under the surface. A client may be very difficult with a receptionist not because the bill is high or he/she has had to wait for their appointment, but actually because they are worried about their ill child, their job or how to pay the next mortgage instalment. The hidden agenda comes to the surface, and although the receptionist will have no knowledge of this agenda she must always be aware that clients can have all sorts of reasons for behaving as they do and take this into account when dealing with them. By appreciating this it will help reception staff to stay calmer and deal better with some of these difficult situations.

There are of course genuinely difficult clients for whom nothing will ever be right, and this would be the case whether they are at the veterinary surgery or the supermarket.

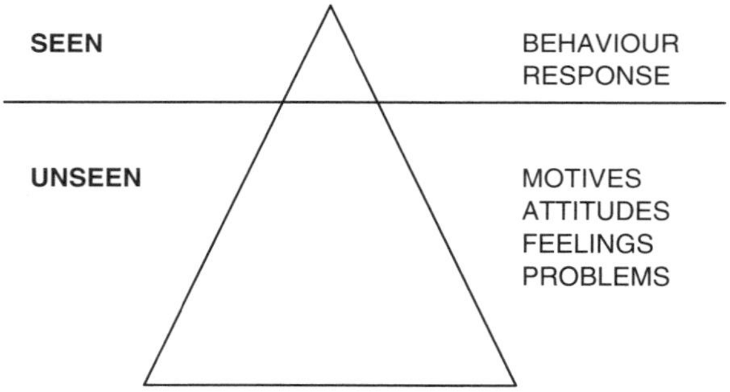

Figure 11.3 The hidden agenda.

Staff need to be taught how to deal with this group of clients.

Staff need to be:

- positive
- friendly
- patient
- calm
- non-argumentative
- emotionally controlled
- aiming for the best outcome, which may not necessarily be a win–win situation
- able to let off steam – away from the reception desk!

EXCELLENCE IN CUSTOMER SERVICE

This is what all practices should be aiming for, and all staff should believe in and be trained to provide. The practice should be committed to excellence in client care and always be prepared to 'go that extra step', for example, by phoning the client the day after their pet has had an operation just to ask how the pet is, sending the letter of sympathy to a client whose pet has been euthanased or perhaps providing a collection service for pets belonging to old people who cannot easily get to the surgery. Staff should be confident in their client care skills, showing:

- *Care* – towards the client
- *Consideration* – they do not always have to agree with the client but they must show consideration towards their feelings
- *Control* – of their own emotions when clients are being really difficult
- *Courage* – when they are in difficult situations and need to be assertive to deal with awkward or aggressive clients.

It is important to develop and maintain a good relationship with your clients, and this is all about good communication, attention to detail and treating the client as you would wish to be treated.

CHAPTER CONTENTS

What is sales and marketing, and what's the difference? 119

Why do we need it? 120
The passive practice 120
The reactive practice 120
The pro-active practice 120
Changes in marketing of professions 120

General marketing principles 121
New, existing and bonded clients 121
Marketing mix 122
Features and benefits 122
Differences between products and services 123

The marketing plan 124

Marketing of products 124
POM products 125
Farm PML medicines 126
Small animal routine healthcare products 126
Pet food 127
Lifecare products 127
General retailing principles 127

Marketing services 127
Marketing clinical services 127
Healthcare programmes 128
Pet insurance 128

Marketing the practice 128

Marketing tools 129
Advertising 129
Practice website 129
The media 131
Community liaison 131
Client's recommendation and feedback 131
Wall-mounted displays 131
Leaflets 132
Client newsletters 132
Practice brochure 132
Personal promotion of services 132
Your database 133

12

Sales and marketing

For many people, 'sales and marketing' conjures up images of slick, pushy salesmen in suits, trying to sell you something you don't want. But some form of sales and marketing activity is essential in practice if your clients are to understand the many ways in which your practice can help them and their animals.

WHAT IS SALES AND MARKETING, AND WHAT'S THE DIFFERENCE?

Marketing is essentially a strategic function – researching the client's requirements, investigating new opportunities, planning and predicting levels of sales. The Marketing Society defines marketing as *'The management process within a company responsible for identifying, anticipating and satisfying customer requirements profitably'*.

Marketing encompasses a wide range of activities, all of which would be regarded as separate divisions in large companies, such as:

- market research
- planning
- sales
- public relations
- advertising.

In a small business such as veterinary practice, it would be unrealistic to separate the various aspects of marketing. During a conversation with a client, your receptionist will be finding out what the client wants, assessing the most appropriate product or service, arranging to supply it, promoting the practice image, and ensuring the client passes this favourable opinion on to all her friends too. If it was a new request, the receptionist would also feed the information back, *'If Mrs X wants this, shall we offer it to all similar clients?'*

WHY DO WE NEED IT?

Historically, all professions have taken a dim view of marketing. Any form of obvious sales, PR or advertising was considered 'touting for business' and appropriate only for tradesmen.

For many years the veterinary practices 'sold' their treatments and medicines by dictating the treatment needed to the animal's owner. The only 'advertising' done was to put up a brass plate beside the surgery door, and then wait for the clients to contact the practice.

As we have seen in earlier chapters, there have been huge changes in the nature and organization of veterinary practice in recent years. A more pro-active approach to our clients is becoming necessary for many reasons, including:

- increase in practice numbers
- reduction in pet population
- crises in farming
- increased specialization
- more discerning clients
- higher public profile of veterinary medicine
- alternative sources of information
- changes in professional regulation
- recognition of the human–animal bond.

Our clients no longer regard all vets as equal, and do not simply go to the nearest one they can find. Good marketing is now essential for veterinary practices to survive and develop.

The passive practice

The passive practice waits for clients to find it and ask for treatment. They rely on unthinking client loyalty and that they will always have sufficient client numbers by random selection.

Once, clients would go to the 'town vet' with a sick animal, and the vet would lay down the law of treatment with little discussion with the owner. These clients would have been very loyal – the same vet may have run the practice for decades, and clients were not so aware of alternatives. They either came back regardless, or if they were really unhappy, would go to the next one on the list.

The reactive practice

Times change, and even the most conservative practice has to react to external pressures. These may be due to changes in legislation, or as a result of client complaints or requests. The reactive practice tends to think it is doing quite well – after all, it is responding to customer demands and that's a good thing, isn't it? Yes and no – any requests/suggestions should of course be taken into account, but by the time the customer has kicked up a fuss they may have already gone somewhere else – and certainly others will have.

A properly co-ordinated marketing plan is essential to help the reactive practice become more pro-active. Unless this happens, staff will become de-motivated. *'We tried puppy parties once but they didn't work.'*

The pro-active practice

The pro-active practice makes an effort to find out the needs of its clients and patients. They regularly review the products and services on offer, and the way they are offered. All marketing is co-ordinated by a plan, and all staff give the same message. They believe in what they are doing, and know why they are doing it.

Table 12.1 illustrates some of the differences in attitude between these three types of practice.

Changes in marketing of professions

Things are changing across all professions.

Opticians have changed the public view of spectacles from an object of ridicule to a fashion accessory. And just take a new look at some of the other professionals that we deal with.

Accountants are split into two sections. Some firms are doing an excellent job in raising their

Table 12.1 Contrasts in marketing attitudes of practices

	Passive	Reactive	Pro-active
Client asks for a product not stocked at the practice	'We don't sell that.'	'I can try to get some for you.'	Displays full catalogue of products available for order
New product/service comes on the market	Ignore it – why change?	Tries it out regardless	Decides if it fits in with the overall plan
Preventative healthcare	Vaccination, worming	Try to keep up with whatever clinics the practice down the road is offering	Uses client feedback to develop new services such as pre-purchase advice
Advertising	Brass plate, Yellow Pages	Accepts all offers of advertising space	Plans strategic advertising
Waiting room decoration	Faded prints of wildlife	Mass of posters and leaflets, some handwritten and out of date/dog-eared	Carefully co-ordinates and regularly updates topical information and displays

profile in the veterinary profession by producing useful fact-sheets, comparative reports and speaking at CPD meetings. But what about the rest? Consider the numerous practices of accountants in your local town. Very few of them admit to doing anything but 'count', and yet there are many out there who could offer excellent business, tax planning and other financial advice. Yet you continue to simply hand them the practice accounts year after year, neither asking for nor being offered anything more. Wouldn't you appreciate it if they took an interest in your business? *'Mr X, we also offer this service,'* or *'Now your practice is a certain size, why don't you try doing this?'*

On the other hand, the legal profession's heavy advertising of 'no win, no fee' and accidental injury services is a much more aggressive form of marketing.

There is a feeling among some veterinary surgeons that any form of marketing is simply not professional, and it is important to recognize that everybody has different comfort zones. As it suggests in a moderately famous book, *'Do unto others as you would like to be done to yourself.'* If you base your marketing on the standard of service you would expect from other professionals, you won't go far wrong.

Let clients know what you can offer, why they might want it, and how to go about getting it. Good marketing must be underpinned by good client care and good veterinary medicine.

Box 12.1 Professional, ethical marketing

Professional, ethical marketing is:
- giving the best care for your patients
- giving the best service for your clients

Professional, ethical marketing is not:
- 'just selling dog food'
- a dirty word for professionals
- advertising and price wars
- selling unnecessary or substandard products and services

GENERAL MARKETING PRINCIPLES

Before looking in detail at the practical aspects of marketing, there are some basic principles that apply across the board.

New, existing and bonded clients

One of the first issues that must be addressed in any marketing plan is deciding who you are marketing to. Are you aiming to market more products and services to existing clients? Or looking to expand the client base by attracting new clients?

It is generally considered to be about five times more costly to make a sale to a new client rather than an existing one. All practices need a certain influx of new clients to at least balance those who move out of the area or lose their animals. In some cases, the marketing strategy may be aimed at attracting larger numbers of new clients, in the case of opening a new branch surgery or relocating the premises.

Within your existing client base, clients can be divided roughly into 'casual' or 'bonded' clients. Casual clients are the ones who turn up every few years when the animal is sick, and frequently switch between vets – not out of dissatisfaction but because they simply don't mind where they go. A bonded client consults the practice regularly for healthcare advice, makes sure their animals are properly vaccinated and wormed – and often brings in chocolates at Christmas time! These bonded clients are more likely to attend healthcare clinics and take up new services the practice has to offer.

Your practice management system software should be able to produce a list of clients that contribute most towards your turnover. It can be a surprisingly short list – figures from Fort Dodge Animal Health suggest that 69% of practice turnover comes from the 38% of clients who have fully vaccinated animals. Looking in more detail at those clients, 48% of practice turnover was derived from the top 25% of those key clients – i.e. less than 10% of the client base!

There are a number of key points to be aware of when considering marketing to these various client types:

- Your top clients are very valuable – so look after them, they will leave a big gap if they leave.
- Bonded clients are more likely to respond to marketing initiatives than casual clients are.
- The more bonded clients you have, the lower your client turnover and the fewer new clients you need to attract to maintain the same client base.
- If you target all your marketing at your top bonded clients they will eventually get sick of it!
- Aim to 'upgrade' your least-casual clients to bonded ones.
- Bear the target group in mind when drawing up the plan: casual clients will probably not respond to an invitation to senior pet blood screening, but may be initially attracted by a budget payment plan.

Marketing mix

This is also known as the P's of marketing. Any marketing plan must involve considering these aspects. The 'original' four P's, which applied to marketing goods, are:

- **P**roduct – what are you selling?
- **P**rice – what is your pricing strategy?
- **P**romotion – how are you going to let customers know about it?
- **P**lace – where are customers going to find you?

The original four have been expanded over the years to include many more P's, applicable to goods and services, such as People, Processes, Physical evidence, Positioning and Pro-activity. Pricing strategies for goods and services are covered in Chapter 16, 'Pricing of fees and products'.

Features and benefits

The client needs to know more than just a list of products and services on offer; they need to know why they might want to use them.

- A feature is a technical description of the product – that is, what the product/service provider thinks is good about it.
- A benefit is why the customer is going to think it's good!

The client is not interested in buying the product or service per se, they are buying the consequences. You might think the selling point of a new ectoparaciticide is that it contains some wonderful new compound but as far as the owners are concerned all they want to know is that it kills fleas quicker than anything else does.

One way of ensuring that you are putting across the benefits is to apply the *'So what?'* test to any marketing points you come up with. You may have to do this several times before you come up with the true benefits of the service. Look at the extract of a practice letter

The Veterinary Practice

Dear Mrs Jones,

We would like to inform you about our wonderful new piece of laboratory equipment, the Analyzer. This will allow us to test blood samples for x, y and z at the surgery.
Please telephone for an appointment if you would like Trixie to be tested.

Figure 12.1 Client letter without *'So-what?'* test.

The Veterinary Practice

Dear Mrs Jones,
We know you want Trixie to stay healthy into her old age.

Our new laboratory equipment will allow us to test Trixie's blood for early signs of ageing. If any of these signs are detected, we can advise you straight away on a special diet for Trixie. This will help control the effects of ageing, and allow her to remain healthy for longer.

We would be pleased to arrange an appointment with you to assess Trixie's ongoing healthcare.

Figure 12.2 Client letter applying *'So-what?'* test.

shown in Figure 12.1. Here we have three main points:

1. The name of the equipment – the Analyzer. *'So what?'* Nothing at all – so leave it out!
2. Test for x, y and z. *'So what?'* So we can pick up early signs of damage to internal organs. *'So what?'* So that we can alter Trixie's diet to keep her healthy for longer. *'Good.'*
3. At the surgery. *'So what?'* So we can give the results to you quickly. *'So what?'* So you don't worry and we can start helping Trixie as soon as possible.

Once you have done your *'So what?'* tests, re-write the letter. Figure 12.2 shows how it might now read.

Always put yourself in the client's position. The 'best' benefits from your viewpoint are not always the ones that make the difference to the owner. There are a number of scientifically-formulated dried brands of cat food sold in many surgeries, which all have numerous benefits in terms of keeping the cat healthier for longer. But when it comes down to it, the benefits that many owners appreciate are the simple things:

- It doesn't smell as awful as tinned cat food.
- It doesn't go off in hot weather.
- You don't have to wash the bowl out as often!

Differences between products and services

Veterinary practices provide a mixture of products and services for their clients, and it is important to understand some of the differences between them. These differences have an effect on the way they are marketed and priced.

Some of the key differences between two common 'sales' in practices – a bag of branded cat food and a bitch spay – are described below.

- ***Products are tangible. Services are not.*** The client understands what a bag of food is, can see it exists, can try out a sample before deciding to buy, and can assess how much is in the bag for the money. However, the spay is not so obvious – the client is unlikely to be aware of what is involved, cannot try it out beforehand, and is not likely to notice any difference to the animal afterwards.

- ***Products are more easily comparable between providers. Services are not.*** It is quite easy for the client to decide where to buy a bag of cat food, as the food will be the same in both places. The degree of client care, surgical expertise, anaesthetic monitoring and post-operative care will vary considerably between practices, even though the final outcome – a neutered bitch – will be the same (hopefully!).

- ***Services are inseparable from their provider. Products are self-contained.*** The way in which the client and animal are treated as they arrive on the morning of the operation, and the care provided as the animal is returned to the owner, are all part of the service. Whilst the attitude of sales staff will have an effect on the decision to return to the practice, the bag of cat food is identical whoever sells it.

• ***Unsold services cannot be kept to sell later. Products can be.*** If a practice has not filled all the operating time available, that time cannot be charged for – ever. A bag of food will remain on the shelf until sold. Although a rapid turnover would be more beneficial to the practice, there is a long time-slot in which the product can be sold.

These differences mean that the marketing of products and services provide different challenges to practice staff.

- The ease of comparison with retail products means they are generally more price-sensitive than services.
- The intangible nature of services makes it vital that a well-informed member of staff gives a full explanation of what is involved. This is essential for the client to fully understand what is on offer.
- Client care is paramount in any marketing situation, but will have a greater effect on sales of services than of products.
- Financial projections must take into account the 'lost time' when services are not 100% subscribed to.

THE MARKETING PLAN

Marketing, like any other practice management activity, needs to be planned. If this is not done, then the practice will show the signs, such as:

- tatty, out-of-date posters advertising products that you don't sell
- literature promoting services your staff know nothing about, or 'We haven't done that for years.'
- display stands with out-of-date products
- sending reminders to dead pets
- inconsistency – a 'neutering clinic' suddenly trying to promote senior pet checks.

It is important that your marketing plan follows on from your overall practice business plan. The business planning process is covered in detail in Chapter 7, 'How are you going to do it?' This 'master plan' will have looked at the overall objectives and ethos of the practice, assessed the range of products and services currently provided, and identified a number of marketing objectives, for instance:

- To provide at least two client education clinics by March 200X.
- To investigate the potential for increasing sales of equine worming products.

Each of these marketing objectives can then be planned in detail covering aspects such as:

- What product/service are we selling?
- What are our targets in financial terms?
- What is the target client base?
- Which people are going to be involved?
- Is there a need for training?
- How much are we going to sell it for?
- Where will it happen? – Is there a need for more display or clinical space?
- When will it be sold?
- How is it going to be advertised?
- How will we decide if it is a success?

There is no single plan template which can be used in every situation – it will depend upon whether you are planning a product or a service, whether you are launching something new, or trying to increase uptake of an existing product or service. Figures 12.3 and 12.4 give examples of the sort of steps you could take planning the two marketing objectives given above.

As with any practice project, it is easy to read an article, or attend a conference, and be fired with enthusiasm to 'do' marketing. Make sure you plan to have the time, resources and staffing level to carry any project through. There is nothing so dispiriting to support staff than to be given the go-ahead to run a clinic, then given no time, money or opportunity to carry it out.

It is essential that the overall practice business plan be used to guide the general direction of marketing activity, to ensure all areas of the practice are heading in the same direction.

MARKETING OF PRODUCTS

Different products need to be marketed in different ways. There are many ways in which products can be categorized in practice, but the main ones

Primary objective	To provide at least two client education clinics by March 200X.
What type of clinic?	Examine client database for key target groups – e.g. cat/dog owners; young or older pets Conduct a client survey to find out what sort of educational clinics they would be interested in attending
Plan clinic no1	**Kitten care**
Define the product/service	What topics should be covered? How many sessions should there be?
Logistical planning	Who is going to run it? Where? When? What do they need?
Identify target market	Use computer system to find owners of new kittens and pregnant queens
Price	Is there a charge? How much?
Promotion	Design leaflets Inform all staff of project External promotion? – pet shops, local papers
Monitor progress	Client feedback sheets Staff feedback Information from computer system
On-going planning	For next time!

Figure 12.3 Sample marketing plan for client education clinics.

are by species, i.e. large animal, canine or exotic products; or by legal drug category. The legal implications of the categories of GSL (General Sales List), PML (Pharmacy and Merchants List) and POM medicines are explained more fully in Chapter 20, 'Pharmacy and dispensing'.

Products marketed in veterinary practice include the following:

- prescription only medicines (POMs)
- animal healthcare products for farm animals and domestic pets
- food
- accessories.

POM products

These are generally needed by the animal for the immediate treatment of a disease, and thereafter necessary for its continued wellbeing. Traditionally owners used to be in a 'captive' position, with very little choice over the type of medicine their animal was being prescribed.

Objective	To investigate the potential for increasing sales of equine worming products
1) Identify current levels of sales	Data from stock control system
2) Estimate potential sales	Number of horses registered with the practice × annual product use × price per dose
3) Set targets	Realistic increase on figure in 1)
4) Analyse factors affecting current sales	SWOT analysis Poor staff knowledge Prices too high Client ignorance
5) Deal with any weaknesses identified in 4)	E.g. Staff training Pricing strategy Client education
6) Monitor results	Data from stock control system
7) Review plan as necessary	

Figure 12.4 Sample marketing plan for increasing sales of horse wormer.

Several factors are now having an impact on the supply of POM products:

- Owners are becoming better informed about price and efficacy of drugs.
- Cascade regulations are restricting the range of drugs available.
- Development of new drugs is on-going.
- The threat continues of losing the privilege to dispense.

In farm practice, there are various add-on services which vets can offer to make the farmers' lives easier – disposal of waste medicines, keeping records of batch numbers, medicines record books.

Farm PML medicines

Practices face heavy competition from farm merchants in the sale and marketing of these products.

Some farmers will know exactly what product they want, how to use it, and are only shopping on price. Others will welcome your advice on the best product to use, and may allow you entry to sell other products and services to complement it – e.g. faecal egg counts. Of course, some will take your free advice and then go and buy the cheapest merchants' product, but that's life!

There are ways to stay competitive: look to stock vet-only products, which are harder to compare on price. For smaller farmers, the vet's ability to buy large packs and dispense can give a real advantage on small volumes of wormer.

Small animal routine healthcare products

These are mainly flea and worm preparations, and can fall into a variety of legal categories, POM, PML and GSL, so you will need to be careful about how you display them and market them.

Here you are competing with the supermarket and pet shop. Generally we know our products can win hands down on efficacy – we just need to convince the owners! Veterinary surgeries have a huge advantage in terms of trained, knowledgeable staff who have the time to talk over the options with the owners. You might spend half an hour with a client, just to sell a pound's-worth of worm tablet, but take the long-term view that if you've done the job well, that client will be in several times a year for the next 15 years.

Make it easy for them to buy from you. Nurses are used to flea spraying and giving worm tablets to animals; the owners are not. '*Would you like me to give Fluffy her worm tablet now?*' will be a huge relief to the owner, and will keep them coming back in the future.

Pet food

Marketing pet food, like anything else, relies on selling the benefits to the owner. But you don't need to get overly technical, unless the owners ask you. Often the simplest recommendations are the best. A veterinary nurse saying '*I feed my cat on it*' will be the most effective way to convince owners to try it than all the rest. And don't just rely on practice staff to pass the word – one advantage of a full waiting room is that everybody else joins in too.

Pet food sales were worth over £1.5 billion in 2000, and this is reflected in the TV advertising budget. Practices are most likely to succeed if they concentrate on selling non-supermarket brands and premium products.

Lifecare products

A veterinary practice is unlikely to want to sell, or have space to sell, the range of pet-care products available in supermarkets or pet shops. The sensible option is to stock a small range of good quality items.

Make sure you have all the basic requirements for a new puppy or kitten. Other products stocked might include items of real benefit to the pet – grooming equipment, behavioural 'toys', dental chews and engraved name tags.

Your wholesaler's comprehensive catalogue should allow you to easily order in special items to customer requests. Practices can be pro-active and make up a colour catalogue of items available to order.

General retailing principles

Whatever type of product you are selling, there are some basic principles to take note of:

- Site displays where clients can see them and browse easily.
- Always make sure the price is clearly displayed.
- Make sure shelves are free from dust.
- Remove any out-of-date or damaged products.
- Keep shelves full – customers don't like to take the last item left.
- Products sell best from eye-level shelves.
- People tend to scan shelves from left to right, so put new products to the left.
- Rearrange the product displays enough to keep people looking at them in a new light, but not so often as to infuriate the person who comes in each week for the same thing!
- Make sure your displays are robust and simple – clients will be put off buying from racks which look as if they are about to collapse, or destroying a 'shop window' display.
- Your staff should know how to use all products on display, and the pros and cons of similar items.

MARKETING SERVICES

When vets first think of marketing services, it is in relation to the 'add-on' services that the practice may offer. This is mainly because they assume that clinical services do not need selling – they expect the owner to come to them for treatment, and then simply accept what the vet recommends. But marketing principles apply just as much, if not more, to clinical services as to educational and healthcare programmes.

Marketing clinical services

Many of your clients will never see beyond your waiting room and consulting rooms. Is it surprising that they might assume that, like a GP's surgery, any major work has to be done elsewhere? Make sure your clients are aware that you have in-patient facilities, X-ray equipment, surgical and other specialist facilities that you may offer. This raising of awareness can be done in many ways – by using practice brochures, display boards or open days. The upsurge in TV coverage is opening clients' eyes to the scope of behind-the-scenes work which does go on in veterinary practices.

If you have achieved Veterinary Hospital status, make sure your clients are aware of what this means.

Healthcare programmes

Preventative healthcare programmes have been part of farm animal practice for many years, as the economic benefits of ensuring the on-going health of the livestock are substantial. Unfortunately, routine, 'non-essential' work has been hit badly by the recent crises in farming.

In small animal practice, vaccination has long been accepted as a preventative measure. However, it is only recently that the benefits of the accompanying health check have been actively marketed, mainly due to fear of losing the vaccination business completely. A reluctance of some practitioners to feel that there is value to a health check as opposed to a disease diagnosis may account for the relatively slow acceptance of companion animal healthcare programmes. They don't feel that saying *'Yes, Bozo is perfectly healthy'* is anything to shout about. Yet the pet owner wants to be complimented that their animal is fit and healthy – and preferably that he's the best, most fit and healthy dog the vet has seen that week.

Many healthcare education clinics can be run by veterinary nurses and support staff, which allows them to extend their job roles and actively generate income for the practice.

Preventative healthcare and other client support programmes increase the contact between all the practice staff and the client. They can relate to each other in a non-stressful situation, so that when the chips are really down, the client has a much more trusting view of the practice. Common programmes include:

- herd health visits
- cattle foot trimming and lameness visits
- puppy and kitten 'parties'
- training and behavioural counselling
- geriatric health checks
- dental check-ups
- nutritional advice and 'podgy pet' clubs
- pet loss support
- schools liaison.

Pet insurance

Pet insurance is marketed through the practice, even though the practice does not ultimately provide the final service. As with any product or service sold by the practice, staff should know details of:

- amount and extent of cover
- premiums and any discounts for multiple pets or OAPs
- any exclusions applied, either at inception or after future treatment
- the excess the client will have to pay – fixed, percentage, or based on animal age.

Do not simply leave an assorted pile of leaflets on the waiting room table. The owner does not want to sift through piles of different policies to find the right one. The odd one might, and it is a good idea to keep a small stock of all the available companies' literature in a file. But generally, the owner wants the surgery to recommend the policy that they feel to be 'the best'. Note this can be very different from 'the cheapest'. The practice will know from experience which companies pay promptly after a claim, and which seem to find every excuse to send follow-up enquiry letters and avoid paying at all.

It also makes the practice's burden of form-filling easier, dealing with one set of paperwork. You develop a good relationship with the insurance company staff, both in the claims department and sales. Queries are more likely to be satisfactorily resolved with a good working relationship.

MARKETING THE PRACTICE

Marketing products and services to your existing clients is all very well and good, but first of all you need to secure them as clients.

They need to:

- know your practice exists, then
- decide to go to your practice rather than any of the others, and
- continue to want to re-visit your practice.

Public awareness of the practice can be raised by a number of advertising and PR methods, which are covered in more detail below.

Direct recommendation and a convenient location are two of the key reasons why clients might initially choose one practice out of a selection. Retaining those clients, and developing them into loyal, bonded clients, should result from providing excellent client and clinical service whilst giving good value for money.

The number of different marketing tools available to practices is increasing rapidly. No one can afford to advertise everywhere, and cover all the PR opportunities, so it is important to find out which ones work well. Make a point of finding out from new clients how they found out about you, and use the results to plan future marketing. Some practice management systems have space to record this information on the client records.

Client care and practice accessibility are discussed in Chapter 11, 'Client care'.

MARKETING TOOLS

Marketing efforts can be divided roughly into three categories:

- Advertising – including signage, Yellow Pages, website and other advertising
- Public relations – using local media, community liaison and client recommendations.
- Client information – provided by displays, leaflets, brochures, newsletters and staff.

Underpinning the use of all these methods, enabling effective targeting and feedback, is:

- Your database – client and animal data, sales data and financial data.

Advertising

This can include almost any means of letting the animal-owning public know you are there, and what services you offer. It is well to remember that the most effective ways are often those which cost the least – word of mouth, and a decent sign on the door.

The Yellow Pages are the traditional place for veterinary practices to advertise, and the fact that the RCVS directory of practices lists more practice names beginning with A than any other letter (including one starting Aa) suggests that the race to be top of the listings is still on! However, once you get beyond the simplest entry, the cost of keeping up with other practices in the area can get very high indeed. Yellow Pages salesmen can be very adept at playing one practice off against another in the bid for more column inches sold!

Practices are also bombarded with offers of advertising space from a wide variety of other sources. There are always ones you succumb to out of guilt or public-spiritedness, such as the parish magazine, or local animal charity newsletter. But there are a lot of advertising scams which many practices fall for – space on a local business calendar, or in various brochures or directories which may or may not exist. The best defence against these is to have a practice policy on which publications the practice will advertise in, and give a firm 'No' to anyone else.

The RCVS Guide to Professional Conduct gives strict guidelines about ethical advertising of the practice, medicines and fees.

Practice website

The internet is an increasingly popular means of finding products and services, and this applies just as much to looking for veterinary practices as finding a plumber. A practice website is fast becoming an expectation of clients, not simply a flash gimmick.

The website may be simply based on the practice brochure, or may contain much more information. The client can browse at their leisure, to look at news sections, search for lost and found pets, and read about staff members and the equipment the practice has.

The difficulty many practices face is deciding how to go about getting a website. Some of the more IT-literate practices have written their own, others have used commercial website designers or sites provided by a variety of small business services. There are a growing number of veterinary website providers, who manage to keep costs down for the individual practice by slotting their details into a generic template. This can then be customized further, should the practice need it. Like any business service, it is important to follow up references from other practices using the same source – there are some unscrupulous so-called web experts out there taking advantage of inexperienced e-businesses.

Most web-novices tend to concentrate on getting the content of their website perfect – and of course that is extremely important. But when it comes to getting the best return from your site, a number of other, often overlooked, factors are a prime consideration. Your website must:

- be easy to find. Your potential clients and many of your loyal supporters won't be looking for you by the web address. If an internet search engine doesn't place you in the top ten results for 'vet x-town' then they won't bother looking any further. There are a number of techniques that web designers use to ensure sites are found easily, and are ranked highly on the final results.
- load quickly. The attention span of a web-surfer is probably less than that of a small child! If a web page does not load in a few seconds they will give up and look elsewhere. Fancy graphics and lots of photos look good, but check they don't slow your site down to a crawl.
- be kept up-to-date. A great-looking practice website will soon lose the impact of its first impression if the 'news' section is dated 18 months previously!

Once those three vital aspects of your website are in place, then you can concentrate on other design factors. Popular sections of veterinary practice websites are:

• ***Location maps*** – your potential clients must be able to find you for real! You can either include your own directions, or a link to one of the web-based mapping utilities.

• ***Staff profiles*** – photographs of staff members, with a short description of their place within the practice, will help clients to feel part of the practice.

• ***Virtual tours*** – your website is ideally suited to showing clients a room-by-room tour of the practice, displaying the facilities and care offered. Large animal practices can show photographs of work 'in the field'.

• ***News section*** – not only must clients find the website, they should be encouraged to re-visit it. A visible news section could contain new information about the practice, veterinary news in general, local Crufts winners, etc. Your seasonal practice newsletter can be included on the website as it is produced.

• ***Fact sheets*** – information on pet-care can be displayed and provided in a downloadable format.

• ***Children's area*** – easy-to-read information for children on aspects of animal care.

• ***E-shop*** – web-based shopping is becoming more popular. Most of the sites produced by veterinary web companies or wholesalers offer an e-shopping facility.

• ***Links*** – a good links page will ensure that clients look at your site first, whenever they are trying to find animal-related information on the web. Obvious links include animal charities, good animal healthcare sites, breed societies, and organizations such as RCVS and DEFRA. You might want to include community-based links such as local schools and other useful information such as weather forecasts!

• ***Practice contact point*** – ideally an e-mail address! But if you do publicize your e-mail, make sure someone is checking it regularly – if the practice does not respond to queries for a week, it will not provide a good impression.

The demand for longer opening hours is one of the issues that practices are facing. A practice website may be part of the solution – it could provide information on routine enquiries such as worming and flea control, allow clients to order repeat medication, and even be developed to allow on-line booking of appointments. All this, and more, would complement the existing services provided by the practice, not replace them.

The media

Why pay a fortune for a small boxed advert, when you can have much better exposure free? Local and even national newspapers love animal and vet stories. One of the best ways of raising awareness of your practice is to contact the papers with stories about rescued wildlife, staff awards or practice achievements such as Investors in People. The practice can ask the paper to print photographs of lost and found pets, increasing the caring image of the surgery. Developing a good relationship with the paper will also help get the practice name included with stories about your clients' achievements at Crufts or agricultural shows.

Other media links can include a regular 'vet's column' in the paper or 'ask the vet' slot on local radio. And don't forget to invite them all, including your local TV reporters, to your open days.

Major events such as National Pet Week and Pet Smile Week provide the practice with plenty of marketing opportunities involving the local media.

Community liaison

Local schools are good liaison opportunities for the practice. Most primary schools have a 'pets' corner' or the like, and secondary schools may be involved with more detailed animal-based projects. Schools liaison is an ideal job for veterinary nurses and other members of the practice team. The teachers will appreciate the input of the local practice, and the value to the practice can be considerable. The children's families may already have pets, or may be persuaded to have a pet as a result. The children themselves will eventually become potential clients. The RSPCA are conducting research into the causes of animal cruelty, and it will be interesting to see if improving animal care and welfare education to younger children can help avoid later problems.

Local agricultural and pet shows normally need a 'show vet' to provide emergency cover, and you might also be asked to judge some of the classes.

Client's recommendation and feedback

Recommendation of the practice by an existing client is the best advertising and PR a practice can get. If you routinely ask new clients how they found the practice, you can identify your best 'ambassadors'. Some practices reward these key clients by sending cards or flowers, but a simple 'thank you' is the most important. Client recommendation does not just help bring you new clients; it can be a good marketing tool in the waiting room too, as they start discussing things like pet food, educational clinics and other practice services.

Because your clients' opinions are so valuable to the practice, it is essential to find out what they are thinking. The results of client surveys, focus groups or other feedback sources can help you to plan new services and improve standards of client care. This is covered more fully in Chapter 11, – 'Client care'.

Wall-mounted displays

Displays in the reception can communicate information very effectively to clients, if they are well presented. Displays should look professional, be eye-catching and simple and contained within a notice board or discrete area.

It is a mistake to try to provide too much information in a display; a simple message is sufficient. If they require more details about the product/service being promoted, they can ask at reception or be given a leaflet.

Most veterinary companies are very pleased to provide high-quality posters and display material, and in-house computer publishing packages can be used to produce very high quality display material. Displays can be tied in with topics featured in the practice's client newsletter, if one is produced, so that the message is more firmly driven home.

Displays can reinforce information from open days; behind-the-scenes displays of surgical areas could be placed in the waiting room – either on the wall, in an album, on video or computer display.

And don't forget – by all means show off all the fancy bits of kit, and great facilities, but also make it human (and animal). Make sure you include photographs of nurses caring for the patients, of in-patients all snuggled up in kennels with their favourite comforter, of patients going home with their owners after surgery.

Hand-written posters or scraps of paper with 'lost and found' animals are simply not acceptable any more. Most clients are now capable of producing something half-decent with a computer, and they will be even more critical of your offerings.

Leaflets

It is very easy to go overboard producing dozens of different client leaflets on numerous veterinary and pet care topics. Although each leaflet may be well produced and full of very useful information, if their distribution is not handled with care the client may well begin to drown in the deluge of information. Handing out too many leaflets to clients can be just as bad as not providing any.

As with displays, they must be produced professionally. Manufacturers' leaflets can be helpful for product promotion/explanation, while material produced in-house will be needed to promote services.

Client newsletters

Quarterly client newsletters are now produced by many veterinary practices. Most are produced in-house and then printed externally, although there are companies who will customize a standard newsletter for your practice. Most are also seasonal, i.e. Spring, Summer, Autumn and Winter Newsletters.

The function of the client newsletter is to inform clients of the services and products you provide and to encourage them to use your practice more. The cost of producing a newsletter can be high, and even if a veterinary company sponsors it there is still a considerable amount of time involved on behalf of the practice in its production. The practice should be looking for a return on the newsletter in terms of increased sales, and the manager needs to be measuring uptake of products or services promoted in the newsletters.

The newsletter is also a useful PR exercise – in many cases it will contain a profile of a new member of staff or other changes within the practice. It needs to be an interesting read for the client and the mix of veterinary information, pet care and practice internal news is a good combination. As with the displays and the leaflets, the newsletter must look professional. It should not be a few pieces of photocopied A4 paper stapled together, if you are trying to project a good image to your clients.

Practice brochure

The practice brochure has long been one of the principal methods of providing clients with information about the practice, and as such does its job very well. The problem with many brochures is that the information they contain can quite quickly become out of date as new services are developed and staff changes are made. Nevertheless the brochure is an effective way of promoting the practice. Clients like to have a copy, and most visitors to the practice will pick up a brochure on arrival in the reception area. The brochure also goes to form part of the introductory client pack, and its presence in the reception area adds to the professional look of the practice. There are a number of companies who will help practices produce a brochure, although it could be produced entirely in-house and then sent for external printing.

Personal promotion of services

The personal approach to providing client information is vitally important. Very little can better the personal recommendation of a product or service by the veterinary surgeon, nurse or receptionist. This personal approach will reinforce other sources of information; clients are far more likely to read a leaflet or handout if they are also told why it will be of interest to them, and how they can benefit from the information provided.

All staff should be involved in promoting the practice to the clients. Receptionists are in an ideal position to tell clients about new services and explain more about the displays or leaflets in the reception area. Nurses, especially those running clinics, have a 'captive audience' to whom they can give information. The veterinary surgeon should be playing their part in the consulting room by giving clients information about nurses' clinics, puppy parties, new products, special offers on necessary treatments such as flea and worm control, and so on. In fact the whole practice team should be actively communicating relevant information to their clients.

Your database

A practice can offer new services, attract new clients and provide excellent client care very well without a computer. But some form of practice management computer system is essential for this marketing to be targeted and the effects monitored. Supermarket and high street 'loyalty' cards have not become popular simply because they reward the customer with a few points, but because the retailers can build a picture of customer buying habits to develop their marketing plans. Your computer system can use the information from clinical and stock control records to help your marketing in just the same way. It should be capable of:

- providing the basic client and animal details to be used in personalized mailshots – addressing the letter to the animal is becoming more common!
- categorizing clients by animal species, frequency of visit, products used and income generated.
- identifying how much income is generated by each of the products and services that are currently offered by the practice.
- producing figures for comparison with other practices in marketing indices.
- allowing year-on-year comparisons of income and sales categories.
- being searched for almost anything! Can it produce a target list of neutered, vaccinated canines over 8 years old that have not had any laboratory tests in the last year?

Computer systems are expensive, but used properly they can be the key to developing the practice. Above all, marketing depends on having excellent standards of clinical expertise, product knowledge, staff training and client care.

CHAPTER CONTENTS

Why have financial accounts? 135

Accounting basics 136

What is a profit and loss account? 136
Turnover 137
Cost of sales 137
Expenses 138
Net profit 139

What is a balance sheet? 139
Assets 139
Liabilities 141
Capital 141

Interpreting financial accounts 141
Previous year comparisons 142
Gross profit percentage 142
Cost of drugs and disposables as a percentage of turnover 142
Expenses as a percentage of turnover 142
Net profit percentage 142
Veterinary surgeon income as a percentage of turnover 142
Current ratio 142
Acid test 143
Gearing 143
Stock days 143
Debtor days 143
Return on capital employed 144

13

Understanding financial accounts

The financial accounts of the practice are a little bit like laboratory results – a long list of figures which mean nothing at all unless you have an idea of what the normal range should be. Even then, there is a huge variation in what is 'right', and changes in trends over time can be even more important than absolute values.

This section is not intended to tell you how to draw up practice accounts – there are plenty of books and courses on accountancy which cover that side of things in detail. However, it is important for practice managers to understand what the figures in financial accounts mean, where they come from, and some simple ways to interpret them.

WHY HAVE FINANCIAL ACCOUNTS?

The main purpose of financial accounts is to report in a regulated and standard way to meet the statutory and legal requirements of bodies outside the business, such as the Inland Revenue and Register of Companies. They will be used as a starting point for calculating the tax liabilities of the business owners, assessing the value of the practice, or the risk involved in lending the practice money.

Of course, they also allow business managers to see how things are going, and there are a number of valuable pointers that can be picked up from these accounts. The key problem restricting their use as a management tool is one of timeliness. A year's set of accounts may not be produced for four months after the year-end.

By this time the information at the start of the period is sixteen months out of date! If you have to wait that long before realizing there is a financial problem, then there is not much hope of doing something about it. Computerization has revolutionized bookkeeping and accountancy. Practices that do much of their financial record keeping in-house can get an on-going idea of how the practice's accounts are developing over the year.

ACCOUNTING BASICS

Before going any further, there are some accounting principles to explain.

VAT is not included in reports of income and expenditure for a practice. The VAT element of fees charged is simply being collected by the practice on behalf of the government, and should not be regarded as practice income. The VAT that the practice is charged on expenses can normally be deducted from the amount paid to HM Customs and Excise, and is not a charge to the business.

Most businesses use the accrual system of accounting. This means that income is accounted for at the time the goods are sold or service provided, not when it is paid for. Similarly expenses are shown as they are incurred, not when the bill is settled. Further adjustments may need to be made to expenses, and these are explained later.

The content and layout of the reports contained in the financial 'accounts' are governed by accountancy regulations. The two key financial statements are:

- Profit and loss account
- Balance sheet.

WHAT IS A PROFIT AND LOSS ACCOUNT?

This report shows the income generated by the practice, and the amount of that income which is left after deduction of the costs and running expenses incurred. The exact format of a profit and loss account will vary between sole traders, partnerships and limited companies, but the principles remain the same.

A simplified profit and loss account is shown in Figure 13.1. Technically, this is called a 'Trading and Profit and Loss Account'.

The first section is the 'trading' part. The top line shows the VAT-exclusive amount of work done for clients between the accounting dates. Depending on the preferences of your accountant, it may be described as 'Sales', 'Turnover', 'Fees' or similar.

The 'Cost of sales' figure shows the costs directly involved with producing the turnover. In veterinary practice this is normally made up of the cost of drugs, disposables and other retail

Smith & Jones MsRCVS

Trading and Profit and Loss Account
for the year ended 31st December 2001

	£	£
Turnover		450,000
Less cost of sales		(155,000)
Gross profit		295,000
Less expenses		
Bank charges	3,000	
CPD	1,500	
Depreciation	9,000	
Heat and light	3,500	
Interest expense	3,000	
Insurance, professional fees	4,000	
Motoring	8,000	
Postage, stationery, office	6,000	
Rents and rates	20,000	
Repairs	5,000	
Subscriptions and sundries	6,000	
Telephone	4,000	
Wages	90,000	
		(163,000)
Net profit		132,000

Figure 13.1 Simplified profit and loss account.

products. A full calculation of cost of sales is normally included in the trading and profit and loss account. This calculation is explained later.

The amount left after this stage (the Trading Account) is called the gross profit.

The other running expenses of the business are then itemized, with the final 'bottom line' giving the net profit of the practice.

Turnover

In a computerized practice, the turnover figure will be based on the figures for chargeable work done in the period. Other fee income, which may not directly be invoiced through your practice management system, may have to be added to produce the final figure. This might include things such as 'ministry' work in large animal practice.

Some practices, especially those without sophisticated computer systems, may try to estimate their turnover figures from cash receipts or banking. Whilst it is very important to keep track of cash flow in the business, your turnover figure will bear no immediate relationship to the amount of money paid into the practice bank account. There are three main reasons for this:

- Money banked includes VAT, whereas the turnover is net of VAT.
- Money banked is simply the money paid to the practice during the period, and is no reflection on the actual work done. Payment may be made for work done in previous periods, and current work may remain unpaid.
- The money banked may include other items, such as income tax refunds or drug company rebates, which are not part of practice turnover.

The relationship between turnover, payments and debtors is illustrated in Figure 13.2.

In this simple example, a practice is paid £60,000 in a month. But £15,000 of that sum relates to outstanding fees not paid in a previous period, and £13,750 of work in the current period has been unpaid. The gross work done in the period is therefore £58,750. But this sum includes VAT, currently at 17.5%. This must be deducted to give the true turnover for the period of £50,000.

Cost of sales

Most, if not all, of the Cost of Sales figure is made up of the cost of drugs and consumables sold or used by the practice. The accrual principle means that the 'cost of goods sold' figure should be literally the cost of the goods sold to generate the turnover specified. This is not the same as the cost of goods bought within the same period. Figure 13.3 details the cost of goods sold calculation that would have been included in the Cost of Sales section of

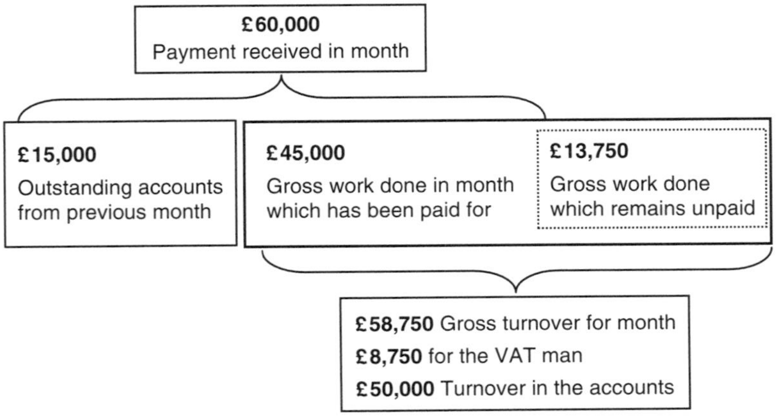

Figure 13.2 Turnover, debtors, payments and VAT.

the Trading and Profit and Loss Account in Figure 13.1.

The practice started the accounting period with £40,000 worth of stock. During the course of the year, goods worth £130,000 were bought. However, the cost of stock sold during the period is much higher than that, as there is only £15,000 worth of stock left at the end of the year.

Other direct costs may be included in the cost of sales section, such as laboratory and cremation fees. Some accountants may regard professional salaries as direct costs of sales.

Expenses

A lot of the expenses are very simple. Items such as stationery, CPD, repairs, and bank charges are charged for on a month-by-month basis. The figures shown in the accounts will simply be the VAT-exclusive charges incurred for the accounting period. Note that, just as in the income situation, the important date is when the service was provided, not when the bill was paid.

Opening stock value	£ 40,000	
Add cost of purchases	£130,000	
	£170,000	
Less closing stock value	(£15,000)	
Cost of goods sold		£155,000

Figure 13.3 Cost of goods sold.

It is not always so easy to understand where some of the figures for other expenses have come from. Insurance, rents, rates, subscriptions and utilities such as electricity and telephone may have to be adjusted to conform to the accruals concept. This is because these expenses tend to be charged annually or quarterly in advance, arrears or even a mixture of both. Calculations must be carried out to identify the portion of the expense attributable to the accounting period.

An example showing adjustments made for insurance expense is shown in Figure 13.4.

Accountancy fees are a real 'chicken and egg' issue – since the fees incurred drawing up the accounts for a particular period are not known until the accounts have actually been done! The fee is normally added in by the accountant as one of his final steps.

Depreciation is not an actual expense, in the sense of money changing hands. It is intended to be a measure of the reduction in value of an item, such as a car, that occurs as a result of its use in the business. In other words, a car might be worth £10,000 at the start of the financial year, and only £7,500 at the end. The difference of £2,500 is the depreciation. Even though the practice has not actually paid that amount of money, it is still a cost of running the business for that period of time, and is therefore shown in

Insurance bill on 1st August 2001, for 12 months is £3,420

Financial year-end is 31st December 2001

The insurance bill is paying in advance for 7 months of 2002

The amount prepaid for 2002 is (£3420/12) × 7 = £1995

Insurance amount charged to the accounts is calculated:	
Amount prepaid in 2000	£ 1,575
Plus insurance paid in 2001	£ 3,420
Less amount carried forward to 2002	(£1,995)
Insurance charged to 2001 accounts	£ 3,000

Figure 13.4 Accrual of insurance costs.

the profit and loss account as an expense. Accountants will use a formula to determine the amount of depreciation to be applied each year.

Some of the money paid out by the practice during the year will not be shown in the list of expenses at all, such as:

- VAT – as explained earlier, the practice simply collects this money on behalf of HM Customs and Excise, and passes it on to them.
- Money paid to, or on behalf of, the owners of the business, e.g. partner's drawings, or contributions to their tax/National Insurance payments.
- Purchases of long-lasting capital items of equipment, such as cars, computers, an X-ray machine or dental de-scaler.

These last two will be dealt with in more detail in the section about the Balance Sheet.

Net profit

This is the figure most used by tax offices, bankers and other outside agencies. It may bear little relation to the overall health of your practice finances. It is quite possible to have good profits but absolutely no money. The very top line of the P&L account – turnover – is the amount of chargeable work done for your clients. If they do not pay you, then you will be forced to borrow, or not pay your suppliers. As mentioned above, the net profit figure also does not take account of some spending. A profitable business can still run into trouble if it spends too much on capital items, or the owners take too much money for their own use. So always remember, the bottom line profit is not real cash.

To get another view of the business, you must also look at the balance sheet.

WHAT IS A BALANCE SHEET?

A balance sheet is a snapshot of the practice finances on a particular date, normally the last day of the financial year. It is a statement of what the practice is theoretically worth to the owners. It lists what the business owns, money it owes to others, and what is owed to it.

A simple balance sheet for a practice partnership is shown in Figure 13.5. The layout of the balance sheet may vary, depending on the preferences of the accountant, and any changes in accountancy standards. However, the principle is always the same – at some point the assets and liabilities are shown to balance.

Assets

An asset is something which belongs to the business. Most people have no difficulty in identifying cash, equipment or cars as assets, but may initially find it odd that the debtors of the practice are assets too! The money they owe to you belongs to the practice.

Assets are divided into two main groups on the balance sheet – Fixed Assets and Current Assets. Current Assets consist of cash (or cash equivalents) and items that are likely to be converted into cash within 12 months, such as trading stock.

Common current assets include:

- cash in hand
- bank balances
- stock
- debtors
- prepayments – e.g. the prepayment of insurance which was discussed earlier.

Fixed assets are generally items that the business expects to have for over a year, and may include:

- the practice buildings or land
- goodwill
- motor vehicles
- fixtures and fittings – the equipment and furniture within the practice.

When the practice buys a fixed asset, such as a piece of equipment, this is not shown as an expense on the profit and loss account. Instead, the cost price of the equipment is added onto the balance sheet as a fixed asset.

Some assets have an obvious value, such as cash, or the total amount owed by debtors. Stock is generally valued at cost price, although damaged or outdated stock should be regarded as worthless.

Smith & Jones MsRCVS

Balance sheet at 31st December 2001

	£	£
Fixed assets		
Land and buildings		90,000
Goodwill		6,500
Fixtures and fittings		36,000
Motor vehicles		15,000
		147,500
Current assets		
Stock	15,000	
Debtors	12,000	
Prepayments	3,250	
Cash	450	
	30,700	
Less current liabilities		
Creditors	18,000	
Accruals	750	
Overdraft	3,000	
	(21,750)	
Net current assets		8,950
Total assets less current liabilities[a]		156,450
Long-term liabilities		
Bank loan		(37,500)
Total net assets		118,950
Partners' equity and capital		
A. Smith		66,246
B. Jones		52,704
		118,950

[a] Fixed assets + net current assets

Figure 13.5 Simple balance sheet for a practice partnership.

Fixed assets are harder to value, and accountancy conventions use a historical cost basis – in other words, things are listed as the value that was paid for them. Practice buildings and goodwill remain at the same value each year in the accounts, regardless of the state of the property market. However, if the business is about to change ownership, these assets will be re-valued.

The valuation, and even the existence, of goodwill can be a contentious issue in the veterinary profession. Goodwill is basically the difference between the overall value of a practice as a whole, and the value of the business assets such as premises and fittings. In other words, it is the added value of buying an existing practice instead of starting up a new one from scratch. Goodwill is not a visible 'thing' that can be seen or physically measured. It is an example of what is known as an intangible fixed asset. Valuation of goodwill is a complex issue, and is influenced by quantitative issues, such as the profit-generating ability of the practice, and qualitative factors, such as client loyalty.

Some fixed assets will wear out over time. These assets, such as cars and equipment, have their value reduced each year by an amount called depreciation. The calculation of depreciation varies depending on the type of fixed asset – cars and computers lose value more quickly than furniture and fixtures. This devaluation of the asset is transferred to the profit and loss account each year as an expense. The asset value shown in the balance sheet will be the cost value of the item, minus the total depreciation that has been applied to it. Your accountant will normally show full details of the depreciation calculations as a note to the balance sheet.

Liabilities

The liabilities shown on a balance sheet indicate how much the business owed to others on the balance sheet date. Just as assets are divided up into fixed and current assets, there are two categories of liability.

Current liabilities are amounts that the practice must pay within the next 12 months. They include items such as:

- VAT due to be paid
- tax/National Insurance contributions due to the Inland Revenue
- trade creditors – wholesalers, laboratories and other suppliers
- accruals – such as rent paid in arrears
- overdrafts – unlike a loan, these are repayable on demand.

Long-term liabilities are sums owed by the practice, which will not be repaid within the next 12 months, including:

- bank loans
- long-term finance for cars and equipment
- mortgages.

Capital

The third type of entry on a balance sheet sets out the practice owner's stake in the business. The total capital of a business is the difference between the sum of the assets and liabilities. In effect capital is a special sort of liability – it is what the business owes its owners.

The layout of the capital section will vary depending on the structure of the business.

In the case of sole traders and partnerships, each owner's share is divided into two main sections – a capital account, representing their long-term investment in the practice, and a current account, detailing their share of profits, drawings taken from the business and balance remaining.

For limited companies, the owners' investment is shown on the balance sheet as share capital. Directors are paid a salary, which is shown as an expense on the Profit and Loss account. The operating profit is then either distributed to the shareholders as dividends, or retained to add to company reserves.

INTERPRETING FINANCIAL ACCOUNTS

Figures extracted from a set of accounts are meaningless on their own.

For instance, you can only assess a net profit figure by either comparing it with previous profit figures from the same practice, or by relating it to other information about the practice, such as number of partners. A four-vet practice with a single owner would show a much lower net profit figure than the same practice where all four vets were partners.

Other parameters, such as stock asset value, can be interpreted by comparing with other figures from the same set of accounts – in this case, the value of stock purchases.

Financial interpretations which require further practice details, such as numbers of veterinary surgeons, will be covered in Chapter 14, 'Management accounts and financial planning'. Other accounting ratios, which can be determined solely from the published financial accounts of the practice, are looked at below.

Some worked examples are shown in Figure 13.6, at the end of this chapter. Many of these ratios can be compared between practices as well as with previous practice performance.

Previous year comparisons

All figures can be compared with their previous year value, and differences noted, both in absolute and percentage terms.

Growth figures, such as percentage increase in turnover and percentage increase in profits, can be compared with industry figures reported in veterinary business publications.

Gross profit percentage

This is the gross profit figure expressed as a percentage of practice turnover. Before comparing figures with external sources of data, it is vital to know the basis used for calculation of the gross profit in each case. A practice which includes laboratory and cremation costs in its 'cost of sales' will have a relatively lower gross profit percentage than one which only includes stock items.

$$\text{Gross profit percentage} = \frac{\text{Gross profit}}{\text{Turnover}} \times 100$$

Historically, large animal practices have derived a larger portion of their income from drug sales than small animal ones. Consequently, the gross profit percentages of large animal practices have tended to be lower than those in the small animal sector. This distinction is gradually becoming less marked as the increase in retailing in small animal practice has tended to decrease their gross profit percentage. Many practices, large and small animal, are also seeking to increase their proportion of fee income and reduce their dependence on drug sales.

Cost of drugs and disposables as a percentage of turnover

Not all practices calculate their gross profit in the same way, and so comparisons of gross profit percentages have to be made with care. The cost of drugs and disposables as a percentage of turnover is more tightly defined.

Expenses as a percentage of turnover

Sometimes expense costs may be quoted as a percentage of turnover, for instance CPD, wages or bank charges.

Net profit percentage

This is the net profit expressed as a percentage of turnover. This figure is useful to compare with previous years in the same practice to track overall profitability. It is of limited value for comparison with other practices because it is affected by the ratio of partners to assistants.

Veterinary surgeon income as a percentage of turnover

In this case, assistants' salaries and locum fees are added to the net profit figure. The resulting percentage of turnover allows comparison between practices irrespective of the number of partners and assistants.

The above figures are all reflections of the profitability of the practice. It is equally important to assess the on-going stability of the business. In order to determine the risk of the practice running out of cash, we can look at some measures of liquidity.

Current ratio

The current ratio of a practice is the ratio between its current assets (stock, cash, debtors) and current liabilities (creditors, overdraft). It gives an indication of the practice's ability to pay its immediate liabilities.

$$\text{Current ratio} = \frac{\text{Current assets}}{\text{Current liabilities}}$$

The resulting ratio needs to be at least 1:1, with a result of 1.5 : 1 being a reasonable figure. In other words the practice will have current assets valued at one and a half times its current liabilities.

Inappropriate use of overdraft facilities instead of arranging a long-term bank loan will be highlighted by this test.

Acid test

The current ratio may leave you feeling secure, but in reality, if some of your liabilities needed immediate payment you could still have a serious problem. The main reason for this is that one of the current assets, stock, is not immediately convertible to cash. The acid test ratio (sometimes called the quick or liquid ratio) does not include the stock value, and is therefore a much more stringent test.

$$\text{Acid test} = \frac{\text{Current assets minus stock}}{\text{Current liabilities}}$$

Both of these ratios will fluctuate during the course of a month, as suppliers are paid, and also between months. The liabilities will increase towards the end of a VAT quarter, for instance. It is important to be aware of this, and to be consistent with your timing when comparing the results with previous figures for your practice.

Gearing

The current ratio and acid test measure the short-term liquidity of the business. A more long-term view is given by looking at the gearing ratio. This measures the proportion of borrowed money financing the practice.

$$\text{Gearing} = \frac{\text{Borrowings}}{\text{Capital}} \times 100$$

There are a number of factors that make this ratio difficult to interpret. Unless the practice has been recently bought or had a change of ownership, the valuation of practice property and goodwill are unlikely to be realistic. This in turn means that the capital value may be significantly understated.

There are several ways of defining gearing, depending on exactly what is covered by the term 'borrowing'. Some sources may use total debts, others may only include long-term finance. Similarly, the capital may be taken to mean only owners' (partners or shareholders) capital, or may be taken as owners' capital plus borrowed capital (long-term loans).

Other ratios can be used to highlight some internal management issues.

Stock days

Stock sitting on the shelf is not earning money, and is also tying up valuable cash that could be used elsewhere in the practice. The stock days calculation allows you to work out the average number of days stock you are keeping.

$$\text{Stock days} = \frac{\text{Stock value}}{\text{Cost of stock sold}} \times 365$$

A sensible target to aim for is 30 days. The stock days figure can be seasonal, especially in large animal practice, when stock levels may be much higher at some times of year. This may happen at turnout or housing time, when there is a peak demand for many routine herd health products.

Debtor days

Monitoring the average time that debtors take to pay the practice gives valuable feedback on your credit control systems. The correct way to calculate your debtor days is to divide your outstanding debtors by the value of your sales on account.

$$\text{Debtor days} = \frac{\text{Debtors' value}}{\text{Credit sales}} \times 365$$

However, the value of your credit sales is not available from your balance sheet, and can be quite a difficult figure to extract from your sales records. A simpler ratio, which gives you the average time taken for *all* your clients to pay, can be used instead.

$$\text{Payment time for all clients} = \frac{\text{Debtors}}{\text{Turnover}} \times 365$$

In a pure large animal practice you may be able to assume that all of your turnover is generated from account sales, and this sum will give you a true debtor days figure. But be aware that in a practice with a large amount of cash sales, a small number of very bad debtors could easily be masked using this simple formula.

The value of debtors shown in the accounts will include the VAT element that they owe, whereas the turnover is shown excluding VAT. The figures used in the ratio should be adjusted so that they are equivalent – i.e. deduct the VAT due from debtors, or add VAT onto the turnover before doing the calculation.

Finally, you might want to look at why the practice owners are in business at all!

Return on capital employed

One of the objectives of owning a veterinary practice is to achieve a good return on the money that has been invested. The profitability of the practice can be assessed by showing it as a return on capital employed (ROCE).

$$\text{ROCE} = \frac{\text{Net profit before interest}}{\text{Capital employed}} \times 100$$

In the case of sole owners or partnerships, the net profit should first be adjusted by deducting a notional salary for the partners to reflect the veterinary and management work they carry out. As with gearing, there are various ways in which this ratio can be calculated. The capital employed normally includes both owners' capital and long-term loans.

A similar calculation is the return on equity (ROE). Here we are looking at what the owners actually receive in relation to their investment.

$$\text{ROE} = \frac{\text{Net profit}}{\text{Owners' capital}} \times 100$$

These returns should be greater than the return on a risk-free investment such as a building society account. A negative return indicates that the practice profits are not sufficient even to cover a notional salary for the partners.

If the accounts show an out-of-date valuation of property and goodwill, the capital value will probably be underestimated. In this case both of these return on capital ratios will be artificially high.

Analysis of Smith & Jones MsRCVS			
Gross profit %	$\frac{\text{Gross profit}}{\text{Turnover}} \times 100$	$\frac{295{,}000}{450{,}000} \times 100$	= 65.5%
CPD as % turnover	$\frac{\text{Expense type}}{\text{Turnover}} \times 100$	$\frac{1{,}500}{450{,}000} \times 100$	= 0.33%
Net profit %	$\frac{\text{Net profit}}{\text{Turnover}} \times 100$	$\frac{132{,}000}{450{,}000} \times 100$	= 29.3%
VS income	$\frac{\text{Net profit + VS wages}}{\text{Turnover}}$	$\frac{132{,}000 + 20{,}000}{450{,}000} \times 100$	= 33.8%
Current ratio	$\frac{\text{Current assets}}{\text{Current liabilities}}$	$\frac{30{,}700}{21{,}750}$	= 1.41
Acid test	$\frac{\text{Current assets - stock}}{\text{Current liabilities}}$	$\frac{30{,}750 - 15{,}000}{21{,}750}$	= 0.72
Gearing	$\frac{\text{Borrowing}}{\text{Capital}}$	$\frac{37{,}500}{118{,}950} \times 100$	= 31.5%
Stock days	$\frac{\text{Stock value}}{\text{Cost of goods sold}} \times 365$	$\frac{15{,}000}{155{,}000} \times 365$	= 35 days
Debtor days	$\frac{\text{Debtors (ex VAT)}}{\text{Credit sales}} \times 365$	$\frac{10{,}212}{112{,}500} \times 365$	= 33 days
Average payment time	$\frac{\text{Debtors (ex VAT)}}{\text{Turnover}} \times 365$	$\frac{10{,}212}{450{,}000} \times 365$	= 8.3 days
ROCE	$\frac{\text{Net profit + interest}}{\text{Capital employed}} \times 100$	$\frac{45{,}000}{156{,}450} \times 100$	= 28.8%
ROE	$\frac{\text{Net profit}}{\text{Owners capital}} \times 100$	$\frac{42{,}000}{118{,}950} \times 100$	= 35.3%

Notes: Vet surgeon salary – 1 part timer @ £20,000 p.a.
Debtor days – 75% of turnover is paid at the time
Assume owner's notional salaries £45,000 p.a.

Figure 13.6 Worked examples of practice accounting ratios.

CHAPTER CONTENTS

Management accounts 147

Figures derived from the financial accounts 149
Average turnover per veterinary surgeon 149
Expenses per veterinary surgeon 149
Net profit per partner 149

Figures derived from income analysis 149
Fees and drugs 149
Income categories by service 149
Specific services 150
Income by client base 150
Average transaction fee 150

Other figures 150
Staff ratios 150
Case volume – by service category and client base 150
Client turnover 151

Financial management 151

Budgeting for profit – will we make any money? 152
Budgeting for turnover 152
Budgeting for expenses 153

Budgeting for cash – can we stay afloat? 154

Budgeting for capital expenses – can we afford to buy? 156
Payback period 157
Return on investment (ROI) 157
Net present value (NPV) 158
Financing the expenditure 159

14

Management accounts and financial planning

The makeup and interpretation of financial accounts has been explained in Chapter 13, 'Understanding financial accounts'. These figures can give the practice manager some very useful information about the financial performance of the practice, but their use is hampered by several problems. The information contained within the accounts is out of date, and they are not sufficiently detailed to enable targeted management decisions to be made. Also, one of the main purposes of the Profit and Loss account for sole traders and partnerships is the calculation of tax liability for the owners. In some cases 'creative accounting' will attempt to maximize apparent expenses, thereby minimizing the potential tax payments. Many advantageous expenses, such as partners' wives' wages, can find their way into the accounts, and can distort the true practice performance.

MANAGEMENT ACCOUNTS

The law says you must produce financial accounts – but why bother with management accounts? Their purpose is to give the manager the information they need to monitor practice performance and make decisions. Management accounts can also be used to give employees motivation and feedback about specific projects within the practice, for instance tracking income arising from nurses' dental health checks. The key requirement is that the figures are up-to-date and meaningful.

In this computerized age it is easy to fall into the trap of compulsive gathering of data, and this can easily reach an overload situation. Some of the printouts available from practice management computer software can look very impressive, but in reality, what does Figure 14.1 mean?

The management reporting process converts this data into useful information. This may be done by adding up different income groups, for instance. The data from Figure 14.1 could be used, in conjunction with other figures, to produce the reports shown in Figure 14.2.

Do not underestimate the costs of data and information. Some of the raw data about your practice finances and clients may not appear to have cost anything specifically, as it may have been gathered as an aside to the basic keeping of clinical records. However, there may be a huge cost in employees' time in converting it to useful information. There is no point spending time and money producing data and reports that no one can understand or has time to act on.

The key is to make comparisons – the figures are meaningless on their own. Your management accounts may include ratios and monthly, quarterly, or year-to-date figures that may be compared with the previous period, or the equivalent period the previous year. Another useful way of presenting data is to use a moving annual total (MAT): this is effectively the previous 12 months' data. As a new month is

	Oct	Nov	Dec
Examinations-Farm	£66.03	£141.00	£179.94
Consultations	£2,227.89	£2,694.63	£2,333.44
MAFF	£0.00	£0.00	£157.00
Examinations Equine	£141.50	£177.50	£35.50
Postage & Packing	£1.50	£0.00	£2.50
Credits	£0.00	£0.00	–£3.00
Cons after hours	£210.00	£259.22	£362.50
Rabbit work	£153.80	£61.20	£99.10
Primary dog vaccines	£389.76	£475.50	£358.30
Primary cat vaccines	£322.99	£404.67	£381.46
Nurse clinics	£53.20	£23.45	£10.50
Equine surgery	£0.00	£153.45	£35.20

Figure 14.1 Raw financial data – income breakdown.

	This quarter	Last quarter	£ change	% change
Consultations	£8,650	£8,235	+ £325	+ 5%
Laboratory work	£6,333	£5,507	+ £826	+ 15%
Vaccination canine	£5,935	£6,340	(– £405)	– 6.4%
Vaccination feline	£4,540	£4,235	+ £305	+ 7.2%
Anaesthesia	£4,140	£3,943	+ £197	+ 5%
Surgery	£3,572	£3,402	+ £170	+ 5%
Radiography	£1,276	£1,251	+ £25	+ 2%

Figure 14.2 Breakdown of top 80% fee income.

added, the equivalent month the previous year drops off the end. This evens out seasonal fluctuations, whilst being more up to date than figures based on financial or calendar years.

So what information do you put in management accounts? There is no official specification for internal management accounts – they are whatever you need them to be. The trick is to find something measurable, present the information in an understandable format, and be able to use the information. A management accounting report will contain figures drawn from a number of sources.

FIGURES DERIVED FROM THE FINANCIAL ACCOUNTS

Ratios derived solely from the financial accounts were looked at in Chapter 13. Some figures in the financial accounts can be interpreted by comparing them with other data about the practice. Even if the practice does not have any sophisticated level of information system, some useful figures can be extracted from the statutory accounts. One of the most common ways to interpret accounts is to compare figures with the number of veterinary surgeons in the practice.

Average turnover per veterinary surgeon

Simply dividing the overall practice turnover by the number of full-time equivalent veterinary surgeons is one of the quickest ways of producing data that is easily comparable between practices. It also allows you to compare with previous data for the same practice if there has been any change in vet numbers.

Expenses per veterinary surgeon

Running costs per veterinary surgeon can be another useful comparison to make. Expenses such as motoring, support staff salaries and CPD tend to be directly dependent on the number of veterinary surgeons in the practice.

Net profit per partner

One of the difficulties in interpreting the net profit figure from sole trader or partnership accounts is the effect of the ratio of owners to employed veterinary surgeons. Dividing the net profit by the number of partners will give an easily comparable figure.

FIGURES DERIVED FROM INCOME ANALYSIS

Unless you have a clear idea of how the practice income is made up, you have little chance of planning how to improve it, or identify where any deficits are coming from. In the 1998 BVA/SPVS practice survey, 44% of the respondents could not provide a basic income breakdown into small animal, farm and equine categories of fees and drugs. On the other hand, there are now over 140 practices regularly contributing very detailed data on income and client activity to the Fort Dodge Index scheme.

Fees and drugs

At the very least, practices should be able to identify how much of their income is derived from professional fees, and how much from the sale of medicines and other products. In the light of the Marsh report into dispensing, how can a practice assess the implications of the loss of the privilege to dispense if they don't know how much income comes from drug sales?

Now that waiting room sales are making up an ever-increasing portion of some small animal practices' income, it makes sense to break down the 'drugs' figure into veterinary and non-veterinary goods.

Income categories by service

Practice management computer systems should allow you to divide your work into categories, such as consultations, surgery, diagnostics, medicines and pet care sales. Setting up these categories should be thought out carefully – too much detail can be as bad as too little. Some work will always be included in a 'miscellaneous' category, but make sure that doesn't get too big. There is no point categorizing your income if you end up with 10% that you can't identify! As illustrated earlier in Figure 14.1, the raw data from these reports is not immediately useful, and will usually need some form of manipulation in a spreadsheet to come up with some final comparisons. Many practice management systems will export their data directly to a spreadsheet, making this process much easier.

Some income categories will be very small, and there is little point including everything. A breakdown of the top 80% of your income will be adequate for routine reporting.

Specific services

In some cases you might want to look at the details of specific income groups, for instance the makeup of your consultation income. It can be interesting to see whether the relative turnover derived from first, second and repeat consultations reflects what appears in the appointment book!

Income by client base

In a mixed practice, income can be divided into that from small animal, farm and equine clients. For a more specialized practice, this breakdown will be more detailed, such as dog and cat income; or work done for racing stables, trekking stables and private owners. These figures can help track targeted marketing activity, or be used to assess the viability of certain sectors of the practice; for instance does the amount of large animal work being done justify the expense of specific drugs, facilities and equipment needed to do the work?

Average transaction fee

The average transaction fee is a measure of the average spend per client visit. It can be broken down by client category, and also divided into fee and drug components. These figures can be used to highlight differences between different client sectors. The June 2001 Fort Dodge Index report shows that the median spend per dog visit is 20% higher than the spend per cat visit. This can have important implications when the balance of client base may be shifting, such as the trend from dog towards cat ownership.

OTHER FIGURES

Management accounts are not restricted to financial values – other practice parameters can be used to track performance and provide feedback to managers.

Staff ratios

The ratio of support staff to veterinary surgeons varies between types of practice. Large animal practices tend to have relatively fewer support staff since the veterinary surgeons spend a large proportion of their time out on their rounds, and a ratio of 1:1 is common. In small animal practice, much higher staffing levels of around three full-time equivalent support staff for each vet are common. This ratio will vary between practices, depending on the roles of support staff and their contribution towards the practice. Too low a ratio might indicate that veterinary surgeons could be wasting their time performing tasks better suited to nursing staff, whereas too many support staff could be an indicator of excessive staff costs.

Case volume – by service category and client base

Practice income depends both on fees per visit and number of visits. Simply monitoring income alone could mask changes in caseload. If major changes have been made to the fee structure, then it is vital to measure the effect this has on volume of work. Monitoring case volume will also help decisions about increasing staff levels. Do you really need another vet, or do you just need to be better organized?

Client turnover

Every practice will lose old clients and gain new ones. Figures for client retention and turnover will allow you to monitor the balance and plan marketing requirements.

Do remember that management reports have to be readily understandable and easily acted upon. A detailed dissection of every practice activity will sit on the shelf gathering dust, and is a waste of time and money. Users will not take in a routine report containing more than about ten different parameters. Remember to tailor your reports to their purpose, such as those in the following categories.

Routine practice performance

Quarterly or monthly comparison with previous period or year's figures:

- turnover per vet
- caseload
- fee income
- drug income
- gross profit %
- veterinary surgeon income as a % turnover
- debtor days.

Re-organizing support staffing levels

Comparing figures with the previous year and published veterinary standards for:

- number of full-time equivalent veterinary surgeons
- support staff: veterinary surgeon ratio
- nurses' caseload
- staff costs as a % of turnover
- staff costs per vet.

Overheads economy drive

Comparing figures with the previous periods or published standards for:

- variable costs per veterinary surgeon – e.g. motoring
- fixed costs per hour – e.g. premises costs
- individual costs as a % of turnover
- specific absolute comparative costs, e.g. electricity £ per month.

Review of equine sector performance

Quarterly or monthly comparison with previous period or year's figures for:

- equine fees/drugs
- equine income analysis – e.g. visits, examinations, vaccinations, surgery and drugs
- equine caseload.

Simple staff feedback

Monthly comparisons or MAT figures:

- graph for example of dental numbers and income.

FINANCIAL MANAGEMENT

Financial management is essential to move the practice forward. Simply sighing over the annual accounts and going back to doing what you always have done will only get you what you got last time, if not less! Financial goals must be set, worked towards, and deviations accounted for.

Financial management involves:

- analysing where you are
- setting objectives
- planning how to get there (budgeting)
- analysing your progress
- revising the plan when necessary.

The financial and management accounts should give you plenty of information about the current state of the practice, and any underlying trends to date.

Almost every aspect of practice activity will have some impact on the financial planning process. When drawing up budgets and forecasts, you will need to consider a wide variety of objectives such as:

- desired profit levels for the practice owners
- target fee positioning in the marketplace

- standards of facilities and professional care to be provided
- staffing levels and pay structures
- specific targets, such as amount of turnover spent on re-investment or training
- the structure of the practice – number of partners, or whether to incorporate.

There are several different financial plans which need to be drawn up:

- profit and loss budget
- cashflow forecast
- investment planning.

Use reports comparing your actual figures with the budget to check whether things are on target. This needs to be checked at least quarterly, if not monthly, to enable discrepancies to be spotted and dealt with before they get out of hand.

You may need to review practice policies, such as changing suppliers, to bring the actual figures back in line with budget. On the other hand, your budget may have been based on erroneous assumptions, and might need to be adjusted for the rest of the year.

A budget is not a static document, and even with the best planning in the world, no budget could anticipate the arrival of some of the recent farming upheavals. Government legislation can also have a dramatic effect. It may affect the income side, such as the threat to the sales of medicines; or cause extra expenses, such as those due to health and safety legislation. There may also be positive effects, and the pet travel scheme has provided new opportunities for many practices.

BUDGETING FOR PROFIT – WILL WE MAKE ANY MONEY?

Budgets cannot be drawn up by one person working in isolation. The manager will need to involve the people who are responsible for generating and spending the money. If, for instance, a head nurse is responsible for ordering and maintaining surgical instruments, then she should be involved in setting the budgets for that part of the practice. Spending budgets which have simply been imposed by higher authority tend to be resented and ignored, whereas if staff have had some input into the process they are more likely to understand the need for restraint and will feel that they have done their bit. Similarly when budgeting for income, don't just assume vets can cope with doing 10% more work – ask them what they think they can do. If they have helped to set their targets, they will feel more involved and are more likely to work hard to achieve them.

Traditionally, practices have budgeted for expenses, hoped for income, and viewed the profit as what happens to be left at the end! Practice income should be planned and managed just as the expenses are, and a more targeted approach to income budgeting is part of the planning process.

Budgeting for turnover

The veterinary marketplace is changing very rapidly, and it is no longer sufficient to just add an inflationary and growth percentage onto previous figures.

Practice turnover depends on two things – caseload and fees. Fee setting and the concept of price elasticity is discussed in detail in Chapter 16, 'Pricing of fees and drugs.' To actively budget for turnover, you need to look in detail at how the practice income is made up, and also include any planned changes. Ideally your practice management system should be able to export detailed sales data to a spreadsheet. These figures should include the number of procedures done, and the average price charged for each. The income breakdown can then be examined in detail, estimating the change in case volume and price for each sector. Projected case volume multiplied by the new price will give you the expected turnover. A small section of such a planning spreadsheet is illustrated in Figure 14.3.

Planning income in this way reflects the objectives of the practice. If there is an intended shift towards more specialized work, then the fees may be increased whilst caseload goes down.

Actual figures				Budgeted income				
Procedure	Old turnover	Sales volume	Average sales price	% change volume	% change price	Projected sales volume	New sales price	Projected turnover
Consultation	£35,000	2,500	£14.00	+5%	+5%	2,625	£14.70	£38,588
Puppy vaccination	£6,250	250	£25.00	−10%	+3%	225	£25.75	£5,794
Pre-anaesthetic checks	£1,000	50	£20.00	+300%	+5%	150	£21.00	£3,150
Pet food	£50,000			+10%	+3.5%			£56,925

Figure 14.3 Budgeting for turnover.

The impact of new services can be assessed, and the effects of changing demographics of the pet population and farming industry allowed for.

Product sales should also be included in this planning sheet. It would be impossible and unnecessary to try to budget for sales of each item individually. The products can be divided into groups, such as small animal medicines, pet food, large animal PMLs and intramammary preparations. The percentage change in sales volume for each group can be estimated. This may be directly linked to changes in caseload, e.g. small animal medicine sales could be expected to rise by the same rate as the increase in consultation numbers. Price rises are likely to be based on manufacturers' price increases by inflation. The projected product sales will be the existing sales multiplied firstly by the projected increase in sales levels, then by the expected selling price increase.

Budgeting for expenses

This has long been the traditional face of budgeting in veterinary practice. At its simplest, expense budgeting involves looking at historic costs, estimating how much they will increase by, and thus arriving at the next year's budget figure. However, costs should not simply be accepted as inevitable and each expense centre should be questioned before allocating it a budget. For instance, do you continue to budget for car tax, insurance, servicing and fuel for each of the assistants' cars, or do you change practice policy to paying them a mileage rate?

Expenses can broadly be divided into fixed and variable costs, and these need to be budgeted for differently.

Fixed costs remain at the same level, regardless of the practice turnover or caseload. These include expenses such as business rates, rent, insurance, equipment leasing, heating and lighting. Fixed costs are only truly fixed for a range of turnover – at some point, increasing turnover would necessitate increased size of premises and therefore costs. Staff wages are fixed for a much smaller range of activity – the practice may well employ more nurses or vets as they get busier.

Variable costs change directly with turnover or caseload. Bank charges will increase as the turnover going through the bank account goes up, and car mileage charges, cremation and laboratory fees and cost of goods sold will go up as caseload increases.

Looking at previous years' figures will help to assess these variable costs as a percentage of turnover. When budgeting using a spreadsheet, these percentages can be set as a formula, so as to automatically update as you change the budgeted turnover. If the income has been budgeted for in detail, then the cost of goods sold, cremation and laboratory costs can be estimated by working backwards from their respective projected income figures.

Cost behaviour can also be divided into controllable and uncontrollable costs. The practice is stuck with its rateable value, and the RCVS fees have to be paid. On the other hand, costs such as heating and lighting can be controlled, both by shopping around for suppliers and reducing

Original figures		**Option 1, Decrease fixed costs by 5%**	
Turnover	100,000	Turnover	100,000
COGS (20%)	20,000	COGS (20%)	20,000
Fixed costs	50,000	Fixed costs	47,500
Profit	30,000	Profit	32,500
		Increase in profit of 8.3%	
Option 2, Increase caseload by 5%		**Option 3, Increase fees by 5%**	
Turnover	105,000	Turnover	105,000
COGS (20%)	21,000	COGS (no increase)	20,000
Fixed costs	50,000	Fixed costs	50,000
Profit	34,000	Profit	35,000
Increase in profit of 13.3%		Increase in profit of 16.7%	

Figure 14.4 Strategies for increasing profits.

wastage. The exact definition of controllable costs will vary depending on the authority of the person drawing up the budgets.

When calculating budgets, you have to start somewhere. There are two main strategies:

- top down
- bottom up.

Top down budgeting involves starting with your budgeted turnover, estimating your costs and then assessing the resulting net profit.

Bottom up budgeting takes another viewpoint. First decide on the desired profit, then estimate the relatively fixed expenses. The sum of these two sections of the budget will give the gross profit figure required. Finally, you need to work out the level of income and associated variable costs needed to meet that gross profit. It may be necessary to repeat the cycle a number of times if you feel that substantial increases in workload, necessitating further expenses, are involved.

Do bear in mind there are several strategies to increase profits:

- decrease expenses
- increase sales volume
- increase fees.

The effects of these options are illustrated by Figure 14.4.

In practice, most budgets will be a mixture of all of these, but it is interesting to note that most budgetary effort tends to be aimed at decreasing costs, which produces the least effect on the bottom line.

The finished budget should be presented in a monthly format, taking account of seasonal variations. Although an overall budget may be sufficient for persuading financial institutions to lend the practice money, a monthly breakdown is essential to compare the budget easily with the actual figures.

BUDGETING FOR CASH – CAN WE STAY AFLOAT?

Formulating a profit and loss budget to give a nice profit is one thing, but do not forget that cash flow is vital. In an extreme example, if you had to pay all your costs up front, and none of your clients paid you, then no matter how much profit there was on paper, you wouldn't find life very easy. By drawing up a cash flow forecast alongside the profit and loss budget, you can identify any 'thin' periods or strategic times to invest. On a very basic level, this can mean simply foreseeing a cash crisis in enough time to rearrange the overdraft without incurring unauthorized borrowing fees.

The cashflow forecast is based on the profit and loss budget, but there are some important amendments to make:

- Take account of debtor and creditor terms.
- Figures must be shown inclusive of VAT.
- VAT payments must be provided for.
- Include capital expenditure and partners' drawings.

Your final budget should list the turnover and expenses on a month-by-month basis. But the cash relating to these activities will not necessarily be received or spent in the same month. Information about debtor days should be used to anticipate when income will be received, and the expense payments adjusted by your normal creditor terms – for instance wages will usually be paid in the month they were incurred, whereas the wholesalers will be paid a month later. Some payments such as rent may be made quarterly. Cash flow forecasts can be used to illustrate the effects of improved or worsening fee collection strategies.

Figures in profit and loss accounts are always shown net of VAT, but the payments in and out of the bank are gross. All the income and expenses shown in your cashflow should therefore be recalculated to include any VAT elements.

The VAT itself will have to be paid to the Customs and Excise, and this should be included at the appropriate interval, usually every quarter.

The profit and loss budget will not include capital payments and partners' drawings, so these will need to be added to the bottom of the cashflow forecast.

Finally, the cashflow forecast needs to show your projected cash balance. The opening bank balance should be entered at the start of the period, and then carried forward for each month by adding inflows and deducting the outflows.

Part of a summarized cashflow forecast is shown in Figure 14.5.

The cashflow will highlight the ups and downs of practice funds. Many expenses are regular

	Month 1	Month 2	Month 3	Month 4
Income	£42,000	£43,560	£45,050	£42,400
Drugs	(£14,170)	(£15,345)	(£14,876)	(£14,500)
Cremation costs	(£578)	(£564)	(£592)	(£524)
Rent & rates	(£800)	(£3,400)	(£800)	(£800)
Telephone	(£1,000)			(£1,000)
Capital expenses			(£350)	(£350)
Drawings	(£7,000)	(£7,000)	(£7,000)	(£7,000)
VAT		(£12,765)		
Opening balance	*£3,567*	*£9,337*	*£1,912*	*£9,994*
Inflows	£42,000	£43,560	£45,050	£42,400
Outflows	(£36,230)	(£50,985)	(£37,018)	(£37,964)
Closing balance	***£9,337***	***£1,912***	***£9,994***	***£14,380***

Figure 14.5 Extract from a cashflow forecast.

monthly payments, but some are not. You may wish to alter the payment cycle of some expenses to even out the cashflow, or make provision for investing any excess cash available. By looking at the overall ups and downs over the year, any cash rich or poor months can be identified. This will act as a reminder not to get carried away spending all the bank balance in the good months.

It is also useful to examine an average month's cashflow in detail to get an idea of the daily ups and downs. By changing the due date of your account clients to a few days before the practice has to pay major suppliers, sudden dips in funds may be avoided.

There is no point having a cash flow forecast if you don't check up on how you are doing relative to it. You cannot do this effectively by simply checking monthly bank statements. If you are flush with cash, then you may be missing out on possible interest income for several weeks, and if you are not doing as well as forecast then you may be at risk from unplanned bank charges. At the very least keep a running total of cheques written and banking deposits (not forgetting automated payments and deposits). This will normally err on the side of caution, and cheques will take a certain amount of time to post and clear. To push your account to the real limits of your overdraft, use some form of computer banking. You can see the balance daily, and transfer funds between accounts as necessary. Don't forget that if you gamble to this extent, you cannot afford to be 'too busy' to check up on things.

As with any forecast, you need to identify reasons why reality does not match up. Cash shortfalls will have a knock-on effect throughout the year, and future plans may have to be amended. Don't get carried away if you turn out better than forecast – make sure it isn't simply a matter of timing, a peak followed by a trough, before you go out and spend it all.

Sole traders and partners may have to balance the cash needs of the business with their personal needs. The practice accountant should be able to advise on the most tax-efficient way of apportioning any borrowing. This is a situation in which the owners need to be honest with the manager about what is happening, otherwise conflicts can develop.

BUDGETING FOR CAPITAL EXPENSES – CAN WE AFFORD TO BUY?

The normal objective of capital investment is to produce a return – profit, which you would not have had if the investment had not been made. Sometimes investments are made to meet certain requirements, for instance achieving a hospital standard. This can also be said to produce a return by means of the enhanced status of the practice.

Occasionally investments must be made for legal reasons, such as complying with health and safety orders, or adapting access for disabled people. Finally, new equipment may be bought because the vet 'wants a new toy'! The sums should at least be worked out and the reasons admitted, rather than pretending it's a worthwhile investment.

Several factors are involved in budgeting for capital expenses. Whether it is a new piece of equipment, or opening a branch surgery, you need to know:

- How much will it cost to buy?
- What are the running costs?
- Are there any training costs?
- Are there on-going costs such as maintenance agreements, or extra insurance?
- What is the lifespan of the item?
- How much money will it bring in?
- How much do you think you will use it?
- What will it save? Time, staff costs, materials?
- Will it affect any other services?
- What else could you have done with the money instead?

There are a number of calculations that can be used to assess the viability of capital investment.

The examples that follow are based on a piece of equipment costing £10,000. The annual running costs are £500, and it is expected to have a useful life of 5 years. At the end of that period it will have an expected value of £750. Each use of the machine costs 50 p, and is charged out at £30. The estimated usage is 80 procedures in the first year, rising to 100 in the second year, and 120 a year for the remainder of its life.

Payback period

This calculates the length of time needed for the capital project to generate enough income to pay for itself.

If the cash inflows are likely to be constant for the life of the equipment, then the payback period can be worked out very easily by dividing the initial cost of the equipment by the annual income. In this case, if the equipment was going to be used 120 times per year for the whole of its life, then the payback period would be:

$$\frac{\pounds 10{,}000}{(120 \times (\pounds 30.00 - 0.50)) - \pounds 500} = 3.3 \text{ years}$$

However, life is not normally that straightforward, and the net cash flows will usually vary from year to year. This may be due to changes in usage, and therefore income, or increased maintenance costs as the equipment ages. To allow for this, the net cashflow for each year must be calculated, and the cumulative total used to find the point at which the overall project value changes from negative to positive. This is illustrated in Figure 14.6. This shows that the machine will have paid for itself after just under 4 years. Any income generated thereafter will be net cashflow into the business.

Calculating a payback period is only a very simple way of initially screening a capital project. It takes no account of the overall cash-generating potential of the capital item, nor does it make allowances for the fact that inflation and interest rates will alter the value of future incomes and expenses. However, on a basic level, any equipment that does not pay back its cost during its expected lifespan should certainly be rejected.

Return on investment (ROI)

This method may also be referred to as the Accounting Rate of Return (ARR) or Return on Capital Employed (ROCE).

There are a number of similar ways of calculating this return. One of the commonest ones is to take the average annual profit from the use of the item, and express it as a percentage of the average capital invested.

The average annual profit can be calculated by applying a depreciation amount to the cashflow projections already calculated. The total net cash flow over 5 years, as shown in Figure 14.6, is: £1,860 + £2,450 + £3,040 + £3,040 + £3,040 = £13,230. This forms the basis for the calculation of ROI, detailed in Figure 14.7.

Note that the depreciation is calculated by dividing the loss in value of the asset by its life span. The average capital figure is the average of the initial and final values of the asset. The return on investment can then be

	Cash outflows	Cash inflow	Net cash flow	Cumulative cash flow
Year 0	£10,000		(£10,000)	(£10,000)
Year 1	£500 + (80 × 50 p)	80 × £30	£1,860	(£8,140)
Year 2	£500 + (100 × 50 p)	100 × £30	£2,450	(£5,690)
Year 3	£500 + (120 × 50 p)	120 × £30	£3,040	(£2,650)
Year 4	£500 + (120 × 50 p)	120 × £30	£3,040	£390
Year 5	£500 + (120 × 50 p)	120 × £30	£3,040	£3,230

Figure 14.6 Payback period.

Average annual income:	$\frac{£13,230}{5}$	=	£2,646
Annual depreciation:	$\frac{£10,000 - £750}{5}$	=	£1,850
Annual average profit	£2,646 − £1,850	=	£796
Average capital employed:	$\frac{£10,000 + £750}{2}$	=	£5,375
Return on investment	$\frac{£796}{£5,375} \times 100$	=	**14.3%**

Figure 14.7 Return on investment.

	Net cash flow	Present value factor at 15%	NPV
Year 0	(£10,000)	1	(£10,000)
Year 1	£1,860	0.870	£1,618
Year 2	£2,450	0.756	£1,852
Year 3	£3,040	0.658	£2,000
Year 4	£3,040	0.573	£1,742
Year 5	£3,040 + 750	0.497	£1,884
Overall NPV			**(£904)**

Figure 14.8 Net present value.

compared with the acceptable return that the business would expect to make.

Like the payback period calculation, this is a very simplistic approach, which takes no account of the change in value of money over time. In order to make allowances for the devaluation of money over time, more complex methods of capital appraisal can be used.

Net present value (NPV)

The simple payback period calculation shown in Figure 14.6 treats the £3,040 received in year 5 as the equivalent value to the same amount received in year 3. The net present value method makes use of the concept of discounting. That is, the fact that £100 income received in 12 months' time is worth less to the practice than £100 now.

If, for instance, the practice could achieve a return of 6% by investing its money in a safe place such as a building society, it would wish to have a greater return on new equipment, which is a more risky investment.

Assuming the minimum return the practice would accept is 15%, then the cashflow figures calculated earlier can be adjusted as shown in Figure 14.8. The present value factors shown in the figure can be calculated, but it is more usual simply to look them up in a present value table.

The initial net cashflow multiplied by the present value factor gives the net present value of that money – in other words, if you had £2,000 now and invested it for 3 years at 15% it would be worth £3,040.

The overall NPV of this equipment purchase has turned out to be negative, minus £904. This means that it will not give the practice the required return of 15%.

The NPV calculation can be used to compare a number of different options for the practice – for instance, should they buy a dental scaler, a laboratory analyser or an automatic processor? By analysing the projected cashflow for each, and adjusting them using the NPV, it is possible to see which ones are viable, and which will give the best return. The higher the figure at the end of the NPV calculation, the better the investment is.

The percentage used for the present value factor will depend on current interest rates, the cost of any finance involved, and the overall target profitability of the practice. Even this method does not encompass all the factors that may impact on assessing capital investment. We have based all income and costs on today's prices, and discounted them to take account of devaluation. But in practice, the future costs and fees would have increased by inflation as well. The tax situation of the business will also affect decisions on capital spending, and it is wise to consult your accountant or other financial advisor to ask for help with more complex projections.

With any capital appraisal method, it is vital that the starting data are as accurate as possible. When calculating projected incomes as a result of investment, make sure you take account of services already on offer. In the case of buying a new dental scaler, presumably the practice already has some income from manual dental procedures, and what you need to assess is how that will increase as a result of the purchase. In other cases, buying a new item of equipment may decrease income elsewhere, for example acquiring an ultrasound machine may reduce the income from radiography.

Financing the expenditure

Major investment in practice premises is likely to be financed by a long-term bank loan. The interest rate payable on this loan will need to be taken into account when assessing the return on investment.

Items of equipment may be bought outright, or financed by a hire or lease purchase arrangement. These options have different effects on the cashflow, balance sheet, tax and VAT situation of the practice.

Outright purchase

If the practice has spare cash, this may initially seem a tempting option, as there will be no interest element to pay. But the cash still has to come from somewhere, and make sure it couldn't be doing something more useful before spending reserves.

Hire purchase

The equipment will show as a fixed asset in the balance sheet, and the amount owed to the finance company will show as a long-term liability. The interest element of each payment is shown on the profit and loss account as an expense. The full VAT amount can be reclaimed at the time of purchase. The value of the asset will be reduced by depreciation annually, and this will reflect in the profit and loss account. At the end of the hire purchase agreement, full title passes to the practice.

Leasing

The equipment remains the property of the finance company, and does not show on the practice balance sheet. The practice pays an agreed monthly sum, including VAT, to the finance company. The VAT on each payment is recoverable, and the payments show as a leasing expense on the profit and loss account. At the end of the lease term, there is usually a 'peppercorn' rental payable for continued use of the equipment.

The final decision will be influenced by a number of factors, such as the debt level of the practice, relative finance costs, whether the practice ultimately wants to own the asset, and the residual value of the asset at the end of the finance period. In all cases, shop around for the lowest finance charges, and consult your accountant or financial advisor for more detailed advice on the most appropriate source of finance for the particular investment in question.

If you are planning capital purchases, don't forget to adjust your profit and loss budget and cashflow forecast accordingly.

CHAPTER CONTENTS

Where are you now? 162
How much stock do you carry? 162
How much stock do you use? 162
How much do you lose? 163
How much is it costing you? 163

Where do you want to be? 163
Quantity – to have sufficient stock levels to meet the normal needs of the practice 163
Price – at the least cost to the practice 163

How are you going to get there? 164
Rationalize the range of stock you carry 164
Do not exceed maximum stock levels 165
Review the timing and quantities of your orders 165
Cut stock losses 167
Optimize discounts 167
Communicate! 169

Legislation and stock control 170

15

Stock management

The drug bill is the largest monthly expenditure for most practices. If you can make savings of a few percent here, you can make a significant difference to overall practice profits. Unfortunately, stock is often taken for granted, and its management may be very haphazard. Large animal vets sometimes hoard hundreds of pounds' worth of unnecessary drugs in the boots of their cars. The ordering of stock (at several thousand pounds an order) is frequently left to someone who is otherwise not allowed to buy an extra pint of milk on the practice's behalf without prior authorization.

There is no single best stock management system for all practices. The ideal system for you will depend on several factors, including the type of products sold, space available and volume of sales. A small practice with an all-seeing head nurse may well have very efficient stock control based on gut reaction and knowing what arrived because she unpacked it and what has been sold as she sold it (until she goes on holiday!). A larger practice may only cope by using a sophisticated computer inventory system.

An effective inventory control system should apply to all products bought and used by the practice, not only drugs, but also laboratory supplies, orthopaedic hardware, cleaning materials and computer consumables. Your stock management plan may include drawing up buying strategies over a portfolio of drugs to maximize manufacturer and wholesaler discounts.

This chapter will explore the basic principles of stock management, and give you some pointers to help you review and improve your systems.

As with any aspect of practice management, you need to start with your plan:

- What is your current stock situation?
- What would you like it to be?
- How are you going to get there?

The analysis of the whole of your practice's stock usage can be a major task. Most managers cannot take the time away from normal duties to 'do' stock, and nor would they want to as it would be totally mind-numbing to tackle it in this fashion. The 80/20 rule (Pareto's rule) can be used to help target the most important stock items. The theory behind this rule is that 80% of your results (in this case, stock cost) come from only 20% of your range (products). This information should be available from your practice management system, or your wholesaler. It is that top 20% of your product range that you should spend time analysing initially.

WHERE ARE YOU NOW?

Your stock analysis should look initially at your most important stock items, and should cover:

- How much stock do you carry?
- How much stock do you use?
- How much stock do you lose?
- What is it costing you?

How much stock do you carry?

An accurate assessment of the volume and value of stock in the practice is needed both for the closing stock figure in the annual accounts, and also as a starting point for good stock management. Stock levels may be calculated by manual or computerized methods, and the importance of an audit of stock should not be overlooked.

- ***Manual stocktake.*** Mention the word 'stocktake', and staff will suddenly become very busy doing something else! Physically counting the quantity of stock items must be one of the most tedious jobs in veterinary practice. It is very expensive to do in terms of staff time, and difficult to carry out during the normal working day. As a result, a full manual stocktake is generally only carried out at the end of the practice financial year. This can give a deceptively low figure, as even practices with very lax stock control will tend to cut down on stock ordering just before the year-end.

- ***Computerized stock control.*** If the practice uses a computer system to charge out stock items onto clients' records, then it is a small step to make use of this information for stocktake purposes. If the computer is told how much stock the practice has at the start of a period, it can keep track of how much has been purchased and sold, and can come up with a stock in hand figure whenever it is asked.

- ***Stock audit.*** Most manual stocktake systems in veterinary practice do not involve a stock audit – in other words no checks are made that the final stock figure reconciles with last year's figures plus purchases less sales. Legally this reconciliation is a requirement for some classes of medicines – see Chapter 20, 'Pharmacy and dispensing'.

If you are using a computerized system, then the figures should be periodically checked against physical stock levels. This can be done on a rota basis throughout the year, for instance one shelf a week, and is much less disruptive than a full stocktake. This type of on-going audit will quickly highlight any discrepancies and allow them to be investigated quickly. They may be due to simple mistakes such as errors in pack size on the computer, or signs of more serious theft problems. Valuable or easily pilferable stock may be checked more frequently than standard items.

How much stock do you use?

This should be based on known sales, not purchases. Ideally you should be able to retrieve monthly sales figures from your practice management system. Even if you are not fully computerized, an 'intelligent till' system may be able to give you the information. If you have no means of determining sales, then use the purchase figures from your wholesaler as a rough guide.

Sales figures should be both an annual total and broken down by month. This will allow you to see which products are seasonal in their use.

How much do you lose?

Stock losses arise from three main areas:

- out-of-date stock
- theft
- damage.

One of the objectives of your stock control system will be to reduce these losses, but firstly they must be identified and recorded. Stock losses are a difficult figure to determine, unless you have systems set up to detect and record them. On a purely manual system it may simply be a reflection of the number of out-of-date products unearthed at the annual stocktake, or the amount of food donated to animal charities due to damaged packaging.

One way of tracking stock losses using a computerized system is to have a dummy client called 'stock'. All stock losses discovered can be charged to that client – destocking from the stock control system, and logging date and amount of loss at the same time. If the client is set up to be sold goods at cost value (possible with some systems), then it is also an accurate record of the value of stock lost in the year, and can be taken account of at the year-end.

How much is it costing you?

At this stage we are not so much concerned with calculating the true costs of individual stock items, but are looking at the overall picture.

Bookkeeping records should be able to produce figures for your monthly and annual drug bill. Make sure any retrospective drug discounts are shown as decreasing the cost of purchases, not being added into income.

A more detailed breakdown of purchases by drug category may be available from your wholesaler.

WHERE DO YOU WANT TO BE?

There are two main objectives of good stock management – to have sufficient stock levels to meet the normal needs of the practice, at the least cost to the practice.

Although quantity and price are the two measurable outcomes and objectives of stock control, they need a third aspect – management – to achieve success. Simply ordering more stock at a time will not stop you running out of stock, and picking the cheapest antibiotics will not save you money, unless there is a strong 'juggling' force managing the stock.

Quantity – to have sufficient stock levels to meet the normal needs of the practice

Please note the word *normal* – you will never be able economically to carry stock levels to cope with every eventuality. Some incidences of being out of stock will always happen – the art lies in making sure they have minimum impact on the practice.

If stock levels are too low, you will run out of products unacceptably frequently. At the very least, this will be irritating to staff and clients, and you may lose the occasional sale. At worst, patient care may suffer. Frequently running out of essential supplies is very frustrating and stressful for vets, support staff and clients.

Excessively high stock levels are less obvious on a day-to-day basis. The first sign may be finding increasing levels of out-of-date stock – either because more was bought than could be used within the shelf life, or the product has been superseded. Overstocking substantially increases the cost for the practice, both from storage costs and money tied up in stock.

Price – at the least cost to the practice

Unfortunately, this cannot be achieved by simply picking the cheapest equivalent product from the wholesaler's price list. The cost to the practice of holding stock is made up of both what you pay for it and how much it costs you to get and keep it there. Total stock cost depends on:

- list price of the product
- wholesaler discounts
- manufacturer discounts
- credit terms
- cost of money tied up in stock
- cost of storage space – shelving, heating, refrigeration
- cost of wasted stock – past sell-by date, damage, theft
- cost of ordering/processing orders – staff time and communications costs
- delivery charges
- cost of running out of stock – lost sales/clients.

Good stock management will balance out these factors to find the minimum overall cost to the practice. Ordering more frequently will reduce the cost of keeping the product in stock, but increases ordering costs. Ordering a large batch at once will increase the cost of holding that stock, but may attract extra discounts and also reduce the cost of ordering and of running out of stock. The exact balance point will vary between practices depending on the predictability of their customer base, size of premises, and business terms of their suppliers.

There are some hideously complicated equations used in industry to determine these optimum ordering quantities. In veterinary practice, a good understanding of the issues involved, coupled with common sense, will be quite sufficient.

The 'cost of goods sold' figure in the practice accounts normally only includes the actual stock cost, less any discounts. The other costs of ordering and holding stock are absorbed into staff wages, bank interest charges and buildings overheads, and are much less easily assessed and compared.

HOW ARE YOU GOING TO GET THERE?

There are a few basic strategies for good stock management, which will reduce both the cost of stock and the risk of running out:

- Rationalize the range of stock you carry.
- Do not exceed maximum stock levels.
- Review the timing and quantities of your orders.
- Cut stock losses.
- Optimize discounts.
- Communicate!

Rationalize the range of stock you carry

Before you can work out how much of each product to stock, it makes sense to decide whether you need to stock it at all. Unless the stock and practice are run by a dictatorial senior partner, it is likely that the range of products on the shelves has arrived by evolution rather than rational decision. Refining your product range will reduce costs in several ways:

- Less storage space will be needed.
- Less stock management time will be needed to manage a smaller product range.
- The products you do use will turn over more rapidly, so less risk of short-dated items.
- You are more likely to benefit from manufacturer discount schemes.

This rationalization should apply to the whole range of products, from injectable antibiotics to dressings and cleaning materials. There are three broad ways to whittle down the product range:

- Remove any direct equivalents – different brands of the same formulation.
- Is every pack size necessary? This is particularly relevant with dressings and other consumables.
- Are there a number of different products which do the same thing? Do you need them all? Particular culprits seem to be ear drops and antibiotic tablets.

Many of the decisions can only be made by a veterinary surgeon. Restricting the range of products stocked may affect vets' clinical freedom, and the situation should be discussed at a clinical meeting. Other products such as dressings and disposables may be assessed by nursing staff.

In some cases the final choices will be decided directly by the vets, if there is an outright product of choice. Alternatively, they may provide the practice manager with a shortlist of equally acceptable equivalents, leaving the final choice to be guided by other factors such as price.

Sometimes a wide range of similar products will have to remain, especially in pet healthcare sales. Even if the practice believes there is one 'best' flea treatment, the client will still want the choice of powder, collar, spray, spot-on or in-feed medication.

Make sure that lines to be discontinued are flagged as such, so that they are not inadvertently reordered when they get low. Reception staff should be made aware of any major drug policy changes before they happen, so they can counter 'But he's always had the little blue ones before'. Once a product has disappeared from the shelves, make sure it disappears from the computer too – old habits die hard, and unless physically prevented, many vets will continue to 'mentally' dispense their old favourites many years after they have been discontinued.

Aim to prevent the situation recurring by persuading vets to be sensible with reps' offers! If they do want to try a new product, ask them to be clear what it is going to replace, so that the old drugs are not re-ordered as well as the new.

Do not exceed maximum stock levels

Most practices are on monthly account terms with their suppliers. As a general rule, stock levels should not exceed one month's use of product. Anything above this level is effectively money sitting on the shelf, when it could be doing something much more useful elsewhere. Unnecessary stock worth £2,000 could be £2,000 less of a practice overdraft, or £2,000 more in a business savings account.

This rule will be broken in a few situations:

- *Very infrequently used products:* where less than 12 courses of tablets/doses are used per year, the amount you need to keep in stock will be more than an 'average' month's use.
- *Products with very large pack sizes:* some tablets are only packaged in 500s. If your monthly use is less than this you have no option but to be overstocked some of the time.
- *Special offers and beating a price rise:* some special offers make it worth buying more than usual to gain a substantial discount. Similarly it may be worth buying larger quantities of stocks just before a manufacturer's price rise. Care should be taken assessing the value of these offers, and this is discussed in more detail later in the chapter.

The smaller the practice, the greater will be the effect of the first two situations. Your monthly sales figures can be amended to take account of changes made to product ranges, and then used as maximum stock level guidelines.

Review the timing and quantities of your orders

The 'simple' system of stock ordering involves setting a 're-order level' (how low you let the stock level get before placing an order) and a re-order quantity (how much you order at a time).

These levels are determined by factors such as:

- frequency of delivery service
- delivery charges or minimum order quantities
- space available for storage
- time interval between placing order and delivery.

Your re-order level should give you enough stock to last for the period between orders, plus the length of time it will take for that order to be delivered.

The re-order quantity should be at least enough stock to see you through to the next ordering date. If you order on a daily basis, then obviously you would not just order a day's worth of stock – the re-order quantity needs to be a reasonable amount depending on the space available to the practice. For most stock items this would be one to two weeks' worth of stock,

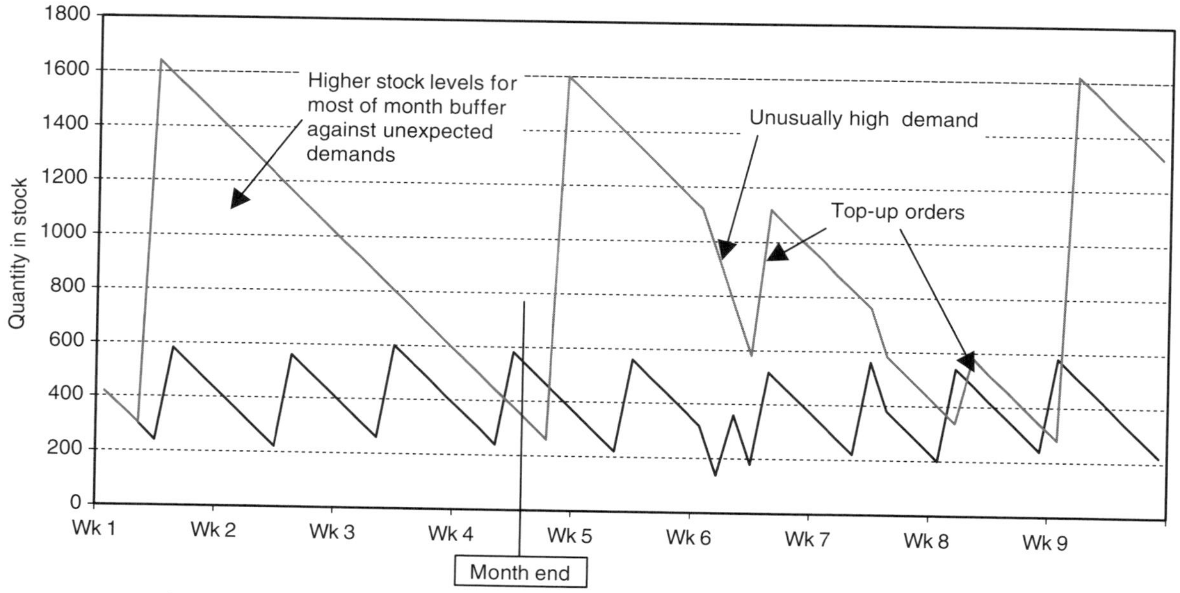

The stock used and ordered is the same in both situations
Lower line: traditional stock control
Upper line: calendar month stock control

Figure 15.1 Effect of different ordering strategies.

but this may have to be reduced in the case of very bulky items such as pet food if storage space is limited. The re-order quantity will be influenced by the pack size of the products.

This simple ordering system is used by automatic computerized stock control systems to generate orders. Each stock item is set up to have minimum stock levels, and re-order quantities. Once the stock level on the computer drops to this minimum, it triggers an order.

If this system is followed rigidly, stock levels should be maintained within acceptable limits – unless there are any unusual demands. But one thing you don't want is a massive order arriving at the end of a calendar month. An item ordered on 30th March will normally be paid for at the end of April. If the order is delayed for a couple of days, until say 2nd April, it won't need to be paid for until the end of May – effectively an extra month of credit. So some form of manual overriding of normal re-order quantities will be normal towards the end of a month.

Some product use is very predictable, and space permitting it makes far more sense to order a month's worth of stock at the start of the month, and top up as required later on. Less time is spent ordering and unpacking, and the wholesaler bill will be the same in either case, as the same amount of stock will have been ordered. Figure 15.1 illustrates some of the differences between these two ordering strategies. You can see that stock levels are generally higher for more days each month with the 'calendar month' method of stock control. This means that the practice is less susceptible to extraordinary demands during this time. If sales are higher than expected, then a 'top-up' order can be made, of just enough stock to last until the end of the month.

This method is not currently supported by computer systems – maybe one day we will be able to set a range of re-order levels and quantities dependent on the time of the month.

Do spare a thought for the delivery driver if you do decide to order a month's supply of everything!

Cut stock losses

Rationalizing the product range and setting sensible stock levels should go a long way towards minimizing short-dated stock. One advantage of the legislation concerning batch number recording is that it has forced veterinary computer suppliers to add batch number recording facilities to their software. This generally records expiry date information as well, and enables reports to be run on stock due to expire.

When unpacking new deliveries, make sure that a system of stock rotation ensures that older products are used before the newest arrivals.

One of the most likely stock items to end up date expired are specialist pet foods, especially disease management diets. They may only be purchased by one or two clients, whose pets are quite likely to die at short notice! It might be possible to ask clients to order from the practice a couple of days before they are due to run out.

All stock should be checked for damage as it arrives from the wholesaler. Liquid preparations and pet food sacks are particularly prone to damage. Proper consideration of manual handling issues will help to minimize later damage to bags through being badly carried or thrown onto shelves.

Proper design of drug storage areas should minimize risk of damage due to bottles falling off shelves or being exposed to extremes of heat or cold.

Maintaining an audit of all stock items using a continuous computer-based inventory is the best defence against stock theft. Look for patterns of disappearance, and pay particular attention to any discrepancies in potential substances of abuse.

Optimize discounts

The manufacturers' list price of a product is often the basis for price comparisons. However, this is normally only a starting point, and determining the true cost of a product may mean battling through several discount schemes.

Wholesaler discounts

Wholesalers will normally offer a 'prompt payment' discount to practices each month. There may be several discount bands, depending on the level of purchases. If the practice uses more than one wholesaler, make sure you are not losing potential discount by splitting your buying power between them. Further discounts may also be available for practices that order electronically.

Manufacturer discounts

Manufacturers love to hide the true cost of a drug under layers of discount. Worst is the pricing of vaccines; it is quite possible to have a scheme encompassing a monthly manufacturer discount given as a wholesaler credit note, a quarterly retrospective discount cheque, free of charge goods, and an annual cash incentive, plus all the usual printing of vaccination certificates, etc. Comparing the price of vaccines can be a mammoth spreadsheet task, which will stop all but the most determined practices from comparing prices.

Company acquisitions and mergers have resulted in a handful of large pharmaceutical companies, each having a very comprehensive product range. The more you buy from any one company, the higher percentage discount band they will give to the practice. The most feasible way to minimize drug costs is to optimize these manufacturer discount bands.

Figure 15.2 shows a typical unplanned purchasing portfolio, with products spread between three different companies. Some of the products have equivalent preparations made by the other companies; only product 3 is unique.

Figure 15.3 is an example of what could happen if purchases are rationalized. By moving the bulk of the purchases to one company, a higher discount is obtained.

	Company A	Company B	Company C	Total
Product 1	£100	Equivalent		
Product 2	£100		Equivalent	
Product 3		£100		
Product 4	Equivalent	£100		
Product 5	Equivalent		£100	
Product 6	Equivalent		£100	
Subtotal	***£200***	***£200***	***£200***	***£600***
Discount	4%=£8	4%=£8	4%=£8	£24
Total cost				**£576**
All companies have the same discount bands – £100=0%, £200=4%, £300=5%, £400=8%, £500=10%				

Figure 15.2 Unplanned purchasing from three different manufacturers.

	Company A	Company B	Company C	Total
Product 1	£100	Equivalent		
Product 2	£100		Equivalent	
Product 3		£100		
Product 4	£100	Equivalent		
Product 5	£100		Equivalent	
Product 6	£100		Equivalent	
Subtotal	***£500***	***£100***	***£zero***	***£600***
Discount	10% = £50	0%=£0	0% = £0	£50
Total cost				**£550**
All companies have the same discount bands – £100=0%, £200=4%, £300=5%, £400=8%, £500=10%				

Figure 15.3 Planned purchasing to maximize discounts.

Of course, in real life it isn't that simple! Equivalent products are not the same list price; different companies do not have the same discount bands. But you can be very effective at reducing drug costs by heavily favouring one manufacturer. And of course, that's just what the drug companies want you to do!

One of the problems with juggling discount bands used to be that it was hard to work out what the discount was going to be until you knew how much you had spent! Nowadays most manufacturers base discount bands on moving annual turnover (MAT), that is, your last 12 months' purchases to date. Each month, the new current month is added on, and last year's equivalent month taken off. This has the advantage that an uncharacteristic poor spending month will not have a catastrophic effect on your discount banding, as it will only alter by a relatively small amount. Conversely, a change in buying strategy can take a while to increase your MAT with a company to climb into the next band – but if you discuss your plans with the company's territory manager they might be able to give you a quick 'step up'!

Special offers

Drug companies and wholesalers will normally top up their basic discount structure with a range of special offers. These are normally administered by the reps at the time of sale. They tend to take the form of either:

- Parcel discounts – a percentage off the price of a mixed selection of goods, or
- Straight discount percentage on a certain quantity of product, or
- Offers of free product if you buy enough – e.g. 2 on 10.

With all these offers it pays to work out the true maths first, as well as the implications of what the drug company is trying to achieve! How good the offer really is depends on four main factors:

- Do you have a use for the product at all?
- How long will it take you to sell that amount of product?
- What % discount is offered?
- What % interest are you having to pay (or not receiving) on the money used to pay for the goods?

Starting with the simplest case, a 10% discount offered on £500 worth of a product that you already use: if you can sell all of it within the first month, then you have not spent any more money than normal, and you will gain from the full benefit of the discount, £50.

If you only sell £100 worth of the stuff in a month, it will take you 5 months to sell it all. Had you not bought the extra stock, that money could have been earning interest elsewhere. At a monthly interest rate of 1%, the interest earned would have been £10. The real value of the discount has therefore fallen to £40.

The higher the interest rate, and longer the period taken to sell the stock, the less the true discount becomes. In extreme situations it can become a loss.

Buying several months' worth of stock is also risky for other reasons. It may go out of date before it can be sold, or may be superseded by a more modern product. Don't forget, the drug companies have a reason for offering these discounts – and they need to shift seasonal or obsolete stock just as much as any other business!

Making sure you understand the true discount offered is also important. A 'two on ten' deal may initially seem like 20% off. But in fact what it means is that, out of twelve products, two are free. The true discount is 2/12, actually only 16.6%.

Other perks

Of course, financial and product discounts are not all that is on offer from your suppliers. Most drug companies support their products with a selection of free promotional literature and display stands. Others offer a bonus or a 'points' system to help the practice buy clinical equipment. Staff education can be a very valuable resource provided by some product manufacturers.

Not everything comes down to scraping the last few percent discount out of a deal. Developing a good on-going relationship with your suppliers, with the knowledge that they will be there to support the practice willingly if there is a problem with a product or supply, can be worth far more.

Communicate!

Good communications between all practice staff are essential for the smooth running of stock management. Clinical staff need to accept the importance of keeping a streamlined product range. It is important that the ordering staff understand the reasoning behind the timing of stock orders. Simply telling staff *'We don't use that product here'*, or *'Don't order anything this week'* will only stir up resentment.

Encourage veterinary staff to take some responsibility by informing ordering staff if they have just used the last packet of X, or if they have just seen a new clinical case which is going to double the normal use of a particular drug.

Vets' cars can be the complete anathema of a stock control system! Communication and pleading with some large animal vets is still needed if they have the habit of clearing the practice shelves into their car boot, only to return the stuff weeks later, when replacements have been re-ordered. Close examination of these car boots (if you were brave enough) might reveal a jumble of bottles, some out of date, lightly covered with various bodily samples, and certainly not stored at the correct temperature. Drug storage legislation and demands by vets' families have gone a long way to literally 'clean up' this problem, and hopefully this worst-case scenario is now in the minority.

Some of your stock control strategies may directly affect the clients. If you introduce a requirement to pre-order repeat prescriptions, be sure to explain the benefits to the client – for example, *'By phoning up first you won't have to wait while the tablets are counted, and we can make sure we have everything you need.'* Similarly, for low turnover animal health products, you may ask farmers to phone in an order the day before they want it: *'If we only get the product in to order, we can keep prices lower for you.'*

LEGISLATION AND STOCK CONTROL

While you are evaluating and planning your stock management, you should also bear in mind the legislation which affects your choice of products, stock control system and how you might store them. These include:

- pharmacy regulations – will affect how medicines are stored and displayed.
- manual handling – will have an effect on the handling of heavy stock items.
- COSHH – may have an impact on the choice of products used.

See Chapters 19, 'Health and safety' and 20, 'Pharmacy and dispensing', for details.

The potential anti-competitive effect of manufacturers' discount schemes is one of the issues of concern to the Competition Commission in their investigation into the supply of POM veterinary medicines. Their report is due to be completed in January 2003 and may lead to changes to the pricing strategy of veterinary suppliers.

CHAPTER CONTENTS

Shopped and non-shopped items 172
Value for money 172

Pricing of products 172
What is the cost price? 172
How much should you mark-up? 173
Margins – what profit are we making? 174
Changes in cost price 174

Dispensing and injection fees 175

Fee setting 176
The fee culture of the practice 176
Fixed-price, time-based or menu pricing? 176
Strategies for fee calculation 177
Managing fee increases 179
Monitoring fees 179

Effects of changing selling price 180

Discounts 181
Know why you are discounting 181
Know what it is costing you 181
Make sure the customer knows what they should have paid 182
Have a practice policy on discounting 182

Surcharges 182
Why are you using them? 182
What will surcharges achieve? 182

Problems arising from prices 183

16

Pricing of fees and products

Fee levels, product prices, and the relationship between fee and drug income can be contentious issues for a practice. On one hand, there is the 'professional clinician' view that a veterinary surgeon should generate his income solely (or mainly) from the application of, and charging for, his professional opinion. On the other hand, the 'holistic' view demands that veterinary surgeons are the best people to advise on the whole care of the animals, and we should be in a position to provide, and make a profit out of providing, any products and services that may be needed.

Most practices, in reality, fall some way between the two extremes. Neither view is right or wrong. The important thing is to be aware of the current balance in your practice and how this fits in with the future plans of the business.

Fee surveys have been conducted over recent years by a number of national and regional veterinary associations, and have been a useful, if limited, source of information for practices trying to rationalize their pricing strategy. However, any idea of a 'national fee scale' is contrary to the Office of Fair Trading's competition laws, so nowadays such surveys have to be very careful not be seen to be a fee recommendation or pricing cartel.

It is important to have a rational basis for pricing of your fees and products, on one hand not to undersell your goods and services, and on the other not to be accused of 'ripping off' clients. The overall pricing strategy of a practice will be affected by factors such as:

- type of practice – first opinion or referral? Mixed practice or specialist?
- position of the practice in the marketplace – budget or exclusive?
- geographical location – effect of overhead and staff costs, local competition, local level of affluence.
- profit level required by the owners.

There are a number of differences between fees and products, which not only affect their marketing (as discussed in Chapter 12, 'Sales and marketing'), but also give rise to different pricing strategies. However, there are some basic principles that affect the pricing of all items.

Shopped and non-shopped items

Customers are more likely to compare the cost of some items than others. These are known as 'shopped items', since the consumer will often shop around to get the best deal. Just as supermarkets take great care to ensure they are competitively priced on shopped items, it is important to be aware of which veterinary services and products are regarded as shopped.

In general, shopped fees in small animal practice are those charged for routine services such as vaccinations, consultations and neutering. For large animal practices, visit fees, equine vaccinations and routine herd health services such as pregnancy diagnosis or de-horning will be shopped.

Non-shopped fees tend to be one-off procedures, such as major surgery.

On the product side, small animal clients will be very aware of the cost of pet foods, but less so of other items such as toys, collars and most drugs. Farm and equine clients will tend to shop around for products that are also available at saddlers or merchants.

Clients may ring round a number of surgeries comparing prices, especially if they are new to the area and they may not have a particular vet. But do be aware, many clients who phone for a price may be simply confirming what to expect before they come down, and are not necessarily looking for the cheapest treatment.

Value for money

Perceived value for money has more of an influence on clients' decision-making than absolute price. A fee for a service provided by a practice with clean facilities and courteous staff will seem much better value than the same fee charged by a scruffy practice with poor client care. It is very important that the practice makes the client aware of what they will get for their money by properly marketing the practice and the services it provides.

Price surveys can only compare absolute fees and drug prices, with little or no reference to quality of service and value for money.

PRICING OF PRODUCTS

The pricing of products is normally much easier than services, for several reasons.

- Products are more directly comparable, either between vets or with other outlets such as saddlers, pet shops or agricultural merchants.
- Products are often given a recommended retail price (RRP) by their manufacturer.
- It is relatively easy to determine the cost of a product.

Most products are priced by adding a percentage mark-up onto the cost price, as Figure 16.1 illustrates.

What is the cost price?

Life would be easy if the cost of a product was simply the manufacturer's or wholesaler's list price. But this list price is often reduced by a

Cost price		£5.00
Mark-up of 50%	$\frac{£5.00 \times 50}{100} =$	£2.50
Selling price		£7.50

Figure 16.1 Using a percentage mark-up to determine selling price.

variety of discount schemes, and increased by the costs involved with holding stock (ordering, storage, wastage, etc.). This is discussed in more detail in Chapter 15, 'Stock management'.

However, when it comes down to it, most product mark-ups are simply applied to the list cost price. This is mainly due to the sheer complexity of many suppliers' discount schemes. At the time of writing, few, if any, computerized stock control systems can take account of these discount structures to work out a true cost price.

It is vital to know whether pricing is based on the list cost or net cost when comparing mark-up percentage figures from practice surveys or industry recommendations. Figure 16.2 shows that while the practice may think they add a 100% mark-up on list price, the true figure could be considerably higher once wholesale and manufacturer discounts are taken into account.

How much should you mark-up?

Some products, especially small animal pet food and pet healthcare products, come with a recommended retail price, or suggested mark-up (over list price). The selling price may even be marked on the packaging.

Other products may be readily comparable with other sources, such as pet shops, feed merchants, even the internet. There is no point getting into a price war with other local retailers. It is most likely that they could drop their prices even lower than you can, and that won't help either side. All you need to reach is the same price, and you can even be more expensive if there is good reason – like better parking, or a delivery service. However, take care if you are more expensive on easily comparable products, as your clients may well assume that all of your products and services are expensive!

But it is the rest of the products that can cause a pricing headache. Prices of prescription products are not so readily compared, and it is not easy to know what other vets are charging. Generally prescription medicines attract the highest mark-ups, with GSL/healthcare products much lower. Surveys by SPVS suggest that POM mark-ups are in the range 50%–100%; however, as mentioned earlier, care should be exercised when comparing these percentages unless the cost price used is clearly defined. Many large animal PML products have very low mark-ups to remain competitive with farmers' merchants.

In the human field, recent legislative changes promoted by the Office of Fair Trading have made it illegal for manufacturers to specify minimum resale prices on over-the-counter drugs, such as painkillers and cold remedies. Pharmacies and supermarkets can now set their own resale prices, introducing competition between them. When the legislation came into force in May 2001 there was an overnight halving of some prices in supermarkets. Although possibly good news for the general public, this is a significant threat to local independent pharmacies.

Practice mark-up of 100% on list price		**The true mark-up**	
List cost price	£5.00	List cost price	£5.00
Mark-up of 100%		W'sale discount 10%	–50p
i.e. $\frac{£5.00 \times 100}{100}$	= £5.00	Manufacturer discount 5%	–25p
		True net cost	£4.25
Selling price	£10.00	Selling price remains at	£10.00
		True profit	£5.75
		True mark-up %	
		is $\frac{5.75 \times 100}{4.25}$	= **135%**

Figure 16.2 The effect of supplier discounts on mark-up percentages.

Perhaps as a result of their 'success' in this instance, the OFT launched an investigation into the pricing of POM veterinary medicines in October 2001. This investigation is separate from the government's review of dispensing. It has primarily been brought about because of differences between prices in the UK and other European countries, but the OFT is also concerned with lack of transparency in prices, and the impact of 'veterinary pharmacies'.

The issue of mark-ups has also become more emotive now that cost price of products is increasing dramatically as more sophisticated veterinary drugs are developed. The 'cascade' regulations also increase cost prices by forcing the switch from relatively cheap generic human drugs, for instance phenobarbitone, digoxin and lasix, to licensed veterinary treatments. A mark-up of over 100% was not going to upset anyone when the tablets only cost fractions of a penny each, but now a lower percentage may need to be applied for high value, high turnover items.

The OFT investigation, along with the Marsh report into dispensing, means that it is important to justify and account for the mark-ups on veterinary products of all types.

But don't forget, buying at one price and selling at another is a standard business activity. You need to make a gross profit on product sales, to contribute towards dispensary staff costs, general overheads, and to generate a profit for the owner at the end of the day.

Margins – what profit are we making?

Many people become confused between mark-ups and margins.

- A *mark-up* is the percentage of the cost price that is being added to produce the selling price – i.e. it is the profit element as a % of cost.
- The *margin* is the profit element expressed as a % of the selling price.

The two calculations are illustrated in Figure 16.3. It is very important when comparing percentage figures for profits on the sale of products that you are aware of whether the figures quoted are margins or mark-ups. Margins are incredibly sensitive to changes in cost or selling price, and it is vital to bear the margin figure in mind when deciding to lower or discount product prices. The maths is covered in more detail later in the chapter.

Changes in cost price

It is essential that there is some system in place for easily recalculating the selling price after cost price increases. In many cases this will be done automatically by the stock ordering software. Other systems may require the use of a monthly price update disk, or manual entry of prices from price lists or invoices. Undetected cost price rises will obviously decrease the profit made by the practice.

What is not always so carefully considered is what to do in the event of a cost price decrease. The list price of products is not normally lowered, but practices may frequently be able to negotiate better discount terms. Those practices who determine their 'mark-ups' over list price are unlikely to suffer, but those who do base their selling price on their true cost, or change to

Percentage mark-up		**Percentage margin**	
Product cost price	£2.00	Product cost price	£2.00
Profit on sale	£1.00	Profit on sale	£1.00
Selling price is £2.00 + £1.00	= £3.00	Selling price is £2.00 + £1.00	= £3.00
Mark-up is £1.00 as a % of £2.00,		Margin is £1.00 as a % of £3.00,	
i.e. $\frac{£1.00}{£2.00} \times 100$	= **50%**	i.e. $\frac{£1.00}{£3.00} \times 100$	= **33.3%**

Figure 16.3 The difference between mark-ups and margins.

Initial calculations		Effect of decreasing cost by 10% while keeping the same % mark-up	
Cost price	£5.00	Cost price £5.00 – 10%	= £4.50
Mark-up 50%	£2.50	Mark-up of 50%	£2.25
Sell price £5.00 + £2.50	= £7.50	Sell price £4.50 + £2.25 **(10% reduction to client)**	= £6.75
Profit on sale of 100 items is: 100 × £2.50	= £250.00	Profit on sale of 100 items is: 100 × £2.25 **(10% reduction in practice profit)**	= £225.00

Figure 16.4 The effect of changing cost price on profitability.

Keep same £ mark-up		Keep same selling price	
Cost price £5.00 – 10%	= £4.50	Cost price £5.00 – 10%	= £4.50
Original £ mark-up of	£2.50	Mark-up is now £7.50 – £4.50	= £3.00
Sell price is now £4.50 + £2.50 **(6.7% reduction to client)**	= £7.00	Original sell price **(no reduction to client)**	£7.50
Profit on sale of 100 items is: 100 × £2.50 **(no reduction in practice profit)**	= £250.00	Profit on sale of 100 items is: 100 × £3.00 **(20% increase in practice profit)**	= £300.00

Figure 16.5 Possible responses to changes in cost price.

a cheaper equivalent brand, may find unexpected effects on their profits from a decrease in cost. The practice will need to decide how much, if any, of that decrease they wish to pass on to their clients.

Figure 16.4 shows the effect of a 10% decrease in cost price. If no adjustment is made to the mark-up, the client will benefit from a 10% decrease in selling price, whilst the practice will lose 10% of its profit.

Figure 16.5 illustrates two possible options the practice could take – keeping the same value mark-up, or keeping the same selling price. Obviously a compromise between the two would benefit both the practice and the client.

Do bear in mind that this mathematical model assumes the same quantity will be sold regardless of price. If a reduction in selling price would increase the sales volume, then this will obviously affect the final profit.

If you regularly switch brands of antibiotic or other commonly-used drugs, it is sensible to make the selling price of all equivalent products the same. This is especially true in large animal practice – the farmer will rapidly query constantly changing prices.

DISPENSING AND INJECTION FEES

The dispensing review and OFT investigation into medicines pricing is highlighting the fact that many practices have been using product profits to offset lower fee prices. Psychologically it seems easier to charge for something tangible like a bottle of pills than for a professional opinion. The consultation fee is both the bread and butter of most practices, and also the fee that many practice owners feel the hardest to charge.

Many practices have tried to reconcile this by using a dispensing or injection fee. Some use dispensing fees as routine, others simply use them when issuing repeat prescriptions without seeing the animal.

These fees can be a sensible way of coming up with a product price – a fixed element to cover the costs of syringes or pill bottles and labelling, and a variable element based on the value of the drug. However, there are some drawbacks.

One danger is that these fees are used to over-inflate the price of the product, whilst keeping the consultation fee low. Another risk is that the existence of a dispensing or injection fee is used to justify both low consultation fees *and* low product prices.

If issuing of prescriptions becomes a reality, then those practices already charging dispensing fees may find it easier to move 'sideways' to charging a prescription fee, than those who do not.

FEE SETTING

Fee setting, like most other aspects of practice management, is not something that can be done once, then forgotten. It is important to review regularly the practice's ideology, its financial income needs, and individual fee levels.

Unlike products, fees are not as easily comparable between practices. A 'Consultation' could mean 5 minutes or 20, with a new graduate or a specialist, in a lock-up branch surgery or approved hospital. This variability can make it much harder to set a fee scale appropriate for your practice. It also makes it very important that price enquiries are never answered with just a figure, but that the prospective client is informed about what exactly is included for that price.

Fee setting involves:

- reviewing the fee culture of the practice
- choosing your pricing methods – fixed price, time-based or menu pricing
- calculating the fee scale
- managing your fee increases
- monitoring your fees and procedures.

The fee culture of the practice

Before individual fees can be devised, the overall fee culture of the practice needs to be established. This cannot be done by any one individual, but must be the result of honest discussion between all members of the management and clinical teams. Failure to do this at the outset will cause tension and frustration between owners, managers and clinicians at a later date.

If you have used a 'bottom up' system of budgeting, you will have an idea of the fee turnover needed. Setting a fee strategy too low in relation to the facilities you provide is not sustainable. In the short-term you might be the 'nice guy', but long-term, not only will your income suffer, but that of your staff, along with your ability to upkeep your facilities and provide a good client service.

If you elect to market yourself as a premium practice then it will be very difficult if you feel you must be affordable for all. Like all things in life, there may be some people who can't afford your fees. Make up your own mind before you are faced with it – what are you going to do in those situations? Maintain contacts with charities that will help, know the requirements of pet-aid schemes, or the location of the nearest PDSA. Be aware of the minimum treatment you need to offer. But operating a two-tier fee structure will be almost impossible.

Fixed-price, time-based or menu pricing?

Whatever method is used to determine the fee amounts, the final figure may be either a fixed-price or determined by a time-based or menu system of pricing.

As fees have increased, and practices have become more aware of the need to inform the client about the various aspects involved in procedures, a variable pricing structure has become more widespread.

At first, the fees for 'perform surgery under anaesthetic' were simply split into anaesthetic and surgical elements. Now it is common to find charges broken down into induction of anaesthesia, maintenance (time-based), surgery and itemized products used. It is possible to take menu pricing too far – although the costs of all consumables and disposables used during surgery should be taken into account, itemizing each element can seem very petty. It is more professional simply to combine them into a 'theatre pack' charge or similar.

Basing procedure prices on a variable rate depending on length and severity of procedure will generally be more profitable than a fixed-price procedure. The cost of a fixed-price procedure can often be worked out on the shortest time needed to do the job, so it will rarely be less complicated or costly than estimated.

Large animal practice often has to deal with multiple procedures at the same premises, for instance pregnancy diagnosis or dehorning. A sliding fee scale is one option for this – with the price per procedure decreasing as more are done. Time-based charging will also compensate the practice for 'messing about' by clients who are unprepared for the vet's visit. On the downside, there is the chance that the farmer is not going to have a friendly chat if they think the clock is ticking!

However, having a variable pricing method (time or menu based) has disadvantages – both when estimating the likely cost to the clients, and when charging out for the work done. It can be difficult for non-clinical staff to give the client an estimate of the cost, and items may be 'missed' off a bill, either by accident or if it is starting to look too large. A surgical record sheet is useful to make sure all fees and drugs used are recorded, and it may be possible to set up your practice management computer system to prompt you for each item in turn.

Most practices will use a mixture of both methods. Routine or shopped procedures may be fixed-price, whilst more complicated or variable surgery may be based on a combination of time and menu pricing.

Strategies for fee calculation

A lot of things in practice continue 'because they've always been done that way', but every so often you should challenge the fundamental basis of your fees:

- Do you have different rates for different species?
  - On what basis is that differential calculated?
  - Do you have a bigger cost differential between a 'cat' procedure and a 'dog' procedure than you do between the same thing done to a Yorkie or an Alsatian?
  - Small children's pets are not 'disposable items', yet do your fees charged suggest it is easier to diagnose a problem in a hamster than a dog?
- Are your visit fees mileage-based, time-based, flat-rate, or divided into zones? Why?

You don't have to change them for the sake of it, but at least be aware of what you are doing and why.

There are a number of strategies for determining fees, including:

- add X% to last year's fees
- cost plus X%
- cost centre analysis
- market driven.

Whatever method you use, one fundamental principle should always apply: review your fee scales several times a year. Even if you decide not to change them, this should be a conscious decision, not simply an omission.

Add 'X%' to last year's fees

This very simple solution is used by many practices. And in some instances it is appropriate. But just take some time to think – what did you base last year's fees on? At least some of your fees should be calculated from scratch each year.

The 'X' is often an approximation of inflation – but veterinary costs are often increasing at a much higher rate. Facilities are upgraded, staff are better trained and consumables become more expensive.

Cost plus X basis

Some 'fees' do have a specific element of product cost, such as vaccinations, microchips or in-house lab tests. The fee may be based on a combination of product mark-up and professional time.

Others are, in effect, re-selling someone else's services. Examples include external laboratory fees and private cremation fees. You may be adding a fixed 'interpretation' or 'arrangement' fee to these, or work on a percentage basis, bearing in mind the RCVS guidelines. *'All invoices should be itemised showing the amounts relating to goods and services provided by the practice, fees for outside services and any charge for additional administration or other costs to the practice in arranging such services shown separately'* (RCVS Guide 2002).

Cost centre analysis

This involves calculating the costs to the practice of carrying out the procedure. This may be specific to one fee item – for instance cryosurgery, or radiography; or may be more general – cost per minute of running the operating theatre.

Use the overhead costs of the building divided by floor area to apportion fixed costs to work areas. Then add in any specific fixed costs relating to equipment used, and divide the total fixed costs by the number of procedures carried out. Variable costs of staff time and consumables are then added to come up with a cost price per procedure. An example of costing laboratory tests is shown in Figure 16.6. The procedure cost can then be combined with desired practice profit margins to determine the fee.

Even if you don't use these calculations to come up with the final fee, at least you will be able to identify the profitability of different types of procedures, or discover which ones are making a loss!

It's worth doing the exercise for all specific areas of the practice – the consulting room, theatre, radiography, kennel areas, etc. Many practices badly undercharge on items such as hospitalization – maybe they simply view it as 'sticking the dog up the back for a couple of days'. If that is all they do, then they shouldn't charge much. But work out what it costs to feed the animal, how much nurses' time is spent in routine care, costs of changing bedding, providing heating, and the capital cost of the kennels. Then you will need to add on the special care needed by some patients.

Market driven

Cost centre analysis may help you to come up with a minimum fee price, below which you would not normally go. In reality, some services are priced above this, and some below. However you determine your fees, it is important to look at your final figure and see how it compares to the marketplace.

Shopped fees such as vaccination and neutering are much more sensitive to market forces than fees for more one-off procedures. The fee culture of the practice will determine whether you aim to keep your fees at the top, middle or lower end of the market range of prices.

Be happy with your fee scale

And that means everybody. There is no point coming up with the perfect profit-generating fee scale if deep down, the partners or clinicians don't feel comfortable with it. If staff are uneasy about fees, then those charges will be missed off,

Fixed costs of running the lab			
Annual cost of Analyser		£4,000	
Overhead costs of premises per year	£20,000		
Amount apportioned to lab (floor area)	1/40th	= £500	
Tests done per year	450		
Fixed cost per test done is therefore	£4,500/450		= £10
Costs per test			
Reagent cost per test			£12
Nurses' time per test	10 mins		£1.50
Total cost per test			**£23.50**

Figure 16.6 Cost centre analysis of in-house lab work.

amended or somehow circumvented. Even if your computer system is secure enough that this cannot happen, you may find staff being overly apologetic for the fees.

Being happy with one's fees involves two main parts – understanding the costs involved and recognizing your self-worth.

You must make sure your receptionists understand the need for the fee scale too. This will involve sharing information with them about the costs of running the practice and providing services.

Managing fee increases

It is far better to increase fees gradually over the course of a year, than in a lump on January 1st.

Firstly, the effect of the increase is seen sooner in terms of increased revenue to the practice. Figure 16.7 illustrates the maths for a procedure charged at £10 at the start of the year, and £11 at the end. If this increase is made as four quarterly increases of 25p, the income to the practice will be over 3.5% more than if it was a single increases of £1 at the year end. You can be sure that the practice's expenses increase gradually throughout the year, so why should the fees not keep pace with them?

Secondly, each individual rise is much less. This is not so much for the benefit of the client, as for the staff. The client who brings their dog in for its annual booster will still see a price rise of £1, whereas the vet will only think of four rises of 25p.

Make sure reception staff are warned of any price increases. Not only do they need to know for telephone enquiries, but also it doesn't look professional if they are as surprised as the client is by the increase.

It is a very dangerous practice to leave fees static for any length of time. Your costs will be increasing continually, and when the fees do have to be made more realistic, there will be a much bigger increase to contend with. This can be an emotive issue, especially for large and mixed practices, many of whom have been very sympathetic towards the recent crises in farming. Many practices have not increased visit and examination fees for some years. You must increase these fees to a realistic level – whether you subsequently discount them or not is another matter. A farmer is more likely to stick with a practice who has increased fees steadily, but given a special 'plague' discount, than one who has maintained the same charges but suddenly has to increase by treble inflation as soon as the crisis is over.

Monitoring fees

As mentioned at the beginning of this section, fee setting is not a 'do once and forget' exercise. You should always keep an eye on the income from, and number of, fee procedures being charged for.

Newly-introduced procedures need to be monitored to see if the uptake goes according to

	Single annual increase of 10%		**Quarterly increase**	
	Fee	Income from 600 procedures/quarter	Fee	Income from 600 procedures/quarter
Year 1 Q1	£10.00	£6,000	£10.00	£6,000
Year 1 Q2	£10.00	£6,000	£10.25	£6,150
Year 1 Q3	£10.00	£6,000	£10.50	£6,300
Year 1 Q4	£10.00	£6,000	£10.75	£6,450
Year 2 Q1	£11.00		£11.00	
Total income Year 1		**£24,000**		**£24,900**

Figure 16.7 The effect of raising fees in several stages.

plan, and major reviews in pricing should be checked on to see if there are any problems.

Numbers of related procedures should be checked on – compare numbers of blood samples taken with the number of blood lab work-ups done. Identify any differences – are clinicians unaware that there is a separate sampling fee, do they think the lab fees are too high and are amending the bill in their own way? Compare the numbers of primary and repeat consultations. Does this relate to the picture of clients coming in? Too far one way indicates clinicians may be charging out lower repeat consultations instead of primary ones; too far the other way suggests either clients are not being asked for check-ups or are not being billed for them.

Keep a check on the average price of procedures compared with the official list price. Are users managing to beat the computer and decrease fees?

Check up on discounts given. There will always be some, but look for patterns – specific vets maybe, or certain procedures. Excessive discounting is a sign that someone is unhappy with some or all of the fees they are being asked to charge.

EFFECTS OF CHANGING SELLING PRICE

The relationship between the price of an item and the demand for it is called elasticity of demand. In general, the more expensive a product or service becomes, the less it will be bought. However, this relationship is not simple.

Where a small change in price causes a larger change in demand, the relationship is said to be elastic. At the other end of the scale, an inelastic relationship means that relatively large changes in price only cause a small change in demand. In general, the most easily comparable fees, i.e. shopped fees, are the most elastic, and therefore more likely to respond to price changes than non-shopped items.

It is very important to be aware of the elasticity of different income groups when calculating the effects of price alterations on turnover. Figure 16.8 illustrates the effect of a 10% price change on the number of elastic and inelastic procedures done.

Even more important is the effect these changes in price and work volume have on profits. If the price of a procedure having a 50% profit margin is reduced by 10%, and this causes

	Inelastic fees (resistant to price change)	**Elastic fees** (sensitive to price change)
Increase price by 10%	Slightly less work (–5%)	Much less work (–15%)
Decrease price by 10%	Slightly more work (+5%)	Much more work (+15%)

Figure 16.8 The effect of price change on volume of work.

	Inelastic fees (resistant to price change)	**Elastic fees** (sensitive to price change)
Increase price by 10%	Slightly less work (–5%) At 50% margin, profits up 14% At 100% margin, profits up 9%	Much less work (–15%) At 50% margin, profits up 2% At 100% margin, profits down 2%
Decrease price by 10%	Slightly more work (+5%) At 50% margin, profits down 16% At 100% margin, profits down 11%	Much more work (+15%) At 50% margin, profits down 8% At 100% margin, profits down 2%

Figure 16.9 The effect of price change on volume and profitability of work.

a 15% increase in sales volume, the profit will still fall by 8%. So you are doing more work, and making less money! The lower the profit margin, the more sensitive the figures are, as shown in Figure 16.9. Be very sure to do your maths before you change your prices!

DISCOUNTS

Running a veterinary practice is not a theoretical exercise, and there will always be some circumstances in which the official price of a product or service is reduced. Discounts are a useful marketing tool, but can cause problems if not properly controlled.

There are a few basic rules of discounting:

- Always know why you are giving a discount, and what you hope to achieve by it.
- Know what it is costing you.
- Never give a discount without showing the client what they would have paid.
- Have a standard practice policy on discounting.

Know why you are discounting

Discounted fees may be offered on new products or services introduced to the practice. This may be theoretically intended to benefit the client, but in reality clinicians or managers are sometimes sceptical of the take-up of a new procedure, and may feel happier promoting it at a lower than target price to start with.

A number of common reasons for offering some form of discount are listed below.

- To help old-age pensioners
- For charitable organizations
- An introductory offer on a new product or service
- A special offer from the manufacturer to pass on to your customers
- To encourage prompt/cash payment
- To encourage bulk purchasing
- To encourage pre-ordering/contracts
- To shift short-dated/discontinued stock.

Many of these might have been introduced as a result of marketing or business planning. The results of the discount scheme can be monitored and reviewed to ensure on-going effectiveness.

Other reasons for giving discounts need to be treated much more carefully, as they often reflect underlying problems within the practice. These may include the following:

- Because vets are unhappy with the price to start with. If this is the case, it needs to be discussed properly in a clinical/management meeting.
- Because vets don't think they did a good job. Do not make a discounted fee an admission of clinical failure.
- Because the original estimate was not made up correctly. You might need to give a discount on this occasion, but staff need to learn to do it right next time!
- Staff discounts. These are a common perk of working in practice, but make sure you know how you will deal with staff members who have a multitude of animals before the issue arises. Many practices ask their staff to insure their pets instead – which has the added benefit of staff having first-hand experience of pet insurance.
- To encourage use of the practice at quiet times. Offering discounted fees to clients who come at less popular appointment times can spread the workload effectively, but be very careful on the perceived value of the service. '10% discount on services on Wednesday afternoons' might make the clients wonder why – is that when the less qualified staff work, or what? It is better to combine this with another reason for discounting – for instance, target your OAPs or charity work during the off-peak times.
- Because they're a friend. This can cause real problems, particularly in small or rural practices – the senior partner may have 'special' friends, but what happens about all the other staff members' mates?

Know what it is costing you

It is vital to be aware of the profit margin and price sensitivity of products and fees in order to assess the impact of discounts. Even a small discount of 10% can have a dramatic effect on profitability. At 33% margin, you will need to do 43% more work to maintain profit levels!

For stock items, rather than simply lowering the price, discount incentives can be given in the form of extra product, such as:

- buy 4, get one free
- free product X when you buy Y
- vouchers off future purchases.

These incentives are useful for several reasons – firstly, the customer tends to think the deal is better than it is. At first sight *'Buy 4, get one free'* looks the same as 25% off, but in fact is only a 20% reduction in price. Secondly, offering more product for the same price will sell more stock – useful if you are trying to shift slow-moving items or short-dated stock.

Linked product incentives are a way of encouraging the client to buy a wider range of items from the practice, and also offer the client a substantial 'carrot' at retail price whilst only costing the practice the buying price.

Vouchers off future purchases will encourage on-going customer loyalty.

Make sure the customer knows what they should have paid

There is absolutely no point giving a discount unless the client knows about it.

In the case of products, make sure the normal price is clear, along with the reason for the discount – 'introductory offer', 'summer sale', or 'clearance'. The client needs to know that the price may be back to normal next week, or that there is no point expecting a long-term supply of something which is discounted as a discontinued product.

Never discount a bill by simply missing off fees, or underestimating the complexity or time taken to do a procedure.

If there is a prompt payment discount, then this should be clear on the invoice – clients will feel disgruntled if they find they were entitled to a discount but did not take it because it was hidden away in the small print.

Have a practice policy on discounting

If there is no standard discounting policy within the practice then this can get very difficult for both staff and clients. If the practice owner regularly gives discounts to their favourite clients, what will happen when there is someone else on duty? Chances are the client will be upset, and the staff member embarrassed.

If staff are allowed discretion in giving discounts, then these must be clearly recorded, and checks made to ensure there is no abuse of the system.

Fees or procedures that are regularly discounted should be examined in detail to see why. Is the official price too high, or the costs not understood?

SURCHARGES

Administration charges, booking fees, surcharges, call them what you may – many practices use some form of fee to encourage prompt payment and/or penalize those who pay late. A surcharge system may be used in conjunction with a discount scheme. Whatever way you use surcharges, you should know why.

Why are you using them?

- As a threat – *'You will be charged £X if you do not pay by dd/mm/yy.'*
- As a routine to discourage sending bills – *'An invoicing fee of £X has been added to your account.'*
- To recoup specific charges, for instance if the client's cheque has bounced, or if you send them to court.

What will surcharges achieve?

If your normal terms of business are cash at the time of consultation, then it will be more effective to concentrate your efforts on training the reception staff and educating your clients to adhere to these terms.

What will you do when account customers simply deduct any surcharges from their remittances? If the system is ignored anyway, does it cause more bad feeling than it solves?

Any surcharge system should be clearly set out in your terms and conditions of business.

PROBLEMS ARISING FROM PRICES

Fees accounted for 50 of the 789 written complaints received by the RCVS in the 12 months to March 2001. Bear in mind that these figures only represent those clients who felt strongly enough to make an official complaint. Some unhappy clients will complain to reception staff or the practice owner, but many will simply not bother returning to the practice.

However, complaints are rarely caused solely by the prices themselves, but are usually a result of poor communications between the practice and client. One of the major reasons for this communication breakdown is that both sides are uncomfortable talking about money when the welfare of an animal is at stake. Practice staff may put off mentioning price until the last minute, and the owner does not wish to seem uncaring by asking 'how much?'

Good management can minimize the likelihood of a complaint about prices; for example:

- Clearly label all displayed products with their price, and keep it up to date.
- Train receptionists to answer routine price enquiries confidently and accurately. They should understand the reasoning behind the practice fee price structure, and be aware of the economics involved. It is vital not to hide costs from the client – if asked to give the price for a consultation, make sure the client understands that there will be extra costs for medication and treatment.
- Ensure that veterinary surgeons explain the financial implications of treatment options. Beware of making assumptions about a client's financial status – the final choice must be the client's.
- Use estimates for all surgical procedures and extended treatments. Have an agreed procedure for communicating with the client if unexpected costs crop up. An estimate should always be a price range, and ideally high enough so that the final bill is pleasantly low! Be aware that a 'quotation' can be legally binding – so always make sure the client understands the difference between a quotation and an estimate – and always use the latter!
- Confirm the extent of cover of insured animals with the insurance company before starting extensive treatment. The owner may think it is insured but could be unaware of any excluded conditions or treatment limits reached. Now that percentage excesses are becoming more common, it is sensible to make sure the client is aware of their contribution.
- Make sure the client knows the payment terms of the practice.
- Produce clear, itemized bills and receipts as a routine – not just when someone has a query. Be sensible with the degree of itemization, and don't go to the extreme of showing each disposable theatre item separately. By all means take them into account when calculating the fee, but simply show it on the bill as 'theatre pack'.
- Never apologize for your prices. You may need to be understanding and sympathetic – *'Yes, it's amazing how it mounts up,'* is fine, but not *'I'm afraid it's rather expensive.'* Use the computer to take the personality out of it. 'This is what the bill adds up to,' not 'This is what I am charging you.'
- Ensure that reception staff can answer any initial queries about the make-up of the bill.
- Draw up an official in-house complaints procedure. This should be understood by all staff. A fee complaint handled well will often result in a very loyal client. A badly-handled complaint will only add insult to injury.

17

Information technology

CHAPTER CONTENTS

What computers can do 186
What computers cannot do 186

The use of computers in veterinary practice 186
Client and animal records 186
Marketing 188
Finance 188
Stock control 189
Communications 190
Human resources 190
CPD and education 190

Choosing and evaluating a system 191
What do you want it to do? 191
Who will supply the system? 192
What software do I need? 192
What hardware do I need to run it on? 193
Where is it going to be installed? 193
How much support and training will I get? 194
How much will it cost? 194

Contingencies 195
Data back-up 195
Power supply 195
Security against hardware theft 196
Minimize risk of accidental damage 196
Dependence on the system manager 196
System monitoring 196
Software security 196
Fraud awareness 196

Associated legislation 197

The information technology field is changing at a tremendous rate. The Chairman of IBM could not have been further from the truth with his famous quote,

> 'I think there is a world market for maybe five computers.'

That was in 1943. And in 1965, Gordon Moore noticed that microchip processing power was doubling every 18–24 months. Amazingly, Moore's Law, as it is known, still holds true even now.

There are major changes in software systems and the companies that produce them – whether it is market leaders being dragged through the American judicial system, or the constant evolution, death and rebirth of specialist veterinary information systems.

This constant change in the computer world means that it is impossible for a book of this nature to set out any detailed technical specifications for computer hardware or software. However, this chapter should give you an understanding of the uses and limitations of computers in veterinary practice. It also aims to give you an idea of what can be achieved, what to look out for, and how to prevent disasters!

As with any management tool, the complexity of the computer system needed will vary from practice to practice. A single-handed vet with a couple of staff will have different requirements from a busy multi-centre practice. Many of the recent advances in veterinary practice management have only been made possible by the use of IT.

What computers can do

Computers have a vast memory and an amazing capacity for doing boring repetitive tasks.

The key feature that makes computers so useful is their ability to take data stored for one purpose and easily reuse it for another purpose at a future date. Computerized clinical records may not at first sight seem much of an advance on hand-written cards (especially as many vets' typing is as bad as their handwriting!). But combine the recording of an animal's treatment with the capacity to automatically log stock items used, generate reminders and run reports on how many cases of specific diseases you have seen, and suddenly it is a very powerful tool.

What computers cannot do

Remember that computers are not intelligent. They are simply machines, and incapable of independent thought (thankfully!). They cannot function in isolation, and only have limited control over the information they receive. Before you curse the system, remember the adage *'Garbage in, Garbage out'* – GIGO.

Computers do not automatically save you time, money or paper. The potential for producing information is increased many times beyond your capacity to analyse and act on it usefully. At one time, turnover was measured by adding up the banking receipts; now it can be analysed down to income from cutting gerbils' toenails.

The paperless office is a possibility, but rarely exists in practice. It is human nature not to be satisfied unless something written down can be seen. A single computer may have a memory equivalent to a whole organization, and full back-up facilities, but no one is happy unless they have a filing cabinet full of hard copy.

Computers can consume vast quantities of materials, money, energy and stress. Make sure they are working for you, not the other way round!

THE USE OF COMPUTERS IN VETERINARY PRACTICE

Computers were first used in veterinary practice for storing basic client and animal data, and producing vaccination reminders. As illustrated in Figure 17.1, information technology now has an influence on all aspects of modern veterinary practice, including:

- client and animal records
- marketing
- finance
- stock control
- communications
- human resources
- CPD and education.

Client and animal records

A simple client and animal database is normally the first requirement for a computerized practice management system (PMS). As well as recording basic patient details, it may include:

- clinical records
- fee calculation and billing
- appointments diary.

It is vital that any system used to manage the interaction between clients, their animals and the practice, helps and not hinders it. Some aspects of computerization simply duplicate information previously recorded on a card system, others improve on the 'old system', or were simply impossible to perform pre-computerization.

Practices should be aware of the need to comply with the Data Protection Act, which now applies even to records held within a manual filing system.

Clinical information

At their simplest, computerized clinical records mimic card-based systems. However, most have

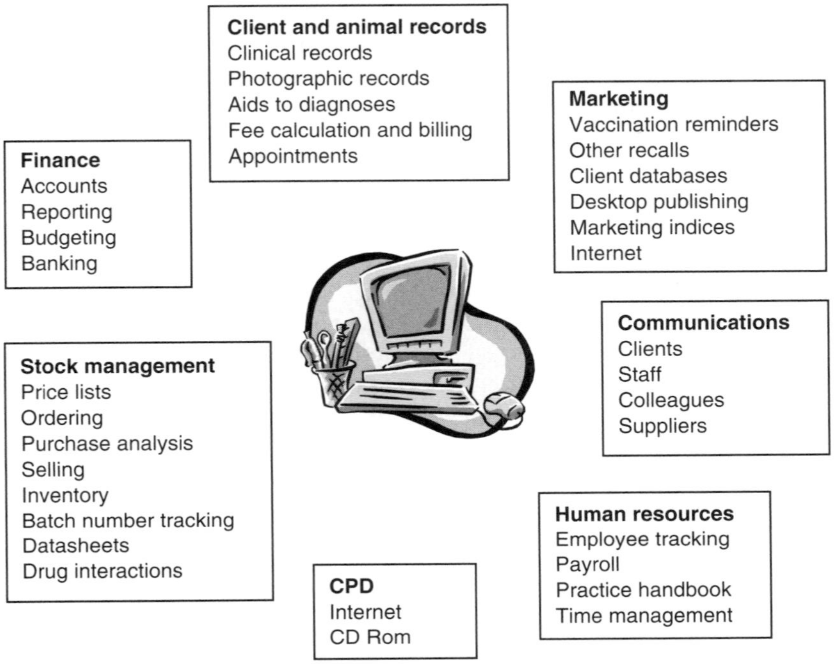

Figure 17.1 Information technology encompasses all aspects of veterinary practice management.

some form of automatically adding commonly-used procedures and drugs onto the client's record, and accurately pricing them. Some vets are reluctant to use the computer for keeping details of clinical records, and use a card system in parallel, even if they use the computer to generate vaccination reminders and invoices.

Clinical protocols included in the system can talk vets through a series of questions/diagnostic stages when investigating cases. This may be of help to new graduates, or to clinics wanting to standardize on treatment methods.

A few years ago, hard disk storage limitations made routine storage of large files such as graphics a luxury. Now, the combination of affordable digital cameras and multi-gigabyte hard drives means that photographic records of cases can easily be attached to an animal's history. This has tremendous advantages, both from keeping track of cases being seen by different vets, convincing owners that a long-term skin condition is slowly getting better, and of course, legal back-up. X-rays can also be scanned and stored on computer, although the resolution is unlikely to be as good as looking on a viewer.

Fee calculation and billing

A computerized medical record/charging system will ensure accurate pricing. The computer provides an independent, impersonal interface between the vet/receptionist/bill and the client. The system should also make it easier to provide accurate estimates for more serious treatment. However, computers cannot stop human error (deliberate or accidental) from missing items off bills.

Having calculated the fees due, the computer should be able to manage the sending of bills – as often as the practice chooses, as well as adding surcharges or allowing discounts as required.

Appointments

The appointment section of a program can be the most crucial part of a practice management system. Vets may feel able to put up with a cumbersome clinical entry system for years, but a busy receptionist faced with a constant stream of clients making and turning up for appointments will soon tell you the bad points. Make sure the system can cope with the number of different vets consulting in your practice. How does it cope with marking staff away? How easy is it to manage a waiting room? It needs to be flexible to cope with busy days and folk who just turn up, and yet rigid enough to prevent routine overbooking.

Using a computerized diary means that a record of a client's appointments and cancellations can be kept – useful in the case of complaints and litigation. If you can show that a client didn't keep several appointments, it is no wonder the animal didn't get better.

Marketing

The practice computer system can be a valuable marketing tool. Once you have your clinical database, it can be put to many uses, such as:

- vaccination reminders
- other reminders and recalls
- personalized letters and handouts
- desktop publishing
- data for input into comparative veterinary marketing indices.

Vaccination reminders were one of the earliest functions of veterinary computer systems. Modern practice has expanded the role of preventative healthcare, and you may want to set up and customize other reminders for animals – such as routine flea treatments, dental checks, weight checks, herd health visits. In an equine practice, the system will need to cope with vaccinations due within a specific date range to comply with Jockey Club rulings on equine flu vaccines.

Computers are also changing what we do with the results of a database analysis. Whereas once it was good enough to simply produce a set of address labels to stick onto reminder postcards, now the only limit is your imagination. Mail-merge facilities make it easy to produce personalized handouts and colourful letters. There are several sources of pre-written handouts in electronic format, which can be edited to the practice's personal preferences.

Anything beyond typing a simple letter by computer was once considered the realm of a 'designer', who had spent years mastering complex software. There is no doubt that when it comes to preparing glossy brochures, or designing a new logo, the services of a professional designer can be worthwhile. But modern word-processing packages are now very powerful, and desktop publishing software is much more user-friendly. Clipart cartoons are readily available from a number of suppliers, and some pharmaceutical companies may be able to supply you with some more specific veterinary diagrams.

Marketing indices, run by a number of veterinary companies, allow comparison of marketing data with other practices. The 'performance indicators' used include figures such as client retention and turnover, % vaccinated animals, average transaction fees and many, many more.

Finance

The development of user-friendly accountancy packages and powerful spreadsheets now allows practice owners and managers to have much more control over practice finance and planning.

Accounts

Small practices may manage their finances by using their bank statements and a file of invoices 'to pay'. However, if you are doing any form of management accounting beyond comparing month-end bank balances, at some point you will be adding up payments made and dividing into drugs and others. Why pay an accountant to sift though piles of raw paperwork when you could enter the information within the practice and gain from the timely information? And if you are doing all that work for internal accounts anyway, why not go the next stage further and adopt a system capable of producing the final accounts? Take advice from your accountant on packages to use. Even if you do not do all the year-end adjustments in-house, you may find significant savings in your accountancy bill if you can send them compatible files by e-mail or disk. Do make sure the software is user-friendly, though; there is no point saving a few hundred pounds on an accountancy bill if the software takes twice as long for your staff to run!

Management reporting and budgeting

Both the practice management system and the bookkeeping/accountancy packages themselves should be able to produce year-on-year comparisons. In addition, both these should be able to export figures into spreadsheet format for further analysis and planning.

Banking

Banking by computer has become very popular, driven by the need for instant information at any time of day. The ability to check the account balances easily, and to know which transactions have been processed, allows tight control of cashflow. Significant savings can be made by juggling payments to keep just the right side of overdraft limits or interest bands. Money can easily be transferred between accounts to maximize the return on any spare funds.

Electronic transactions are generally cheaper than paper ones. Using a BACS system to pay suppliers will save on cheque charges and postage. Accepting payment into your account by direct debit will save on banking time and charges, but is only of any real use if you can see on a daily basis what has come in.

Accepting payments by direct debit or swipe machine reduces the risk of loss or theft of practice funds.

There are two slightly different ways of using computer systems for your practice banking – computer banking and internet banking.

Computer banking involves directly dialling your bank, and transferring information about your account. Your bank will supply you (or sell you!) their specific banking software to install on your computer. This means that you can only access your account from the computer that has this software installed. If you have accounts with several different banks, you need separate software for each one. On the positive side, having the software on the computer means that you can set up all the transactions you want to make before dialling in. Account statements are downloaded to the computer, and can be looked at any time.

Internet banking works quite differently. You log onto the internet through your normal service provider, and then log onto the bank site. The banking software is all held on the bank's own website, so you can access your accounts from any computer or internet café. There is no costly software to buy or clutter up your computer. The downside of this method is that you do not have any access to information and cannot set up payments off-line. It is also susceptible to general slowness/crashing of the internet. At one point, internet banking was viewed as less secure than direct dial-up computer banking, but this is no longer the case.

Some banks offer high-interest current or deposit accounts that can only be run using the internet.

Stock control

Computer systems can be used in all aspects of stock use and management, such as:

- producing price lists
- ordering by direct modem linkup or internet
- purchase analysis
- charging stock items to clients' accounts
- keeping track of inventory
- batch number traceability
- datasheets – formularies as stand-alone CD-ROM reference or integrated into the PMS
- drug interaction warnings
- repeat prescriptions/medication records.

Stock control is covered in detail in Chapter 15, 'Stock management'.

Communications

E-mail and the internet have revolutionized many aspects of communication between the practice and:

- clients
- staff
- colleagues
- suppliers
- external organizations.

E-mail can be used to send client reminders and practice newsletters cheaply and quickly. It is important to have clear guidelines about what constitutes acceptable use of practice e-mail and internet facilities for staff. Be especially careful about anything that may be going out under the practice's e-mail header, as opposed to staff having their own personal e-mail addresses. One risk of e-mails is that the original sender has no control over future use or misuse of their message. One woman hit the headlines in December 2000, after a personal e-mail to her boyfriend was forwarded initially to six of his friends, and eventually reached 1 million recipients around the world!

In October 2000, the Telecommunications (Lawful business practice) (Interception of communications) Regulations 2000 set out a number of situations in which the employer is authorized to monitor communications, including e-mails, without the permission of the sender or recipient. Although you won't want employees to waste hours of their time surfing the internet, do bear in mind that it is cheaper for staff to use e-mail than to make private phone calls during working hours!

The use of e-mail discussion groups allows any number of friends and colleagues to share queries and information. Some very successful groups are now run by a number of veterinary organizations such as the VPMA, SPVS, VCU and others.

The practice website is a powerful marketing and communication tool. As well as letting clients know about the practice, there is potential for more interactive use of the website, such as buying products (on-line pet shop) or booking appointments. Some American clinics even have webcams in the kennel area, so clients can log onto the practice website and observe their pets in hospital.

Human resources

This is probably one of the most recent areas to take advantage of computerization in practices, and can involve:

- employee records
- payroll calculations
- practice handbook
- time management.

Employee management software will help practices to keep track of employee details, salary records, hours worked (important for the Working Time Regulations), holiday planning, appraisal notes, disciplinary records, etc. Remember that the Data Protection Act applies just as much to employee records as to those of your clients.

Payroll may be a stand-alone function, or more likely integrated into either your accounts package, or human resources management system. There is normally an annual fee payable to have the integral tax/NIC tables updated.

Staff handbooks are ideally suited to computerization. The information can be easily updated, and to make life easy you can start using one of the templates available from specialist veterinary suppliers.

Using organizer software with contact management features, you can plan and account for your time, as well as keeping a record of who you contacted when.

CPD and education

Apart from the general use of word-processing for typing up notes and producing portfolios, computers have now revolutionized the whole learning process. The older distance-learning tools of workbooks, audiotape and videos have now been complemented by the use of CD-ROMs and the internet.

The internet can be used both for on-line learning and also for research and hunting for information. Bear in mind that your clients will also be able to look at most of this information too – so be prepared for them when they turn up with stacks of paper and a total diagnosis before you have even looked at the animal.

CHOOSING AND EVALUATING A SYSTEM

Computer systems are now central to the running of a modern practice, and choosing the right one is critical. With practice management systems costing several thousands of pounds for even a basic system, the money involved is considerable. But even choosing the right payroll system at a few hundred pounds cannot be taken lightly. The consequences of the wrong choice include not only wasted money, but also disruption to the practice, staff stress and possible loss of data.

Whether choosing a new system, or reviewing the merits of your current one, involve all the current and potential users of the system in the plan. Keep an open mind – just because your old system did things one way, do not discount one which works differently.

One of the most valuable sources of information is from other veterinary practices. There are a number of email discussion groups, such as those run by the VCU, VPMA and SPVS, which regularly have queries about computer hardware and software. Many practices are very happy to demonstrate their systems in action, and give you their feedback on the good and bad points. Do follow up any perceived inadequacies with the system suppliers, however, as very few practices are totally familiar with all the available functions of their systems.

When choosing a system, there are several aspects to look at:

- What do you want it to do?
- Who will supply the system?
- What software do I need?
- Does it need to be compatible with other software?
- What hardware does it need to run on?
- Where is it going to be installed?
- How much support and training will I get?
- How much will it cost?

What do you want it to do?

Drawing up a system specification can be a 'chicken and egg' situation – it is difficult to know what features you will need until you've used a system that doesn't have them! Depending on previous IT use and knowledge, it should be possible to draw up at least an outline specification, listing broadly what you want the system to do, who will be using it, and basic hardware parameters. For instance, you might be looking:

- For a stand-alone payroll program
- To cope with eight employees
- To run on a single PC.

After further discussion with colleagues and some system suppliers, you might expand the specification to include further features. In this example you may wish to include:

- Absence and sickness tracking
- Employment legislation guidelines.

Think carefully before deciding which features are unnecessary – you might want them in a couple of years' time. Bear in mind any future expansion of the practice:

- How many employees might you have in 3 years' time?
- Might you want to run the system over a network?
- Will it need to integrate with a future accounting package?

Predicting your future use is not easy… .

> 'There is no reason for any individual to have a computer in his home.'
>
> (Ken Olson, President, Digital Equipment, 1977)

Once you have a rough idea of what you are looking for, it is time to draw up a list of possible suppliers to ask for more detailed information and quotations. Shop around – price will be a major factor, but so are service and back-up.

Who will supply the system?

There are several sources of computer software and hardware for veterinary practices.

- ***Veterinary practice management system companies.*** Most veterinary-specific software, and a lot of the hardware it runs on, is supplied by a number of specialist companies. Although some are well-established names in the profession, it is very much a changing market, and new contenders are always emerging.

- ***Veterinary companies.*** Most veterinary wholesalers offer some sort of computer software or hardware. This may be simply a stock ordering and control system, up to a full practice management system. Other companies may provide software relating to their product ranges, for instance to monitor the effect of pet weight reduction diets, or to calculate correct fluid therapy treatment.

- ***Off the shelf.*** High street shops will supply general business software such as office, accountancy or employment software packages. They may also be very competitive sources of general hardware such as printers and windows PCs.

- ***Free software.*** Most of the computer magazines give away free software with each issue. This is often an old (but perfectly adequate) version of the program, with a special upgrade deal to the new one. This can be a good source of graphics and web design packages, as well as some of the less well-known office programs.

- ***Bespoke one-offs.*** Most people have a friend (or offspring of a friend) who is a 'computer nerd' and just loves the challenge of writing a better program than the one you are using. This can be a good way – several commercial systems now available started life as a 'one off for a friend'. But beware, if it was that easy to write a good system, there would be lots more out there. Make sure that the person is capable of doing what they say they can, and protect your position in the case of the final product being inadequate, late or non-existent. Is the person able to provide on-going support for the system – or will he have disappeared by the time you want a new add-on?

What software do I need?

Your initial specification should list:

- What type of software are you looking at?
- What do you need it to do now?
- What might it need to do in 2 years' time?
- Does it need to be compatible with any other software?
- Do you want a text-based or graphical system?
- What operating system do you want the system to run on?

When following up references from other vets, make sure you find out some background about their practice. Just as no two veterinary practices will run in exactly the same way, their ideas of a 'perfect' computer system will not be the same. For instance, the appointment booking features of a system may be perfect in a small practice, but simply can't cope with six vets consulting at once.

Computer magazines feature comparative reviews of off-the-shelf hardware and software. Software compatibility is an increasingly important issue. In the early days, when practice management systems were very basic, integration with other applications was not important. Now that your database can be the key to the practice business, it is vital to be able to use that information in other programs. You may want to send turnover figures to an accountancy package, use detailed income breakdown information in a planning spreadsheet, or export a list of target clients to a word-processor.

Whilst almost all 'office type' software has a graphical ('Windows type') look, practice management systems can be divided into text-based or graphical systems. Both options have their staunch followers, and there are advantages and disadvantages of either. In the end, like most things, it comes down to personal preference. Supporters of text-based systems will claim that they are faster to use, and less cluttered to look at than graphical systems; on the other hand, users of graphical interfaces feel they are more modern looking, and more intuitive to use by people already familiar with the ubiquitous Windows-based products.

As well as looking at which software application to choose, you will need to consider which operating system (OS) to use. The OS is the special software that the computer needs to exist at all. It allows the computer to communicate with all its internal widgets, and to interpret instructions from the application programs. Although the average user will never need to know any details about using the OS, apart from how to start it up and shut it down, the choice of OS will have a significant effect on the software and hardware needed.

The three operating systems commonly used to run veterinary practice management systems are Microsoft Windows, Unix and Theos. Most of the general business and office packages you look at will be designed to run on one of the Microsoft Windows operating systems (there are several different versions of Windows). But choosing your practice management system (PMS) software will also involve deciding which operating system you will be using. In some cases, the choice of PMS will determine the operating system; in others, you may decide to only look at systems that will run on a particular OS.

Hybrid systems are becoming more common, in which UNIX- or Theos-based systems can integrate with Windows PCs on the same network.

What hardware do I need to run it on?

> 'Computers in the future may weigh no more than 1.5 tons.'
>
> (Popular Mechanics, forecasting the relentless march of science, 1949)

> 'It would appear that we have reached the limits of what it is possible to achieve with computer technology, although one should be careful with such statements, as they tend to sound pretty silly in 5 years.'
>
> John Von Neumann (ca 1949)

Computers have obviously come a long way since these statements were made. Your initial specification should outline:

- Do you want a stand-alone system or a network?
- How many terminals or workstations do you require?
- Do you need printers for documents, labels, receipts, or barcodes?

After initial enquiries, you might decide to add some extras:

- scanner
- digital camera
- handheld units for farm/home visits
- CD writers
- barcode reader.

And you will need to refine some of your initial outline:

- What type of printer? – Dot matrix, inkjet, laser or thermal? Black and white or colour?
- What sort of terminals – Windows workstations, or simple terminals? This will be partly determined by the choice of operating system (or vice versa).

The detailed specification of hardware must take the software into account. Even the best software will perform badly if it is installed on inappropriate hardware. Practice management system suppliers will advise you on the optimum specification, and may often supply it themselves. Off-the-shelf software will specify minimum hardware needed to run the application.

Where is it going to be installed?

Computers and all their bits and pieces can take up a lot of room in a surgery, especially in older premises which will not have been designed with computers in mind. In some cases, the space available will dictate the choice of hardware. This might involve using UNIX terminals (consisting of only a keyboard, monitor and possibly a small 'brainbox') instead of Windows PC workstations; or opting for flat screens.

Veterinary surgeries are not the ideal environment for computers. The main server is best kept in as clean an environment as possible, out of range of animal hair and spilt liquids. An office area is normally the ideal choice. Make sure it is easily accessible for changing back-up media, but not in a place where it might accidentally be switched off.

Consulting room terminals are often just plonked on the only shelf space available. But give some thought to whether the vet is going to be standing or sitting when using the screen. Think about the position of the screen relative to the patients – do you want the client to be able to read what is being typed on the screen? Do you want to have to turn your back on them while typing? Consulting room keyboards are exposed to the dangers of 'flying cats' and inquisitive children – consider having a sliding-away keyboard. Protective keyboard 'gloves' will minimize the risk from liquids, hairs or bloody fingers. If you have a Windows-based system, remember that the mouse does not like hairs and sticky residues. It might be worth considering alternatives such as an optical laser-driven mouse in some areas of the surgery – they have no balls ('castrated mice' – doubly applicable in veterinary surgeries)!

All terminals and workstations will need to be examined as part of your Health and Safety assessment to ensure compliance with the Display Screen Regulations.

If you are planning any upgrades to the premises, it is important to consider the computer system, for instance provision for network cabling and power supply. There are never enough electric sockets for all the computer hardware!

How much support and training will I get?

Whenever any new equipment is bought for the practice, staff will need training in how to use it. This applies just as much to computer software as to surgical or diagnostic tools. If staff are not properly trained to use the system, they will not get the best use out of it, and may even cause serious errors.

In the case of office or business software such as accountancy packages, your local college may have a suitable selection of evening or daytime classes. Specialist practice management systems will have their own training staff visit the surgery.

But don't forget, computer system training is not a one-off need when you buy the system. To continue to make the most of any software, new staff will need to be trained, and full advantage taken of any upgrades to the system.

All suppliers will offer some degree of software and hardware support. It is vital that the critical parts of your system are protected. Make sure you know who to contact in the case of an emergency, and how much cover you have. What will happen if you have a problem during a Saturday surgery? How long will it take to get a replacement screen? Try to find out from other users what their experiences have been – is it easy to get through to speak to a member of support staff? Do they fix the problem promptly?

Make sure all your support contracts are up to date, and that you are not still paying for hardware items you might no longer use.

How much will it cost?

Your planning process should include a budget for IT. It is important that you research all the costs involved with the practice's computer system. These will include:

- purchase costs of hardware and software
- extra costs for installation and cabling
- training costs
- software and hardware support contracts
- replacement equipment or software upgrades not covered by contracts
- consumables, such as printer ink, toner, back-up media, paper and labels.

The rapid changes in the IT field mean that you should budget for regular replacement of key items of the system. Whilst keyboards and simple terminals may last for many years, it is likely that the main server will need to be replaced by a faster, more powerful model after only 2–3 years.

Any equipment in veterinary practice must earn its keep, and the computer system is no different. Although your IT budget may appear high, you should be able to identify ways in which the computer system contributes financially towards the practice as well. These will include helping to save money (e.g. saving staff time or analysing drug purchases to negotiate better discounts) and also by generating income (by correct pricing and improved marketing).

CONTINGENCIES

Any record system, computerized or not, needs to be protected from both accidental and intentional theft or damage. Be the ultimate pessimist and try to think of some of the disaster scenarios that could affect your computer systems. Power failure, telephone line disruption, theft or accidental damage are common ones. Then plan how the practice can be least disrupted by these events. Make sure anyone in a position of responsibility knows where the plans are – they don't need to phone you to find out what to do. Some example contingency plans are shown in Figure 17.2 at the end of the chapter.

Your plans may include the following:

- data back-up system
- safeguard power supplies
- security against hardware theft
- minimize risk of accidental damage
- dependence on the system administrator
- system monitoring
- software security
- fraud awareness.

Remember that for a plan to be useful, it must be put into action – and computer systems are the biggest fans of Murphy's Law – it *will* crash on the only day you don't have a back-up!

Data back-up

All computer records must be backed up regularly onto some sort of removable media. How often is regularly? That depends on how much data you can afford to lose and how much time it would take you to restore it. Most practice management systems come with automated daily back-up procedures, but these still need some form of user input: the back-up media must be changed each day – the ideal rotation is to use a different set of media for each day of the week. This way, if it takes a few days for you to notice a data corruption, you are less likely to have overwritten your last good back-up.

Back-ups should be stored safely, preferably away from the surgery. Do not simply leave the tapes or disks sitting on top of the computer – how are they going to help you in the case of fire?

Simply taking back-ups is not enough – you need to test them regularly. Ask your system support team how to do this; you don't want to discover that your rigorously taken back-up is as much use as a scratched record when you need to use it.

Don't forget to back-up all your other programs, such as office documents and e-mail – even the waiting room display posters that took hours to design are not easily re-created.

Part of your contingency planning might be to routinely print out information such as the day's appointment lists each morning.

Power supply

Too much or too little electricity will cause problems for computers. The bare minimum protection should be an anti-surge electrical extension cable in between the mains socket and computer server. Ideally computer equipment should be on a separate ring main, so that power surges from other equipment (e.g. fridges starting up) will not disrupt the supply to the computer.

An Uninterruptible Power Supply (UPS) will normally smoothe the incoming voltages as well as providing some degree of emergency power. Note the term *emergency* – the UPS will not allow you to run the computer on battery power for any substantial period of time. It will only either protect you against a quick dip in supply, or provide enough power to complete a controlled shutdown of the system in the case of a full power cut. Be very wary when you see Electricity Board road gangs outside the surgery!

Security against hardware theft

Computer equipment is often a target for thieves. The general security of the surgery should be up to a good standard anyway, but devices are available that will securely fix the hardware to desks. Thieves are usually after the processors in the main server unit, so this is the key part of the system to protect.

Turning monitors off at night will lessen the temptation to thieves by preventing that telltale glow from within the building, as well as saving energy.

Minimize risk of accidental damage

As mentioned previously, take care with the siting of computers. Years ago they used to live in air-conditioned rooms – nowadays they get less respect than the TV and video! Keep equipment out of range of the over-enthusiastic floor-moppers, or dog leg-cocking height. Think about other hazards too – could there be danger of flooding from above (water tank overflowing) or below?

Regular cleaning of system peripherals and the main server by suitably experienced operators will reduce build-up of pet hairs and other debris. Well-meaning poking around in printers with bent paperclips or surgical forceps will probably do more harm than good!

Computer equipment should be tested at suitable intervals to comply with the Portable Electrical Appliance regulations.

Dependence on the system manager

The person who looks after and controls the computer system can be a godsend, but be aware of how much knowledge rests with any one person. It is not always practical to have two people fully up to speed with all the systems used in the practice, but at the very least, all user manuals and instructions should be accessible, and the system manager should write down all systems of work. If any major passwords are changed, then any software support personnel should be made aware of them; otherwise there is little they can do to help you.

System monitoring

One support feature offered by many practice management system suppliers is some form of remote system monitoring via a modem link. They will compile information on parameters such as available disk space and system speed, and alert the practice if they diagnose a problem.

Most systems will need some form of database maintenance to remove old or spurious data: ask your supplier how best to do this.

Software security

Consult the system suppliers to make sure your set-up is as safe as possible from accidental loss of data. Password-protected access levels should be used so that only suitably-authorized staff can edit or delete records.

Any system that has any form of interaction with any other computer, via floppy disks, back-up media or a modem, is at risk from computer viruses. Microsoft Windows-based systems are most at risk, but virus checker software is readily available. This can be regularly updated over the internet for a small subscription. Users of other operating systems should ask their suppliers for the most appropriate virus protection if necessary.

You may need to take security measures against unauthorized remote access to your system via the modem (hacking). Systems with a continuous internet connection, or ones which will accept incoming modem connections (often needed by your software support engineers) are most at risk, but even normal dial-up internet access can be corrupted. There is a wide variety of 'fire-wall' software available to combat this threat.

Fraud awareness

Fraud and theft by employees is a situation which most practice owners think won't happen to them. But it is surprisingly common. It may take several forms, including:

- theft of information
- 'cooking the books' – stealing money directly or indirectly
- theft of time – playing computer games or surfing the internet
- theft of consumables
- malicious damage to the system by employees.

Client database information may be 'stolen' by employees going to work in a competing practice, or misused as part of a separate business venture such as dog grooming. As well as wanting to protect the interests of the practice, you have a responsibility under the Data Protection Act to protect the security of your clients' data. It should be made clear to all employees that misuse of any practice data is a disciplinary offence.

Nowadays most financial records are held on computer, and therefore improving your computer security and working practices should help to minimize the opportunity for fraud. Unauthorized staff should not have access to alter financial amounts on clients' records, and all editing, even by a senior partner, should be annotated with the reason for the change. A secure computer system should have the facility for an audit log, which records all transactions and changes to them. If fraud is suspected, this audit log can help to identify when changes were made. Till drawers can be set to interlink with the computer system, only opening when a sale has been made. Receipt printers should be used as standard practice, so the client has a record of their payments.

Access to accounting or banking software should be tightly controlled by password protection. Systems of work should be used so that no single person has entire control of money transfer transactions.

In large office-based companies, significant amounts of employees' time is wasted by playing computer games or personal e-mailing/surfing the internet. This is less likely to be a problem in veterinary practice, particularly amongst clinical staff using text-based systems with few other programs installed. However, as internet-based learning becomes more popular, access to this temptation is increasing. Your staff should be made aware of whether personal use of these facilities is acceptable, and if so, whether they are restricted to use outside normal working hours.

Any office consumables are at risk from theft, and computer supplies such as floppy disks, printer cartridges and paper can have a tendency to 'walk'.

There is always the chance that a disgruntled employee may attempt to seek revenge by sabotaging the computer system. This is a very real threat in highly IT-based industries, but is less of a risk to veterinary practices. Good system security in the form of password protection and back-up facilities should minimize the risk. Worth checking your insurance policy, though!

ASSOCIATED LEGISLATION

Computer equipment, and the use of information technology in practice, is subject to a number of areas of legislation. These are covered in more detail in chapters 18 and 19, including:

- Data Protection Act
- Display Screen Regulations
- Portable appliance testing
- Telecommunications (Lawful business practice) (Interception of communications) Regulations 2000.

Useful information

Telephone numbers
- Computer hardware support ....
- Computer software support ....
- Electricity supply board ....
- Local electrician ....

Location of fuse boards ....

Electricity supply board customer ref. number ....

Main problems and possible solutions

Appointments – not knowing who to expect	Routinely print off expected appointments each morning **Or** Ruled paper to write down clients as they arrive for their appointments, receptionists to apologize for any confusion and offer tea/coffee/alternative appointment if running late.
Recording clinical findings	Supply of cards for recording clinical notes – receptionists to fill in owner and animal names from appointment printout or as clients arrive, and give to vet.
Dispensing medication	Supply of dispensing labels pre-printed with statutory information.
Pricing work done	Printed price lists for stock and fees – one per consulting room and reception desk Invoice pads (duplicate carbon or NCR) Receptionist to staple copy invoice to clinical record card.
Receiving money	Receipt pads (duplicate carbon or NCR) Manual credit card slips in case of total power failure Receptionist to staple copy receipt to clinical record card.
Client forms	Supply of blank estimate sheets, euthanasia and operation consent forms, prescription sheets, etc.

Standard procedures

- Every morning, print off day's appointment lists
- Every month, print off full stock price list
- After every quarterly price rise, print off fee price list.

Price lists, record cards, receipt and invoice pads, credit card slips, supply of forms, pens and calculators to be kept in red plastic box behind reception.

Figure 17.2 Example of a contingency plan in case of computer failure.

CHAPTER CONTENTS

Record keeping 199
Filing systems 200
Data Protection Act (1998) 200
Archiving records 201

Credit control 201
Make sure people know they are expected to pay at the time 202
Make sure they know how much they are expected to pay 202
Make it easy to pay 202
Send bills promptly 203
Follow-up unpaid bills quickly 203
Allow clients to ask for help 203
Outside debt collection agencies 203
County court action by the practice 204
Writing off the debt 204
Consumer credit licences 204

Office equipment 204
Equipment care 204
Lists of suppliers and consumables 205

Telecommunications 205
Telephone systems 205
Out of hours services 206
Mobile communications 206
Broadband and the internet and e-mail 206
Telecoms (lawful business practice) (interception of communications) Regulations 2000 206

Premises management 207
Building and maintenance work 207
Utilities management 207

Security 209

18

Office management

General office management covers much of the behind-the-scenes work involved in running a practice. This includes:

- record keeping
- credit control
- office equipment
- telecommunications
- premises management.

RECORD KEEPING

Every organization must keep records of its activities, both for use internally and for external bodies. In many cases, there are statutory minimum requirements for the keeping of records, laid down by various government and professional organizations. A veterinary practice will have records concerning:

- client details
- clinical information
- sale and purchase of medicines
- financial transactions, including those relating to VAT and tax
- employee information, including payroll, interview notes and other employment info
- health and safety – including records of radiation dose, servicing and testing of equipment.

There is no point having records if they cannot be found when needed. A well-organized filing system is essential.

Filing systems

A good filing system will allow information to be easily filed and retrieved, whilst keeping it secure from loss or damage. Filing cabinets are the normal way of storing paper records. In order to set up the most appropriate filing categories, try to envisage the circumstances when you might need to retrieve the information. Often each filing drawer will contain a broad category, such as 'Employment' or 'Premises'. Within that drawer, individual files will divide the category into smaller sections, such as individual employees' files, year-end PAYE returns, and so on. What seems a logical division to one person is not always clear to the rest of the practice staff. It is sensible to produce an index to your filing system, which will help staff to find and file documents in the appropriate place. Much information is now stored on computers, which allows instant retrieval of data and the capacity to categorize information under several headings.

The filing system will also need to be categorized by security level. Some records, such as supplier details, will be available to all staff; whereas others, such as disciplinary records, should be only accessible to authorized users.

The collection, storage and use of data is governed by the Data Protection Act (1998).

Data Protection Act (1998)

The 1998 version of the Act came into force on 1st March 2000, replacing the 1984 Data Protection Act.

The Data Protection Act has two main requirements. Users of personal data (i.e. data relating to a living individual who is identifiable from the data) should notify the Information Commissioner that personal information is being held, and must comply with eight principles of Data Protection. The eight principles state that data must be:

- fairly and lawfully processed
- processed for specified, limited purposes
- adequate, relevant and not excessive
- accurate
- not kept longer than necessary
- processed in accordance with the data subject's rights
- kept secure from unauthorized access or accidental loss of data
- not transferred to countries outside the EEA without adequate protection.

The data subject is the person about whom data is being held. They have the following rights under the act:

- To be informed upon request of details held about them by a particular data controller
- To prevent processing likely to cause damage or distress
- To prevent the processing of their data for direct marketing
- To request that decisions are not made solely by automated means based on their data, such as credit ratings
- To be compensated if they have been caused any damage by contravention of the Act
- The removal or correction of any inaccurate data about them.

Every user of personal data, whether it be held on a computer or in a manual filing system, must comply with the data protection principles. What this means practically is that you have a duty to ensure that data you hold about your clients, staff or suppliers is accurate, no more detailed than necessary, and is not held for longer than necessary. It is also your responsibility to hold that data securely: this can involve making sure staff do not have unauthorized access to records, and also taking care that visitors to the surgery do not see data belonging to other persons. For instance, this could happen if the computer record of the previous client, which might contain notes about their credit control status, was visible in the consulting room when the next client came in.

You should also bear in mind that your clients, staff and other individuals have the right to request a description of the data which you hold about them, and what you are using it for. This information must be supplied in permanent form, and if any of the information is not intelligible without explanation, the data subject should be given an explanation of that information. It is not uncommon for veterinary practices to make coded notes about various aspects of client behaviour on their records, both manual and computerized, and this right to inspect should be borne in mind when making notes of this kind.

Individuals have the right to request not to receive direct marketing information from organizations holding their data. You are advised to inform clients that their data may be used in this way, and give them the opportunity to decline, when they are first registered. The line between clinical care and direct marketing is getting more blurred as time goes on, and practices would be wise to bear the Data Protection Act in mind during their marketing activities.

Notification involves letting the Information Commissioner know what data you hold, what you do with it, and who else it may be disclosed to. There are some exemptions from the requirement for notification, which cover core business activities. Further information on exemption and the Data Protection Act can be obtained from the Information Commissioner's website, www.dataprotection.gov.uk.

Archiving records

Keeping unnecessary records is a waste of valuable time and space. If the data concerns individuals then this is also contrary to the principles of the Data Protection Act. All filing systems, manual or computerized, should be cleared out periodically, and out-of-date records removed. Some records must be kept for a minimum period of time:

- PAYE – Pay records must be kept for at least three years after the end of the tax year to which they relate.
- VAT – HM Customs & Excise state that business records relating to VAT should be kept for 6 years.
- Tax records – the Inland Revenue states that partnerships and sole traders must keep records for 5 years from the latest date for sending back your tax return. Company records must be kept for six years from the end of the accounting period.
- Health and Safety – Some records must be kept for long periods, whilst others have no formal requirement. Records of RIDDOR reportable injuries must be kept for 3 years.
- Recruitment records – ACAS recommend records be kept for 6 months in case of discrimination challenge.
- Medicines – The bound book used for recording Schedule 2 drugs must be kept for 2 years after the last entry. Various regulations concerning the keeping of records about the administration, sale and supply of veterinary medicines to food-producing animals state that records should be kept for 3 years. However, the BVA Code of Practice on Medicines encourages veterinarians to maintain records of medicines sold to all animals. It also states that records should be kept for at least 6 years in case of civil action for damages.

The regulations concerning the maintenance and keeping of records are subject to change, and the advice of the appropriate authority should always be sought before irretrievably destroying records.

CREDIT CONTROL

Credit control is a major headache for veterinary practices. It is a regular topic in practice management journals and CPD meetings, and is also much discussed on eGroup forums.

There are some basic steps that can be taken to minimize the problems experienced by your practice. These include ensuring that clients:

- know they are expected to pay
- know how much to pay
- can pay easily.

Many of the credit control problems in practice stem from the reluctance of vets and practice staff to discuss fees and payment. Consequently the client is often given no information about payment terms, or may be told, *'Don't worry about that now'*. Staff training is essential to ensure that all practice members are confident about discussing the financial aspects of veterinary care. A practice policy on payment and credit control will make sure all staff give the same message to clients.

Make sure people know they are expected to pay at the time

Practice owners and managers become very frustrated by clients who don't seem to think they need to pay at the time. *'They would have to pay for pet food at the supermarket; why do they expect us to send a bill?'* is a common cry. One answer is that retail outlets have very obvious tills, cashiers and 'please pay here' notices! Veterinary practice generally has a mixture of 'cash' and 'credit' clients. Small animal owners who see other clients coming to reception to pay their monthly account may become confused. Use of a computer system can also lead clients to believe that work is being 'added to their account'.

Your terms of business should be obvious. A simple notice asking for payment at the time of treatment should be clearly visible in the waiting and consulting rooms. If billing fees or other charges may be incurred by non-payment, then this should be made clear too. Written terms and conditions of business should be given to all new clients, and may be included in the practice brochure. They should include:

- payment terms
- any fee or charges added to overdue accounts
- credit control policy and methods – e.g. use of agencies
- who to contact if the client has a problem with paying for treatment.

Make sure they know how much they are expected to pay

The selling price of retail products on display should be clearly marked. The price may be on the goods themselves, or on the shelf upon which they are displayed.

Clients should be reminded of the price of standard services, such as vaccinations, as the appointment is being made. Many treatments or surgical procedures are not easy to price until they have been done, but clients should always be given an estimate range of prices.

If the client is insured, make sure they realize what is covered and what the excess will be.

Make it easy to pay

Review the positioning of your reception desk – is it too easy for clients to go straight from the consulting room to the practice exit? Once the client is at the payment point, do the receptionists have time to deal with outgoing clients as well as incoming ones? In a large practice there may be scope for separating the functions of reception and payment.

Make sure there are no possible reasons to turn down a payment – keep sufficient small change in the till, and accept both credit and debit cards. Remember to use credit cards as credit. If the client claims they have no money, then ask them for plastic.

Never turn a payment down – especially in a crowded waiting room. You and the pet owner might know that the pet is coming in for treatment every day that week, but the ten people who overhear the client being told to pay later don't know that.

Have a system in place so that any accounts not paid at the time have a note from the person responsible for the transaction explaining why payment was not taken.

Promoting and adhering to a strict payment policy can prevent many debts. However, this is not always possible in practice for many reasons, including the ethical need to provide first aid treatment, and the need to maintain client service. In these cases, and with genuine credit customers, good management of accounts receivable is needed to prevent bad debts. This should include:

- sending bills promptly
- following up unpaid bills quickly
- allowing clients to ask for help.

Veterinary surgeons do have the right to hold an animal until outstanding fees have been paid, but the RCVS guide to professional conduct points out that it is not in the best interests of the animal to do so, and that the practice will incur additional costs. This right should only be exercised in extreme cases and after discussion with the RCVS.

Send bills promptly

Clients who don't pay, for whatever reason, should be given a bill as they leave. Remind them courteously that your terms are payment at the time. You may be able to take credit cards over the phone once they get home.

Account clients should be billed promptly at the end of the period. If their month-end bill arrives two days later, it implies that the practice is 'on the ball' with its credit control. A bill turning up three weeks late will make them think they can get away with paying late.

Follow-up unpaid bills quickly

The longer a debt remains unpaid, the harder it will be to collect. It is vital to maintain the impression of efficiency. If your bill stated payment in seven days, then send a follow-up letter on day eight.

If a bill remains unpaid, do not repeatedly send the same follow-up letter each month. That will imply that you do not have a more effective method of ensuring payment. Some practices like to take a personal approach and telephone debtors who have not responded to the first follow-up letter. A second follow-up letter should be sent after a specified period, informing the clients that the matter will be referred to a credit control agency or county court.

Allow clients to ask for help

Some clients will have a genuine problem in paying their bills. Ideally, they should have the chance to mention this before treatment starts, but this does not always happen. Your credit control system should always be carried out in a courteous and professional manner, and should give the client the option to discuss their situation with you. In many cases, there are charitable organizations which may be able to help with some of the bill.

After a couple of follow-up letters and phone calls, further action will be needed. Speed is of the essence – the longer you leave it, the less chance of recovering the money. The common options are:

- outside debt collection agencies
- County Court action by the practice
- write off the debt.

Outside debt collection agencies

Many practices make use of external credit control agencies. These organizations often help the practice by providing sample payment request letters, and, when requested, will take over recovery of the debt. Sometimes the threat of referral to an external agency is sufficient to persuade slow payers to come up with the money.

The persistent bad payer may well have numerous county court judgements outstanding. A collection agency will use information about the debtor's circumstances to ascertain the chances of recovering the debt. Agencies will use a number of techniques, from telephone calling to County Court action, to pursue the debt. Most agencies charge on a commission basis, with extra fees for court actions.

Take care when selecting a credit collection agency. Some are very good, and will do everything they claim to, but there are some rogue companies out there too. Don't rely on written submissions from companies you have never heard of. Ask them for references from other local companies or vets, which can be followed up. The various veterinary eGroups are a good forum for finding out information such as this. In particular, be sure to check:

- the costs and commission rates
- whether there will be any costs if action is unsuccessful

- how long they take to pay their money to the practice
- their manner of dealing with people. Debtors are still your clients, and you will want them to be dealt with firmly but politely.

Check with your local Trading Standards Office if you are unsure about the credentials of any debt collection company.

County court action by the practice

The practice can do everything a debt collection agency does. Bad debtors are infuriating to practice managers and owners, and care must be taken not to get too personally involved. Do not spend excessive amounts of time or money on chasing debts out of righteous indignation! Set a limit below which you don't bother to follow-up. Also remember that you are unlikely to be successful if the client has no money or assets.

The Small Claims Court forms are straightforward to fill in, and make it simple to move from one step to the next. Be aware that the client does have the option to dispute a claim, and if there are any doubts about the success of treatment it may be prudent to seek advice from your professional indemnity insurer before proceeding.

Advice about the Small Claims Court can be found at www.courtservice.gov.uk.

Writing off the debt

There are cases when the only option is to write off the debt. This is often when the client has no money, or the amount is less than the cost of recovering it. VAT relief on a bad debt can be recovered from HM Customs and Excise, provided the debt is 6 months overdue and has been written off in the practice accounts. The requirement to inform the debtor that this has been done was revoked in the April 2002 Budget. This change will come into effect following Royal Assent of the finance bill.

Whatever the outcome of your debt recovery procedure, the practice may no longer wish to deal with the client. The RCVS Guide to Professional Conduct 2002 states that *'In the case of persistently slow payers and bad debtors it is acceptable to give them notice in writing (by recorded delivery) that veterinary services will no longer be provided.'*

The practice may also consider obtaining creditworthiness reports on new clients before doing large amounts of work on account for them.

Consumer credit licences

Most credit offered by veterinary surgeries is exempt from the need to have a consumer credit licence. In particular, a licence is NOT required for normal trade credit. This may be either 'running account credit', for example for the farmer who runs up an account but is asked to pay it in full at the end of each month; or 'fixed sum credit' – such as for the small animal client who has a large bill for an operation and is allowed to pay in up to four payments within a year.

Payment of over four instalments can still be accepted without need for a licence, provided that it is only used in very unusual circumstances, and is not routinely offered as an option to clients.

One emerging complication for veterinary practices is that of 'Practice Health Plans'. These are arrangements where the practice offers the client a treatment bundle, which may include annual health check, vaccination, worm and flea treatment, dental checks, etc., for which the client pays a fixed monthly sum. These are subject to the Consumer Credit Act, and a licence would be required. Many of these schemes are administered by third party companies on behalf of the practice. In this case the administering company will have the appropriate licence, and the practice may not need to register.

OFFICE EQUIPMENT

Equipment care

Office equipment has a hard life, being used and abused by most members of the practice, often with no one person taking responsibility. Whilst surgical equipment is normally carefully cleaned after use, and may even have a routine maintenance contract, most office equipment is expected to function with no input whatsoever.

A named person should have responsibility for the maintenance of the equipment, and have a budget to do it. Printers do work better if they are not full of fluff; photocopiers will produce better results if someone cleans the sticky fingerprints off the glass.

Most office equipment can be covered by a maintenance contract. This does allow planning for on-going costs, and ensures a rapid response in the case of problems. However, some smaller items of equipment are effectively regarded as disposable. Items such as printers are often cheaper to replace than to repair.

Manuals for office equipment should be readily available. Simple instructions for common tasks, such as removing paper jams from the photocopier, should be posted in an obvious place close to the equipment.

Lists of suppliers and consumables

Many of the common queries for managers are along the lines of 'How do I...?' or 'Where do we get...?'. It is good office management to maintain a list of all suppliers and part numbers of office consumables such as printer refills and fax rolls. This can be a central list, or simply a label stuck onto each piece of equipment.

Make sure somebody has responsibility for re-ordering supplies – it is amazing how often the last fax roll gets put into the machine, and no one does anything about it!

TELECOMMUNICATIONS

The modern business depends on good communications with its customers, staff and suppliers. Telecommunications covers a wide variety of communications tools, including telephones, mobile phones, pagers, fax, and e-mail.

There is a wide variety of telecommunications options available to practices, and making the right choice is not easy. Prices change rapidly, and many services are offered as a package deal, making direct comparisons difficult. Many services are not available in all areas of the UK, such as high-speed internet connections, some non-BT line providers, and mobile phone coverage.

An excellent starting place for assessing your telecoms needs is the Telecoms Advice website, www.telecomsadvice.org.uk. It is an independent organization, set up in response to a recommendation by OFTEL's small business task force. It contains lots of useful information such as buyers' guides, FAQs, comparisons and helpful advice on choosing systems.

Telephone systems

Customers are getting more demanding, and the telephone system is often their first contact with the practice. If your lines are always engaged, or the client gets 'lost' in the queuing system, they will soon choose to go elsewhere. Even if they only want to book a routine appointment, they may be worried about what would happen if they should have a real emergency. It is also important to have a good system for communication between members of the practice, within the building or out on call.

Once, a simple telephone system with one incoming line was sufficient for many practices. The increase in client contact necessary for appointment systems, post-op call backs, and other client communications, coupled with the use of fax and internet, has made this inadequate. Your practice management computer system may need a dedicated line of its own to communicate with branch computers or to allow remote access by the software support company. Staff time is valuable, and the use of a dedicated ex-directory line will ensure that staff can make calls without having to wait for the main practice lines to become free. It will also mean that staff out on call or at a branch surgery can easily contact the main surgery without having to wait. However, you should make a point of phoning your practice on the normal outside line occasionally to assess the level of service.

Modern telephone systems can handle a number of incoming lines on the same number, but do remember that simply adding more incoming lines is not the answer to client service if you don't have enough receptionists to answer them! Call management systems can allow the client to choose the department of their choice, such as reception, accounts, small animal or large. Systems are available which allow callers to hold, whilst giving them further information about the practice. When choosing a system, bear in mind what you like or loathe about the telephone systems of your suppliers. If canned music annoys you, it will probably do the same to your clients.

Within the surgery, make sure your system makes it easy to locate and call other members of staff, whether it is for internal communications or for putting an outside caller through to them.

Out of hours services

The use of answerphones for out of hours call minding is being superseded by a variety of call divert options. The seamless operation of these means that message handling centres several hundred miles away from the practice can handle calls. Bear in mind that any out of hours call handling system must comply with the RCVS guidelines on 24 hour care.

Computer software can take the place of much telecoms hardware. Fax and answerphone functions on a PC can replace bulky items of equipment, halting somewhat the proliferation of electronic boxes in the modern office!

Mobile communications

Mobile phones and pagers have revolutionized large animal practice in most areas, although coverage is still poor in many rural areas. Although call charges have dropped over the years, the variety of operators and tariffs still make choosing the most appropriate one far more difficult than it should be. Many trade and other associations offer special deals on mobile rates.

Broadband and the internet and e-mail

ISDN and ADSL technology allow faster internet access and multiple use of the same lines in those areas where they are available. E-mail is covered further in Chapter 17, 'Information technology.'

Telecoms (lawful business practice) (interception of communications) Regulations 2000

These regulations came into force on 24th October 2000. They set out a number of circumstances in which it would be lawful for an employer to monitor, intercept and record communications without the consent of the sender, recipient or caller.

These interceptions are only allowed if the business has made all reasonable efforts to inform every person who may use their telecoms system that communications may be intercepted. The practice should update staff contracts or handbooks with a clause stating that interceptions could take place.

The main circumstances where interception is allowed are:

- to establish facts relevant to the business
- to ascertain compliance with regulatory or self-regulatory rules or guidance
- to ascertain or demonstrate standards which are or ought to be achieved
- to prevent or detect crime
- to investigate or detect the unauthorized use of their systems
- to ensure the effective operation of the system – for example monitoring for viruses.

In addition to the above, the Regulations allow monitoring (but not recording) without consent:

- for the purpose of determining whether or not the communications are relevant to the business
- in the case of communications to a confidential anonymous counselling or support line.

This means the practice is authorized to monitor and record phone calls or e-mails in certain circumstances, for instance to monitor standards of client care and advice. Communications may also be monitored to make sure the business systems are not being abused by private use.

Monitoring may be used as a means of detecting fraud within the practice, or as evidence in cases of harassment or discrimination.

Legal advice should be taken before undertaking any monitoring or interceptions of this nature, since the sender or the recipient of the communication will be able to obtain an injunction if a business makes an interception without the correct legal authority. They can also sue for damages if they can show that they suffered a loss because of the interception.

PREMISES MANAGEMENT

The upkeep of practice premises, and the cost of associated overheads such as heating and lighting, can be a significant element of the practice expenses.

Building and maintenance work

The practice premises will need an on-going programme of maintenance. All aspects of the premises should be considered:

- Grounds – car park and gardens
- Exterior – signage, windows, doors, roofs, gutters and general building fabric
- Interior – flooring, décor, fixtures, fittings and equipment
- Infrastructure – wiring, plumbing, drainage, telephone and computer cabling.

On-going premises and equipment maintenance is essential for several reasons:

- To present a good image to clients
- To comply with RCVS/BSAVA/BVHA practice standards
- To ensure good staff working conditions
- To comply with Health and Safety legislation, such as repairs to unsafe flooring, routine electrical and gas safety checks
- To comply with access requirements for disabled people
- Because contents insurance may be void if locks or doors are not up to a specified standard
- To protect the value of the property.

In other cases, the practice may be wishing to extend or improve the premises.

Routine maintenance work should be planned and budgeted for on an annual basis. If you only redecorate or tidy the garden when it looks as if it needs it, the chances are that your clients will have noticed it needed doing far sooner than the practice did!

Any form of building or maintenance work will involve liaising with the tradesmen involved. Major work may be project managed by the architect involved, but routine or small jobs will generally involve the practice manager or a partner. Your architect should also be able to advise you about building regulations and planning permission.

Some practices will have their 'pet' builder or electrician. Even in these cases, you should obtain a couple of alternative quotations for work. If you are looking for a suitable company to do the work, then make sure you follow-up references. Reliability and attention to detail should be taken into account as well as overall price.

Careful planning of any work is essential to minimize disruption to the normal running of the practice. You will need to perform a health and safety risk assessment, identifying any problems which may be caused by the work, such as making sure any temporary rearrangements in the practice are safe. The contractor should demonstrate to you that he has assessed and managed his own risks.

Utilities management

The costs of electricity, gas, heating oil and water may not have been significant in small practices. As practice size and the amount of electrical equipment in them increases, looking at these costs is becoming much more important. The Climate Change Levy, an extra tax on non-domestic fuel, was introduced in April 2001, increasing costs even further.

There are three approaches to reducing your utilities costs:

- Make sure that you are being billed correctly for what you are already using.

- Buy from the best value supplier and use the correct tariff.
- Reduce your consumption.

Small businesses may only have their utility meters read a couple of times a year, the supply companies basing their bills in the meantime on estimated use. These estimate bills can get seriously out of line with the true readings, either due to seasonal variations or to changes in business operation. While underestimation of your supply may be good for your short-term cashflow, be aware that the day of reckoning will come. Whenever a bill arrives, check it against the meter readings. If you don't know where your meters are, then find out. They are normally located close to the main gas valve/fuseboard/water stop tap, and you should know where these are for safety reasons. Direct debit payment of utilities is nice and easy, and a good way to even out cashflow, but often means that the bills may be scrutinized less carefully.

The gas and electricity market has been opened up to allow competition between suppliers. The main reason many people don't change is that the number of suppliers and tariffs means that choosing the correct one is as complicated as picking the best mobile phone deal. To compare prices you need to know what your usage is from previous bills. You can work out all the maths yourself, or use one of the cost comparison links on the OFGEM (Office of Gas and Electricity Markets) website – www.ofgem.gov.uk.

Methods of reducing consumption can be divided into 'Habits' and 'Hardware'.

Habits

Habits cost nothing but a bit of memory until they become second nature:

- Do not leave external doors and windows open in winter.
- Turn off lights when not in use.
- Do not leave equipment on or on standby longer than necessary for operational readiness. X-ray processors, photocopiers and other electrical equipment all waste power when on standby instead of being turned off.
- Turn off computer screens and terminals when they are not needed, and at night. Although the main server may need to be left running, significant savings can be made by turning off unnecessary peripherals.
- Take care with the kettle! Jug kettles allow you to boil as little water as you need. Avoid the tendency to put the kettle on and then get distracted before making the tea!
- Don't be heavy-handed with the thermostat. Turning it up to full will not make the room heat up quicker.
- Defrost fridges and freezers regularly. Don't leave the doors open longer than necessary, especially with upright models. Batch items to be put into or removed from cold storage, so as not to open the doors more frequently than needed.

Hardware

Energy-saving hardware does require some investments, but the payback periods can be surprisingly quick. The following are examples:

- Low energy light bulbs.
- Energy-saving lighting systems. Lighting links with health and safety in many areas – it is not acceptable to simply turn off lights in many stairwell and corridor areas. Larger practices would be advised to contact a lighting specialist for a system of low-level safety lighting which is then either manually or automatically brightened when the area is in use.
- Insulation of hot water tanks.
- Fitting of thermostatic radiator valves and radiator reflector panels.
- Energy-efficient boilers and control systems require more investment.
- Replacement of washers on leaky taps, and repair other water leaks. Remember that you pay for water twice – once on its way in and once on the way out as sewage charges.
- Ensuring elbow taps are easy to use, otherwise vets don't bother to turn them off!

- Checking the energy rating when buying new electrical appliances.
- Fabric improvements such as an entrance lobby, double glazing, insulation and draft proofing will save considerable amounts of energy.

Grants may be available for many energy saving measures.

SECURITY

There are many threats to the security of veterinary practices, such as:

- general theft from practice premises
- theft of drugs from premises and veterinary surgeons' cars
- assault by clients
- danger to lone workers, whether they be on night duty, making house calls or simply the only staff member at a branch surgery
- theft of cash in transit from the surgery to the bank
- loss or damage or unauthorized access to vital practice data.

In some cases, the security of practice premises and staff needs to comply with various aspects of legislation.

- storage of medicines and controlled drugs
- health and safety aspects of lone working
- requirements of your insurance company.

Health and safety, and the safe storage of medicines, are covered in chapters 19 and 20 respectively.

Your local police force should be able to give the practice advice on security measures, and point out areas of weakness. Areas of attention may include:

- blinds on windows to prevent room content being seen from outside
- window locks
- security bars on windows
- high security door locks and hinges – and make sure the door is good quality too!
- a register of who holds practice keys – make sure ex-employees hand theirs back in
- safes and lockable cupboards for valuables, cash and controlled drugs
- panic buttons in areas where staff may be vulnerable, such as reception
- safe design of reception desks in high risk areas
- minimizing cash movements by using electronic payments where possible
- safe systems of work, and personal alarms for lone workers
- standard written procedures for security measures such as end-of-day locking up, dealing with out-of-hours callers, and employees' responsibilities for security of practice property such as cars, mobile phones and pagers
- staff training in aspects of security and personal safety
- door intercoms to check the identity of callers
- CCTV monitoring and video recording of key areas of the premises
- intruder alarms, which may be routed to the local police station
- external security lighting and fencing.

Care must be taken to ensure that security measures do not compromise fire safety requirements, such as alternative means of escape through windows.

Practice security is a risk assessment in itself. Most security measures are sensible, whatever the practice, but others will depend on the likelihood of danger. A protected, glassed-in reception desk may be necessary in some inner city areas, but would be a barrier to client care and communication in a small, friendly village. There may be specific times when practice security is especially vulnerable, such as when building work is being carried out. At these times it may be wise to employ an external security agency.

CHAPTER CONTENTS

Why be concerned with health and safety? 211

Health and safety legislation 211

Enforcing bodies 212

Responsibility for health and safety 213
Employers' responsibilities 213
Employees' responsibilities 213

The practice health and safety policy 213
Writing the health and safety policy 213

Risk assessments 213
The risk assessment procedure 214
Risk assessment paperwork 215

Control of substances hazardous to health (COSHH) 220

Staff training 221

19

Health and safety

WHY BE CONCERNED WITH HEALTH AND SAFETY?

The simple answer to this is that it is the law and has been since 1974 when the Health and Safety at Work Act came into being. It is also good practice to ensure a safe working environment for all employees: it minimizes the likelihood of accidents and the cost of accidents to the employer. Around 25 million days are lost every year in accidents and ill health caused by work activities. It is estimated that the cost of work-related accidents and employees' ill health is between £3.5 billion and £7.3 billion each year.

HEALTH AND SAFETY LEGISLATION

The aim of all health and safety legislation is to prevent accidents and protect health. The Health and Safety at Work Act 1974, the Health and Safety at Work Regulations 1992 and The Management of Health and Safety at Work Regulations 1999 are major pieces of legislation affecting all businesses.

The Health and Safety at Work Act 1974 placed the responsibility for minimizing/eliminating risks to health and safety with those who create the risks, that is, in most cases the employer. This was in effect self-regulation where the employer was obliged to take the necessary precautions to ensure the health and safety of his/her employees. The 1992 Health and Safety at Work Regulations (sect. 2) state that: 'It shall be the duty of every employer to ensure so far as is reasonably practicable the health, safety and welfare of all his employees.' Together with this piece of legislation came the requirement for employers to carry out risk assessments, and in the same year the first six regulations requiring risk assessments were published:

- Manual Handling Operations Regulations
- Workplace (Health and Safety at Work) Regulations
- Personal Protective Equipment Regulations
- Provision and use of Work Equipment Regulations
- Health and Safety (Display Screen Equipment) Regulations
- Management of Health and Safety at Work Regulations.

Subsequently, other areas requiring risk assessments have been identified:

- fire
- first aid
- electricity
- young people at work
- lone workers
- noise
- new and expectant mothers
- working time
- substances hazardous to health – Control of Substances Hazardous to Health (COSHH) Regulations

ENFORCING BODIES

The Health and Safety Commission (HSC) is the body which oversees and encourages health and safety. It produces health and safety reports, investigates accidents and acts in an advisory capacity to the Government on health and safety issues.

The Health and Safety Executive (HSE) is the enforcement body of the HSC. It inspects places of work, investigates accidents and cases of ill-health and enforces good health and safety standards by advising, ordering improvements, or if necessary prosecuting those who have failed to carry out health and safety duties. Inspectors have the right to enter any workplace without giving notice, although normally notice of a few days is given. On a normal inspection an inspector would expect to look at the workplace, the work activities, employer's management of health and safety and to check that he/she is complying with the law. They will expect to see paperwork backing up your health and safety procedures.

The inspector may offer guidance and advice, talk to employees and health and safety representatives and take photographs and samples of items or areas where he/she has health and safety concerns. If the inspector finds a breach of health and safety law, he/she has a number of actions to take which are based on the severity of the breach of health and safety rules. Where the breach is fairly minor, the inspector will informally tell the employer where the problems are and what action should be taken. If the breach is more serious the inspector may issue an improvement notice telling the employer to comply with the law. The notice will say what has to be done, why it has to be done and a date by which it has to be carried out – at least 21 days are normally given for compliance. Failure to comply with an improvement or prohibition notice can result in fines of up to £20,000. Where the breach of the law involves the risk of serious injury the inspector may serve a prohibition notice which prohibits the activity immediately, and not allow it to be resumed until remedial action has been taken. In very serious cases the inspector may initiate a prosecution against the employer.

Local authority environmental health officers are responsible for enforcing health and safety in places such as shops, offices and places used for leisure and consumer services – hotels, restaurants, etc.

Veterinary practices at present come under the jurisdiction of HSE inspectors. The HSE is there to help you implement health and safety in your practice; they publish large amounts of guidance and advice, carry out research and provide a health and safety information service. Their website (www.hse.gov.uk) also contains large quantities of health and safety information and updates on new legislation.

RESPONSIBILITY FOR HEALTH AND SAFETY

Both employer and employee have health and safety responsibilities under the law.

Employers' responsibilities

- The employers must appoint a competent person to organize health and safety measures in the workplace.
- They must ensure that risk assessments are carried out in all the areas specified by health and safety law.
- They must supply health and safety information to employees and visiting workers.
- They must provide health and safety training for their staff.

Employees' responsibilities

- Employees must take reasonable care of their own and others' health and safety.
- They must co-operate with their employer in health and safety matters.
- They must use equipment and substances in accordance with health and safety training.
- They must inform their employer of any health and safety hazards or lack of protection.

THE PRACTICE HEALTH AND SAFETY POLICY

A health and safety policy is required by any business which employs more than five people. The policy is a written statement on how you will implement health and safety protection at work for your employees, and should be revised when necessary and on a regular basis. All employees should have access to the health and safety policy, have read it, understood it and follow it.

Writing the health and safety policy

The policy should contain:

- your health and safety statement – your statement on how you provide and ensure health and safety for your employees
- the responsibilities for health and safety within the practice – who has overall responsibility and to whom specific responsibilities have been delegated
- the risk assessments which will be undertaken
- how the practice will organize consultation with its employees
- how the safety of equipment will be organized and who is responsible for this
- how the practice will implement the COSHH
- what arrangements there are for providing health and safety information, instruction and supervision
- what health and safety training will be given, and who will provide it
- accident and first aid arrangements
- fire and emergency evacuation procedures
- how the practice will monitor and review its health and safety.

The health and safety policy must be signed and dated by the owner, and a review date set.

RISK ASSESSMENTS

A risk assessment is a careful examination of what in your work or workplace could cause harm to people. The assessment involves identifying the hazards and assessing the risk to employees of those hazards. It is important to remember that just because a substance or activity is hazardous it does not necessarily mean there is a significant risk to an employee. Earthquakes are great *hazards*, but in the UK there is very *little risk* of anyone being harmed by them. Conversely a car itself is a low hazard, but driven at 90 miles per hour on a very busy motorway in fog it becomes a *very high risk* to its driver and everyone else in the vicinity. In brief:

- A HAZARD is anything which can cause harm
- THE RISK is the chance/potential that someone will be harmed by the hazard.

It can be helpful to use a risk rating chart when assessing hazard and risk; an example is shown in Figure 19.1.

PROBABILITY OF HAZARD CAUSING HARM	SEVERITY OF HAZARD	RISK FACTOR	ACTION
PROBABLE 3	CRITICAL 3	6–9 HIGH	IMMEDIATE ACTION
POSSIBLE 2	SERIOUS 2	4–5 MEDIUM	ACTION IN SPECIFIED TIME
UNLIKELY 1	MINOR 1	1–3 LOW	NO PLANNED ACTION
Rate the severity of the hazard on a scale of 1–3, 1 being the least hazardous. Rate the probability of the hazard actually causing harm on a scale of 1–3, 1 being the least likely. Multiply the severity rating and the probability rating for the activity or substance to obtain its risk factor.			

Figure 19.1 Risk rating chart.

The chart gives a general guide to the degree of risk there may be from a hazard, and the kind of action which should be considered.

Ideally all hazards should be removed but in many instances this is impossible, impracticable or totally uneconomic. The HSE recommends the following three actions with regard to hazards:

1. Eliminate the source of the hazard whenever possible.
2. Substitute the source of the hazard if it cannot be eliminated.
3. Control the source of the hazard if it cannot be substituted.

Risk assessments need to be carried out for the areas and activities discussed earlier.

The risk assessment procedure

The following steps are necessary in order to successfully complete a risk assessment:

- Consider the task or situation – exactly what does the task involve, what are the procedures, how long do they take, etc.
- Identify the hazards associated with the tasks/procedures and rate on a scale of 1–3.
- Identify those people who carry out the tasks and who are at risk or exposed to the hazard.
- Assess the probability of exposure to the hazard and rate on a scale of 1–3.
- Assess the risk level – use the risk rating chart.
- Consider whether the hazard is already adequately controlled – i.e. what control measures are already in place.
- Identify any other control measures which are needed – i.e. eliminate, substitute or control the hazard. Control measures may be Local Rules, Standard Operating Procedures, or the provision of personal protective equipment in the form of disposable gloves, safety glasses, face masks, plastic aprons, heavy duty gloves, animal catchers and other equipment which will enable them to carry out their job safely.
- Record all the findings of the assessment.
- Implement the control measures which have been identified as needed.
- Inform all relevant staff of the assessment, its findings, and the control measures which will be put in place.
- Train staff in any new procedures which have arisen as a result of the assessment and the new measures which are to be adopted.
- Monitor and review the assessment on a regular basis, or if there are any changes in the tasks/activities.

There is no single right or wrong way to carry out a risk assessment, but the procedure for the risk assessment should remain consistent for all assessments in the practice. A single general risk

RISK ASSESSMENT FOR ....

ASSESSOR .... SIGNATURE ....

DATE .... REVIEW DATE ....

TASK	HAZARDS	PEOPLE AFFECTED	RISKS	EXISTING CONTROLS	CONTROLS NEEDED	ACTION TO BE TAKEN	SOPs LOCAL RULES

Figure 19.2 Risk assessment form.

assessment form can be used, like the one shown in Figure 19.2. It is important that all staff are involved in ensuring a safe and healthy working environment, and to this end it is highly desirable for staff members to be involved in risk assessments. It is especially important that the individual/s carrying out particular tasks which are to be assessed are involved in the assessment.

A very good starting point for risk assessments is to ask every member of staff to complete a risk assessment form for the work they carry out. This not only provides very useful information but also starts to give the employee some ownership of health and safety responsibilities and acts as one of the employee consultative methods. These forms can be collated to form the basis for specific risk assessments.

Risk assessment paperwork

It is always a good policy to keep paperwork to a minimum but there are some essential documents which must be produced with regard to risk assessments. The risk assessment itself must be documented and filed, as should all reviews of the assessment.

As a result of a risk assessment it may be necessary to produce some general Local Rules for ensuring health and safety. These will cover areas such as when and where eating and drinking can take place, general hygiene and tidiness.

Standard Operating Procedures (SOPs) may also need to be produced as a result of a risk assessment. The SOP is a specific procedure which must be followed to ensure the health and safety of employees. It can relate to an activity, such as the handling of sharps or the handling of substances such as drugs or blood.

There is ample literature, much produced by the HSE, on how to carry out the various risk assessments which the law requires. Below is just a brief guide to the risk assessments you will need to carry out in your practice. The first four assessments are likely to be areas which most practices have already addressed, but it is still important to revisit and revise all risk assessment on a regular basis.

Ionizing radiation (The Ionizing Radiations Regulations 1999)

Most practices should already have in place the required measures to comply with the Ionizing Radiation Regulations. All practices which use X-ray equipment must have Local Rules for the X-raying procedure and be registered with their local HSE as a user of ionizing radiation. The practice must appoint their own Radiation Protection Supervisor (RPS), whose duties are to ensure that any work involving ionizing radiation is carried out in accordance with the Regulations and that Local Rules are observed. A Radiation Protection Advisor (RPA), must also be appointed from outside the practice to monitor and advise on ionizing radiation safety and procedures. Personal dosimeters should be available to and worn by all staff involved in X-ray procedures, and protective clothing such as lead gloves and aprons supplied.

Anaesthetic gases (The Control of Substances Hazardous to Health Regulations (COSHH) 1999)

Anaesthesia can be a serious potential risk to employees, and all precautions should be taken to provide a safe working environment in the operating theatre. There should be an efficient gas scavenging system in operation; ideally an active gas scavenging system should be in use. Monitoring of the environment, both that of the operating theatre and recovery rooms, should be carried out on a regular basis. Gas monitoring tubes can be obtained from a number of sources at a relatively low cost.

Fire safety (The Management of Health and Safety at Work Regulations 1999, The Fire Precautions Act 1971 and The Fire Precautions (Workplace) (Amendment) Regulations 1999)

Practices should appoint a Fire Officer who will be responsible for ensuring the practice and its employees comply with fire regulations. The practice must have fire assembly points, adequate fire-fighting equipment and Fire Rules displayed in the building. Fire exits should be clearly marked and never obstructed, and fire drills carried out on a regular basis and recorded.

First aid (Health and Safety (First Aid) Regulations 1981 and Reporting of Injuries, Diseases and Dangerous Occurrences Regulations 1995 (RIDDOR))

A veterinary practice is considered as a medium risk environment, and as such must appoint a person responsible for first aid if they have fewer than 20 employees. If there are between 20 and 50 employees working on the same site a trained first aider must be appointed. This person must have undergone first aid training approved by the HSE. This would normally be a 3- or 4-day course provided by the Red Cross or St John or St Andrew's Ambulance Brigade.

An assessment should be made of the first aid needs appropriate to the circumstances of each surgery, and should consider:

- workplace hazards and the risks involved
- size of organization
- history of accidents

- remoteness of site from emergency medical services
- lone working.

The practice must have the necessary first aid kits available to staff, and maintain an accident book in which all accidents at work must be recorded on each of their sites. There is no standard list of first aid items which should be kept in the first aid box; it depends on what you assess the needs to be, but the following are recommended by the HSE where there is no special risk:

- a general first aid leaflet, e.g. HSE leaflet *Basic advice on first aid at work*
- 20 individually-wrapped sterile adhesive dressings (assorted sizes)
- 2 sterile eye pads
- 4 individually-wrapped triangular bandages (preferably sterile)
- 6 safety pins
- 6 medium sized (approx. 12 cm by 12 cm) individually-wrapped sterile unmedicated wound dressings
- 2 large (approx. 18 cm by 18 cm) sterile individually-wrapped unmedicated wound dressings
- 1 pair of disposable gloves.

Tablets or medicines should not be kept in the first aid box.

The accident book should record the name of the person injured, the date and time of the injury, what the injury was, how and where it occurred and what action was taken. The entry must be signed by the first aider or the person dealing with the accident. The practice must also comply with the Recording of Injuries, Diseases and Dangerous Occurrences Regulations (RIDDOR). RIDDOR requires an employer to report to the HSE a death or major injury, an injury which involves the injured member of staff being away from work for more than 3 days, a reportable disease or a dangerous occurrence.

The twelve other risk assessments which must be carried out are described below.

Workplace health, safety and welfare (The Workplace (Health, Safety and Welfare) Regulations 1992)

The workplace **environment** must have:

- adequate ventilation
- a temperature which provides 'reasonable comfort' without the need for special clothing (guidelines suggest a temperature not below 16°C)
- suitable and sufficient lighting
- clean floors, fixtures and fittings
- sufficient space to allow safe work (as a guide at least 11 cubic metres of room per person)
- a suitable workstation which allows employees to perform their tasks easily.

The workplace **safety** must ensure:

- well-maintained floors and traffic routes, free of obstructions, e.g. no loose carpet, uneven surfaces, etc.
- handrails on stairs, and unsafe areas are railed off
- windows and transparent areas in doors are made of safety material
- car parks are well signed with safe walkways
- trailing cables are properly tied or fixed
- safe climbing aids are provided.

The workplace **facilities** must provide:

- suitable washing and sanitary areas
- drinking water
- areas for change of clothing
- suitable eating facilities
- rest areas for staff and pregnant staff and nursing mothers.

The workplace **housekeeping** must ensure:

- good maintenance of buildings
- maintenance of safe equipment
- safe disposal of waste materials
- building security.

New and expectant mothers (The Management of Health and Safety at Work Regulations 1999)

Individual risk assessments should be carried out on each new or expectant mother, looking at the work she carries out and the added hazards now associated with the work due to pregnancy. Areas for particular attention will be:

- ionizing radiation
- manual handling
- work with any drugs or animals associated with abortions
- physical nature of the work, e.g. long periods of standing, etc.
- zoonoses
- anaesthetic gases
- workstations and work space.

Young persons (The Health and Safety (Training for Employment) Regulations 1990 and The Management of Health and Safety at Work Regulations 1999)

There are specific regulations designed to deal with the health and safety of young persons under the age of 18. Individual risk assessments should be carried out for any new young employees, looking at all the hazards listed in the regulations and any other areas in the practice which may be considered as a risk. The results of the risk assessment will determine the training the young person requires as well as the prohibited areas of work, e.g. X-raying, the areas where supervision is required and the work areas which will be restricted.

Lone workers (The Management of Health and Safety at Work Regulations 1999)

Lone working has its own associated risks, and in veterinary practice can apply to veterinary surgeons on call at night and weekends and staff on duty in the surgery premises. Working alone, particularly for female members of staff, can place staff at the risk of personal abuse or attack. The lone worker may also be at risk from persons with the intent to rob the surgery of money, drugs or firearms. Driving alone to visit clients at night has the added risk of car breakdown and/or accident. A full risk assessment should be carried out of all the potential and real hazards of lone working.

Personal protective equipment (Personal Protective Equipment at Work Regulations 1992)

Personal protective equipment (PPE) must be provided for all staff if there is no other way of eliminating their personal exposure to a hazard. PPE includes safety goggles, masks, gloves, operating gowns and aprons, as well as lead gloves and lead aprons for X-raying.

Protection for X-raying animals is an obvious example; other areas where protective clothing is required are operations (operating gowns) and dentals (goggles and masks).

Noise (The Noise at Work Regulations 1989)

The employer must assess the levels of noise to which employees are exposed and take steps to eliminate, reduce or control the exposure. In veterinary practice the most likely source of harmful noise is from the kennelling area. If noise levels from barking dogs is above the 'first action noise level', which is 85 decibels, for continuous periods then appropriate hearing protection must be provided, e.g. ear plugs or defenders.

Electrical safety (The Electricity at Work Regulations 1989)

A risk assessment must be carried out on the electrical safety of both the premises and the electrical equipment in use. The practice electrical systems should be installed, modified, and repaired only by a competent electrical contractor as defined in the Electricity at Work Regulations. Fixed electrical equipment must be regularly inspected for signs of damage and regularly examined and tested by approved contractors. Portable equipment (any piece of equipment that is plugged into a wall socket) should be regularly inspected for signs of damage or malfunction, as well as being examined and tested by a competent person. All equipment should be labelled to show the date of inspection/examination and the date when these tests are next due.

Display screen equipment (Health and Safety (Display Screen Equipment) Regulations 1992)

If not used correctly, display screen equipment and poorly designed workstations can result in headaches, eyestrain, neck ache and work-related upper limb disorders. Relatively few veterinary employees are considered as high users of display screen equipment as defined in the Health and Safety (Display Screen Equipment) Regulations 1992, but workstations and equipment and the way they are used should be regularly assessed. The equipment should be of low radiation type, have good contrast and no glare, an adjustable screen and stable image, as well as a legible keyboard and wrist rest if required. The workstation should have adequate lighting and leg room, adequate desk space and an adjustable chair with footrest if necessary. The employer is obliged to provide a free eye test for any high-user employee who should request one.

Manual handling (The Manual Handling Operations Regulations 1992)

Incorrect manual handling causes more than 25% of workplace injuries. All work which involves manual handling should be assessed, and where the risks cannot be eliminated equipment should be provided to aid in the handling. Some of the most common manual handling activities in veterinary practice are lifting heavy and/or large dogs, moving heavy bags of food, lifting the larger gas cylinders and moving/pushing/pulling large/heavy pieces of equipment. As well as providing lifting and carrying equipment, the employer should also provide instructions and training on manual handling.

Work equipment (Provision and Use of Work Equipment Regulations 1998)

All work equipment must be safe for use and suitable for the work for which it is being used. Equipment must be kept in good order and repaired, inspected and maintained regularly. All autoclaves must be regularly examined, tested and certified on an annual basis by an approved contractor as set out in The Pressure Systems Safety Regulations 2000. All staff should be provided with adequate training in the use of equipment.

Stress (The Management of Health and Safety at Work Regulations 1999)

Health and safety regulations require the employer to safeguard the health of their employees, and this encompasses the area of stress, bullying and harassment at work.

Stress is not easy to monitor and is often difficult to identify. The best way to monitor employee stress is by informal methods, individual contact, and appraisals, although sickness, absence and low productivity can also be signs that all is not well. The HSE produces a very good managers' guide called 'Tackling work-related Stress' which is very helpful in dealing with this increasing health problem.

Working time (The Working Time Regulations 1998)

The working time regulations set out hours of work, rest periods, night work and annual leave entitlements, and state that:

- average working time is limited to 48 hours during each 7-day period
- there must be a minimum of 11 hours' rest in any 24-hour period
- there must be a minimum rest period of 24 hours in each 7-day period (48 hours for under 18-year-olds)
- there must be a minimum rest break of 20 minutes if the working day is longer than 6 hours (30 minutes if over 4.5 hours for under 18-year-olds)
- if an employee works at least 3 hours between 11.00 pm and 6.00 am they are limited to 8 hours in every 24-hour period
- all employees are entitled to a minimum of 4 weeks' paid annual leave.

Implementing these regulations in veterinary practice is not an easy task when veterinary surgeons and nurses are in night and weekend duty rotas. The regulations should be read carefully in order to establish just what variable working arrangements can be made.

CONTROL OF SUBSTANCES HAZARDOUS TO HEALTH (COSHH)

The Control of Substances Hazardous to Health Regulations state that employers 'must not carry on any work liable to expose employees to substances hazardous to their health unless a suitable and sufficient assessment of the risks created by that work, and the steps necessary to comply with COSHH, are taken'.

The regulations define hazardous substances as any of the following:

- A substance with an occupational exposure standard set by the HSE. There is a complete list of substances contained in the HSE booklet EH40, which is updated on an annual basis.
- Chemicals listed in CHIP 2 – The Chemical (Hazard Information and Packaging for Supply) Regulations. Chemicals are listed as very toxic, toxic, harmful, corrosive, irritants and environmentally dangerous, and are designated hazard symbols
- Hazardous micro-organisms
- Dust in significant quantities
- Any other substance which may be hazardous.

Employers are required to carry out a COSHH risk assessment on all substances used by the practice, and a person responsible for implementing COSHH should be appointed. The same principles apply to a COSHH risk assessment as to all other risk assessments; hazardous substances should wherever possible be eliminated, and where this is not possible they should be substituted with a safer alternative. If neither of these actions can be taken then adequate control measures must be put in place, such as protective clothing, SOPs, etc.

The COSHH assessment should:

1. identify the hazard
2. identify the personnel involved
3. assess the risks
4. implement control measures
5. inform/train staff
6. monitor and review
7. maintain written records.

There are many ways of carrying out COSHH; how it is done will depend on the circumstances of the practice, but there are four basic rules to follow:

1. keep it as simple as possible
2. keep records
3. involve all staff
4. use common sense.

The particular hazards of a substance can be identified by using CHIP, occupational exposure limits, manufacturers' safety data sheets (MSDS), zoonosis guidance and biological hazard groups, as well as your own knowledge of the products. Each substance must be assessed, but for the purposes of writing SOPs they can be categorized into particular groups by use or action, such as anaesthetics, vaccines, sedatives, etc. Alternatively they may simply be listed and their hazard status noted.

There is one particular group of substances which requires special precautions and treatment, and this is clinical waste. Clinical waste comprises animal tissue, body parts and bodies, body fluids, blood, urine, faeces, swabs, and dressings as well as sharps in the form of needles or other sharp instruments and drugs and pharmaceutical products. All clinical waste comes under COSHH regulations in terms of risk assessment, but there are also legal requirements as to its disposal. Pharmaceutical waste comes under the category of special waste, and is treated in a different manner from clinical waste in terms of the paperwork required. All clinical waste must be incinerated, and any firm collecting it must possess a licence for the transport and disposal of the waste materials.

The actual risk to employees from the substance should be assessed by asking:

- Who uses it?
- How is it used?
- How long are people exposed?
- By which route would the substance enter the body?
- Are there any particular people at risk? The young, the pregnant, asthmatics, etc.?

Actions for controlling any identified risks should then be decided and implemented. SOPs will need to be written for those substances which present a hazard. A SOP for spillage should also be written which details the cleaning up procedures and protective equipment to be used.

The paperwork required for COSHH is as follows:

- A list of all substances together with their risk assessment; this can be done very effectively on a computer spreadsheet, which can then be easily updated when new products are bought
- A set of manufacturers' safety data sheets which can be referred to in case of spillage or contamination
- SOPs for all substances (or substance groups)
- Review documents.

Figure 19.3 shows an example of a COSHH Assessment Form and Figure 19.4 the steps in a COSHH Assessment.

STAFF TRAINING

It is a legal requirement that all staff are provided with the necessary health and safety training. Health and safety information, Local Rules, SOPs and employees' duties may be included in staff handbooks, practice manuals or specific health and safety handbooks. A health and safety notice board can be used in conjunction with these to provide current information on new regulations and procedures.

Formal training is also necessary to ensure employees carry out activities safely, such as manual handling, and can implement emergency procedures, for example fire drills.

New members of staff should have time allocated during their induction period for health and safety policies and procedures to be fully explained, and basic training such as first aid and fire procedures to be given.

This chapter cannot cover in full detail health and safety provision in a veterinary practice. The HSE produces large amounts of very helpful information on carrying out health and safety in your business. HSE publications can be obtained from HSE Books, PO Box 1999, Sudbury, Suffolk CO10 2WA. For health and safety enquiries there is the HSE InfoLine, telphone 08701 545500.

The HSE website, www.hse.gov.uk, provides current health and safety information, details of health and safety legislation and HSE publications. Much of this information can be downloaded directly from the website.

CARRIED OUT BY .... DATE .... REVIEW DATE	
SUBSTANCE	
MANUFACTURER	
METHOD OF USE	
PERSONNEL INVOLVED	
HAZARD TYPE OF EXPOSURE LIKELY ROUTE	
RISK IDENTIFIED	
PERSONAL PROTECTIVE EQUIPMENT IN USE	
CONTROLS IN PLACE	
CONTROLS NEEDED	
SPILLAGE	
STANDARD OPERATING PROCEDURE	

Figure 19.3 COSHH risk assessment.

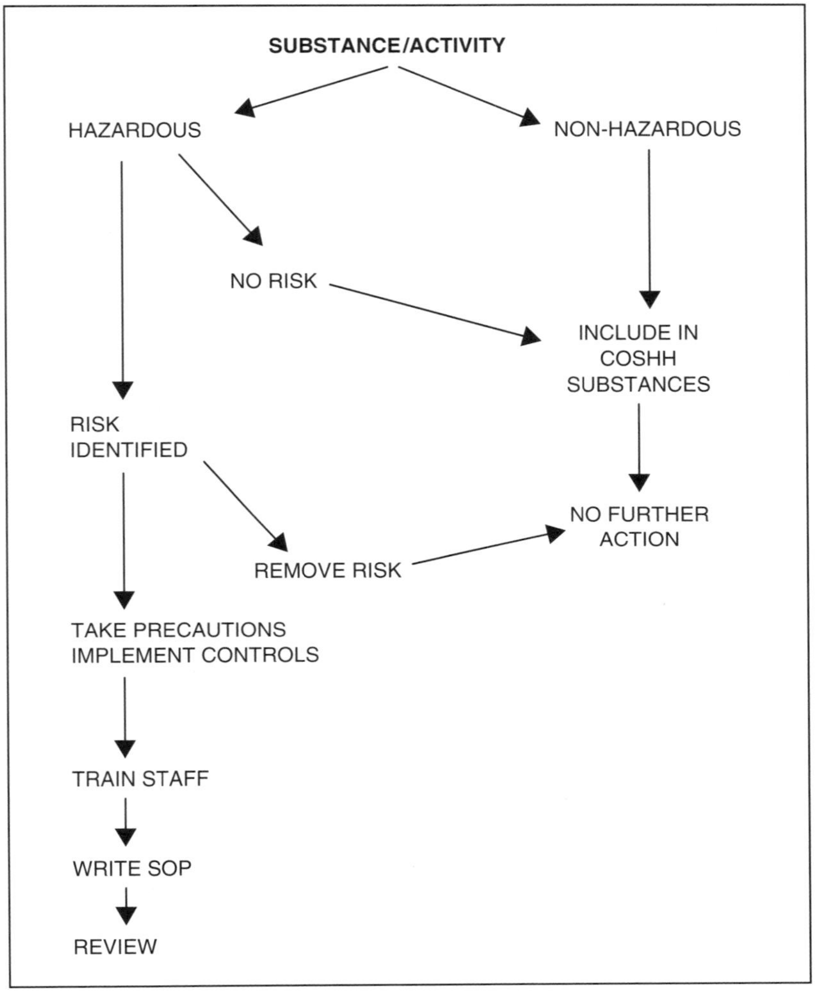

Figure 19.4 Steps in COSHH assessment.

CHAPTER CONTENTS

Drug storage and management 226
Drug categories and controlled drugs 226
Storage conditions 227
Storage of medicines in cars 227
Display of medicines 227
Stock control 228
Personnel 228

Health and safety 228

Dispensing 228
Labelling of dispensed medicines 228
Batch numbers 228
Medicine containers 229
Repeat prescriptions 230
Cascade 230
Returned medicines 230
Waste disposal 231

20

Pharmacy and dispensing

In the UK it is the usual practice for the veterinary surgeon to prescribe and dispense medicines for animals. The Report of the Independent Review of Dispensing by Veterinary Surgeons of Prescription Only Medicines which was published in May 2001 may have some far-reaching consequences for the veterinary profession and may require considerable changes in the way medicines are dispensed and priced in veterinary practices. It makes 14 recommendations, the most important ones being:

- Recommendation – Veterinarians, having once made a diagnosis and prescribed a medicine, should be required to provide a written prescription at either no additional charge or a fee. *This prescription could then be taken by the client for dispensing elsewhere by a suitably qualified person.*
- Recommendation – veterinary practices apply improved business practice in the operation of their pharmacy services with a view to reducing costs.
- Recommendation – the Veterinary Medicines Directorate (VMD) should permit the import of medicines authorized in other member states, provided they are properly labelled and distributed.
- Recommendation – farmers, vets, agricultural merchants and pharmacists should create health plans for farm animals within which medicines can be supplied at cost.
- Recommendation – suitably registered pet shops should be able to dispense cat and dog wormers classified as PML medicines.

- Recommendation – reclassification of medicines into two categories – POMs and GSL. POMs would be further divided into POM (A) – medicines which may be administered only by a veterinary surgeon, POM (B) – medicines which may be sold/dispensed by a veterinary surgeon to animals under their care or by a pharmacy upon veterinary prescription, and POM (C) – medicines which may be supplied by veterinary surgeons to animals under their care or by pharmacists without a veterinary prescription.

It can be seen that these recommendations may put in jeopardy the income derived from drug sales in the practice.

The existing privilege held by veterinary surgeons to dispense veterinary medicines rests not only on the responsible use of medicines, but also on the demonstration of good practice standards of pharmacy and dispensing. It is the manager's role to ensure that high standards are maintained at all times in the practice.

DRUG STORAGE AND MANAGEMENT

Drug categories and controlled drugs

Veterinary medicines are legally classified into five categories: General Sales List, Pharmacy Only, Pharmacy and Merchants' List, Prescription Only, and Controlled Drugs.

1. General Sales List Medicines (GSL).

These are medicines that may be sold without any restriction. A veterinary surgery may sell them to both clients and non-clients.

2. Pharmacy Only Medicines (P).

Few veterinary medicines fall into this category. They may be supplied by a veterinary surgeon for administration to animals under their care or over the counter by a pharmacist.

3. Pharmacy and Merchants' List Medicines (PML).

These are medicines which can be supplied by a veterinary surgeon for administration to animals under his/her care. They may be supplied by a pharmacist to any customer and also by an agricultural merchant who is registered with the Royal Pharmaceutical Society of Great Britain (RPSGB).

4. Prescription Only Medicines (POM).

These medicines may be supplied by a veterinary surgeon for administration to animals under his/her care or supplied by a pharmacist on a veterinary surgeon's prescription. (POM products for incorporation into feedingstuffs are prescribed under a Medicated Feedingstuffs Prescription.)

5. Controlled Drugs (CD).

These are drugs which are capable of being abused and have their own set of rules regarding storage, supply and recording. Under the Misuse of Drugs Regulations 1985, controlled drugs are divided into five schedules in decreasing order of strictness of control.

Schedule 1. This includes cannabis and hallucinogenic drugs such as LSD; these have no veterinary therapeutic use and veterinary surgeons have no general authority to possess or prescribe them.

Schedule 2. This includes drugs such as heroin, cocaine, immobilon, pethidine and fentanyl. They are only available on special prescription, and specific requisition and record keeping is required. A requisition in writing and signed by the veterinary surgeon must be obtained by a supplier before delivery is permitted. Schedule 2 drugs must be entered in a bound register when purchased and also each time they are used. The record must be entered within 24 hours, all entries must be in chronological order and in indelible ink and a separate section of the register must be used for each class of drug. If corrections are made to the entries they should be in the margins or as footnotes, and dated. The date of supply and use of the drug should be noted, as well as the name and address of the owner to whose animal the drug was prescribed, the quantity, strength and reason for use. Any destruction of Schedule 2 drugs must be authorized and witnessed by a representative of the Home Office, and records must be kept in the register. All Schedule 2 drugs must be kept in a locked cabinet, which can only be opened by a veterinary surgeon or a person authorized by the veterinary surgeon to do so.

Schedule 3. This includes the barbiturates and some minor stimulants. Schedule 3 drugs require a prescription and a requisition, but their purchase and use do not have to be recorded. Some Schedule 3 medicines such as temazepam and buprenorphine must be kept in a locked cupboard but there are no special destruction requirements.

Schedule 4. Schedule 4 medicines include librium, valium and benzodiazepines, and are exempt from most restrictions as controlled drugs.

Schedule 5. Schedule 5 medicines include certain preparations of cocaine, codeine and morphine that contain less than a specified amount of the drug. They are exempt from all controlled drug requirements.

Storage conditions

The basic objective of drug storage is to maintain the quality of the veterinary product. The premises where medicines are stored should be a secure building or part of a building dedicated to drug storage, excluded from the public. They should be kept clean, tidy and vermin proof and have storage facilities for medicines which have specific temperature requirements. All medicines should be stored in accordance with manufacturer's instructions. Medicines which must be kept at temperatures between 2°C and 8°C must be kept refrigerated and the fridge temperatures monitored on a daily basis using a maximum/minimum thermometer. The premises generally should have appropriate temperature control so that no products are subjected to any extreme of temperature. Many medicines can be adversely affected by extremes of temperature, humidity and light, and the dispensary premises must have suitable and effective means of heating, lighting and ventilation such that veterinary products are not exposed to any harmful environmental conditions. Medicines which are kept in consulting rooms to which the public have access should be restricted to a minimum, and kept in cupboards or drawers not readily accessible to the client.

Storage of medicines in cars

The same storage requirements apply to car boot storage as to the storage of medicines in the practice dispensary. Only medicines used frequently and daily should be carried routinely in veterinary surgeons' cars, and then only in small quantities. They should be carried in a lockable container or box, the car should be protected against theft, and any medicines should not be on public view. The temperature inside a car boot cannot be easily controlled; in January temperatures may reach below freezing, while in August they may be sub-tropical. It is therefore prudent to store medicines in an insulated storage box, and vaccines should be transported in cool boxes with freezer packs. Lockable medicine boxes also shield medicines from the light and extremes of humidity. Regular checking of car boots and medicine boxes should be carried out by the person responsible for pharmacy and dispensing, to ensure that there are no out-of-date medicines lurking at the bottom of the medicine boxes.

Display of medicines

Prescription Only Medicines (POMs) should not be advertised or displayed to the public. However, the RCVS has indicated that posters advertising POM medicines may be displayed within the practice, especially if they are advertising products, ignorance of which would limit their client education and access to pet healthcare information. Examples of such products are some flea control preparations. P, PML and GSL preparations may be displayed in reception areas, but dummy packets must be used for P and PML products unless they are displayed in a secure cabinet or in such a way that there is no client access.

Stock control

Stock control was discussed in Chapter 15, 'Stock management'. It is a very important part of good pharmacy procedure, in particular the maintenance of minimum stock levels and variety and the careful rotation of stock to avoid drugs becoming out-of-date.

Personnel

There must be a named person in the practice who is responsible for seeing that pharmacy requirements are met and observed. In many cases this named person may also be responsible for COSHH, as the two roles are complimentary. Anyone involved in pharmacy work and dispensing should be suitably trained in drug handling and dispensing as well as the use of appropriate personal protective equipment and cleanliness. It is highly recommended that the practice have a dispensary manual, setting out practice policy, protocols and Standard Operating Procedures for drug storage and dispensing which all personnel involved with drugs must follow. An example of a Dispensary manual outline is shown in Figure 20.1.

HEALTH AND SAFETY

The COSHH Regulations, as well as general health and safety procedures, must be carefully adhered to and there should be Standard Operating Procedures for pharmacy and dispensing as well as specific drugs which are considered to be a risk to staff and clients.

DISPENSING

Labelling of dispensed medicines

Any medicine dispensed from the veterinary surgery must be clearly and correctly labelled. The container or the outer package must be labelled and the labels ideally computer-generated. If labels cannot be computer-generated then they must be written in biro, roller ball or felt tip pen; the use of ink or pencil is not allowed. Ideally the label should not obscure the expiry date of the preparation or important printed information on the manufacturer's label or package. The product information leaflet, which accompanies the product, should be left with the container where appropriate.

The label should contain the following information:

- name and address of owner
- name of animal or description of animal to be treated
- name and address of veterinary surgeon
- date
- medicine name, strength and quantity
- dose to be given and directions for use
- 'For animal treatment only'
- 'Keep out of reach of children'
- for external use only (if applicable)
- withdrawal period for food-producing animals
- any specific warnings for user.

Batch numbers

EU regulation requires that records should be kept for each incoming and outgoing large animal medicine transaction. The information which must be recorded is:

- date
- product name
- manufacturer's batch number
- quantity received or supplied
- name of recipient or supplier

POLICY STATEMENT

PERSON WITH OVERALL RESPONSIBILITY FOR PHARMACY:

NAME..

OTHER PERSONNEL INVOLVED IN PHARMACY AND DISPENSING:

NAME.. ROLE.............................
NAME.. ROLE.............................
NAME.. ROLE.............................
NAME.. ROLE.............................

GENERAL RULES FOR WORKING IN THE DISPENSARY

STOCK CONTROL

DRUG STORAGE

SCHEDULE 2 DRUG REGULATIONS

DRUG ORDERING

DISPENSING

LABELLING OF VETERINARY MEDICINES

THE PRESCRIBING CASCADE

CONSENT FORMS FOR USE OF UNLICENSED PRODUCTS

DRUG BATCH NUMBERS

DRUG WITHDRAWAL PERIODS

REPEAT PRESCRIPTIONS

HEALTH AND SAFETY

DRUG DISPOSAL

Figure 20.1 Dispensary manual outline.

- name and address of prescribing veterinary surgeon.

A detailed audit of all transactions should be carried out on an annual basis. Although small animal transactions are excluded from these regulations, it is good practice to audit small animal medicines on a yearly basis also.

Medicine containers

Containers for veterinary medicines should be approved by the RPSGB. Airtight rigid containers should be used for capsules and tablets, and paper cartons, wallets or envelopes for blister packs and foil strips. It is unacceptable to use plastic bags or paper envelopes as the sole container for dispensed medicines. Amber glass or rigid plastic bottles should be used for oral medicines, coloured fluted bottles for external preparations, and wide-mouthed jars for creams, etc. Discretion should be exercised in the use of child-proof containers as there are occasions when they may be inappropriate if being used to dispense to the elderly or infirm. A sign should be displayed in the reception area indicating that tablets and capsules will normally be dispensed in child-proof containers but that plain containers will be supplied on request.

Repeat prescriptions

Repeat prescriptions for animals may be dispensed under certain conditions. These conditions are normally that the prescription may be given for animals on long-term medication of less than 6 months. Normally the veterinary surgeon will indicate on the client's record that a repeat prescription may be given. Any request for medication for an animal which has not been seen for 6 months should always be referred to the veterinary surgeon.

Cascade

The Medicines Regulations require that product licensed drugs are administered to animals under the care of the veterinary surgeon. There are however situations when off-license prescribing may be permitted, and this requires the veterinary surgeon to follow the rules of the 'Prescribing Cascade'.

When prescribing for non-food animals the following options should be considered:

- Option 1 – use of product licensed for the species and the conditions
- Option 2 – use of product licensed for another condition in the same species
- Option 3 – use of product licensed for use in another species
- Option 4 – use of product licensed for human administration
- Option 5 – use of special product made up under veterinary prescription.

In food-producing animals options 3, 4 and 5 only apply when treating a small number of animals, and in options 2, 3, 4, and 5 the product may only contain substances to be found in licensed products for food animal species. The product must be administered by a vet or under his/her directions, and adequate records must be kept.

If the Cascade is not followed the veterinary surgeon must have written records regarding the prescribing decision. The records must be kept for 3 years, and contain:

- date of examination
- owner's name and address
- number of animals treated
- diagnosis
- product prescribed
- dosage administered
- duration of treatment
- withdrawal period recommended.

It is also wise to have a consent form for owners to sign if a medicine is prescribed off the cascade, with wording such as:

'I understand that... *Name of product*...is a product which is not licensed for use in... *animal species*...but is acknowledged as a product useful in the treatment of... *medical condition of animal being treated*... I have also been made aware of the possibility of side-effects and of the precautions related to its administration. In accepting its use for... *Name of animal*... I accept any attendant risks.'

The form should be signed by the owner and dated.

The welfare of the animal should always override all other considerations but in every case where a non-licensed product is prescribed the veterinary surgeon must be able to justify his/her reasons.

Returned medicines

Once medicines have been dispensed they should not be accepted back into the dispensary and should not be offered for resale. Once the medicines have left the veterinary premises the practice no longer has control over their storage conditions and could no longer guarantee their effectiveness if resold to another client. Many practices will however accept returned unused medicines from clients, which they then dispose of in accordance with the practice waste disposal regulations.

Waste disposal

Pharmaceutical waste is special waste and comprises all items containing pharmaceutical products such as tablets, creams, ampoules and vials. Pharmaceutical waste should not be included with clinical waste for disposal. As already discussed, there are special conditions for the disposal of Schedule 2 drugs. All other pharmaceutical waste should be stored in Doops containers or similar until it is collected for disposal by a licensed waste disposal firm. A record should be kept of all discarded pharmaceutical waste.

More details on pharmacy and dispensing regulations can be found in the BVA Code of Practice on Medicines and the RCVS Guide to Professional Conduct.

CHAPTER CONTENTS

Insurances and pensions 233
Public liability insurance 233
Employer's liability insurance 234
Professional indemnity insurance 234
Buildings and contents insurance 234
Motor insurance 234
Health insurance 234
Locum insurance 234
Partnership protection insurance 234
Pensions 235

Taxes 235
Taxes on goods and services 235
Taxes on income 235

Business structure 236

Ethics 237
RCVS Guide to Professional Conduct 237
VPMA code of ethics 237
Ethical behaviour of members of the practice 237

21

Statutory and ethical aspects of practice

All businesses must comply with statutory requirements concerning their structure, insurance and taxes. Additionally, they may have a specific code of ethics, which governs the day-to-day manner in which their dealings are carried out. This chapter is an overview of the following aspects of veterinary practice:

- insurances and pensions
- taxes
- business structure
- ethics.

INSURANCES AND PENSIONS

There is a wide range of different insurances applicable to the veterinary practice. These include cover to protect against losses arising from:

- liability claims by members of the public, employees and clients
- damage to or theft of property and premises
- inability to work due to illness or death
- other threats to the business.

Public liability insurance

Public liability insurance protects the practice against claims of death, accident or injury to third parties whilst on the business premises. It will also cover the legal costs which may be incurred as a result of these claims.

Employer's liability insurance

All employers must have employer's liability insurance. This will provide cover in case of death, injury or illness of an employee occurring as a result of employment within the business. The practice must display a copy of their certificate of insurance in the premises.

Veterinary practices should check with their insurers as to whether veterinary or work experience students on placement with the practice are covered.

Professional indemnity insurance

This covers for claims made by clients if they have suffered a loss as a result of the veterinary surgeon's actions. It is important to judge correctly the level of cover needed – a practice dealing with racehorses will need higher cover than small animal practice. Professional indemnity insurance is generally provided by specialist insurers, such as the Veterinary Defence Society. These insurers are also a source of useful advice and fact sheets on prevention of indemnity claims.

Buildings and contents insurance

The buildings and contents insurance covers the practice assets against damage or theft. It normally covers a variety of incidental losses such as loss of business as a result of the practice being unable to trade due to an insured risk. It is important that the cover is appropriate and adequate for the business needs. The practice's security arrangements may influence the cover offered or cost of the insurance.

Motor insurance

All practice cars must be insured covering third party liability, damage and theft.

Health insurance

Personal accident/sickness insurance pays a benefit to a person unable to work because of sickness or injury. The policies are arranged for a year, and are renewed at the option of the insurer. There is a maximum limit on the number of weeks that payments are made.

Practice partners will commonly take out Permanent Health Insurance (PHI), sometimes referred to as Income Protection insurance (IP). Unlike personal accident policies, these are arranged on a long-term basis, usually until retirement age. PHI will provide a regular income whilst the insured is certified as unfit to carry out work. There is normally a deferral period of several weeks before the benefits take effect.

Private medical insurance such as BUPA is designed to cover the private medical treatment of illness or injury. Once considered a 'perk' for practice owners, it is increasingly being provided for practice employees as a staff benefit. By enabling staff to have the appropriate treatment as soon as possible, it reduces the burden of sickness and absence on the practice.

Locum insurance

Even if the practice partners have permanent health cover to protect their own incomes, this will not take effect immediately and the practice will still have the added expense of paying a locum to perform the work. Locum insurance should be arranged in conjunction with PHI to ensure that partners' health problems do not cause serious financial problems for themselves and the practice.

Partnership protection insurance

If a partner dies, the beneficiaries of their estate will want to claim their share of the business value. This can cause serious problems if the remaining partner(s) are not in a position to 'buy out' the dead partner's share. Partnership protection insurance is a form of life insurance, where the beneficiaries are the remaining partners of the practice. The sum insured should be sufficient to ensure the on-going stability of the business. In the absence of such insurance, the practice may have to be sold to pay the estate.

The wide range of insurances available to businesses can be very confusing. It is advisable to contact a financial advisor and review the entire practice insurance structure. If various insurance policies have been taken on in a piecemeal fashion it is possible that some areas of cover have been duplicated, leaving unprotected risks elsewhere. A thorough review should enable the practice to benefit from the best cover at the least cost.

Pensions

Pension funds offer a means of investing to provide an income after retirement. The state pension is steadily falling in value in real terms, and business owners and employees are encouraged to make their own arrangements to safeguard their standard of living.

Personal Pension plans were the main options available for practice members until the introduction of stakeholder pensions. Contributions attract full tax relief, but are subject to maximum contribution limits. Other options available to business owners are self-investment pension plans (SIPPs).

Stakeholder pensions were introduced in April 2001. They generally have lower charges than personal pension plans. Employers must offer eligible employees access to a stakeholder scheme from October 2001. There is no obligation for employers to contribute to their employees' pension schemes, but they must provide the facility to deduct the employees' contributions from their payroll and forward the payments to the pension scheme provider.

Planning for retirement is a complex issue. Pension requirements will vary widely depending on family circumstances and other investments. A practice owner will also have to consider the tax implications of selling their share of the business.

Comprehensive financial advice is essential to help you make the best investment for your future.

TAXES

Businesses are subject to a number of tax regimes. These may be taxes on:

- goods and services
- income.

Taxes on goods and services

The most widespread tax on goods and services is VAT. A business must be registered for VAT if their taxable turnover reaches a certain limit. In the year starting 1st April 2001, the registration limit was £54,000. Once a business has registered, it must charge VAT on supplies made to customers. Most veterinary products and services are liable to have VAT applied, with a few exemptions for products such as certain animal foodstuffs.

The practice can reclaim the VAT applied to most goods and services they purchase. A VAT return must be completed on a regular basis, normally quarterly, and any VAT due is paid to HM Customs and Excise. The standard VAT rate is currently 17.5%.

There are other government taxes on specific supplies:

- insurance premium tax (IPT) is currently levied on all general insurance premiums, at a rate of 5%.
- the climate change levy is a new tax on energy supplies (electricity, coal, gas and LPG), charged by the government with the aim of encouraging businesses to reduce greenhouse gas emissions.

Taxes on income

The Inland Revenue collects income tax from employees through the pay as you earn scheme (PAYE). The employer is responsible for calculating this tax, deducting it from the employees' wages and passing it on to the Inland Revenue. This may be done using a manual or computerized system. Employees may also be taxed on employment benefits such as the provision of a company car.

Self-employed individuals (partners and sole traders) must fill in a self-assessment tax return detailing their income and business profits. Tax is normally paid twice a year, in January and July.

Business owners may be liable to pay capital gains tax when they sell their share of the business.

Companies must pay corporation tax on their profits.

National Insurance contributions (NIC) are paid by employees and the self-employed, and are related to the provision of state benefits. There are four classes of NIC:

- Class 1 NIC are paid by employees. They are calculated as a percentage of earnings between the employees' earnings threshold and the upper earnings limit. They entitle the employee to claim a wide variety of state benefits in the appropriate circumstances.
- Class 2 NIC are a flat-rate contribution paid by self-employed individuals. They entitle the individual to claim some basic state benefits such as incapacity benefit, maternity allowance and basic state pension. In the 2000/01 year the Class 2 NIC rate was £2.00 per week.
- Class 3 NIC are voluntary contributions. They can be paid by individuals who are not working, who are not liable to pay Class 1 or 2 contributions, or who have only made very low contributions in a particular year. Class 3 NIC can be used to maintain your contribution records at a sufficient level to be certain of your entitlement to receive state pension.
- Class 4 NIC are paid by the self-employed, in addition to Class 2 contributions, once business profits reach a certain level. They do not count towards any further benefits.

Class 1 and 4 national insurance are paid in the same manner as income tax, via the PAYE scheme and self-assessment respectively. Class 2 contributions are normally paid by direct debit on a monthly basis.

Employers also have to contribute towards National Insurance on behalf of their employees. This is a business cost of employment. The employer's contributions are paid to the Inland Revenue along with PAYE.

There are a number of employee benefits and payments that are administered via the PAYE system, including:

- Statutory Sick Pay
- Statutory Maternity Pay
- Working Families Tax Credit
- Student Loan Repayments.

The rates and circumstances in which these are paid are complex, and beyond the remit of this book. Full details of all tax and National Insurance issues can be found on the Inland Revenue website, www.inlandrevenue.gov.uk.

BUSINESS STRUCTURE

The way in which the business structure of veterinary practice has changed over the years is described in Chapter 1. Currently there are a wide variety of options available to owners of veterinary practices:

- sole trader
- partnership
- limited company
- limited liability partnership
- joint venture.

In addition, there are veterinary practices owned by charities such as the PDSA and RSPCA.

A number of factors affect the choice of company structure, but some key ones are:

- capital funding
- risk
- taxation
- reporting.

A sole trader is personally liable for the debts of the business. Business profits are taxed as personal income under the self-assessment system. The sole trader must pay Class 2 and Class 4 NIC. Although a sole trader must keep sufficient records to enable calculation of tax liabilities, there are no formal requirements to produce accounts or be audited.

In a partnership, two or more individuals contribute their investments to the business. Partners are individually and collectively responsible for all liabilities of the business. As in the case of a sole trader, the partners' personal assets are at risk. The responsibilities and financial structure of the partnership should be covered by a partnership agreement. In the absence of such an agreement, the 1890

Partnership Act takes effect. Partnerships have similar taxation and reporting requirements to sole traders.

A limited company is a separate entity from the individuals who own it. As such, the owners only stand to lose the amount of money they have invested in the business. Their personal assets are safeguarded. In veterinary limited companies, the owners are normally directors, and receive a salary for their veterinary and management work carried out. This is subject to PAYE and NIC as employees. They are only taxed on the income they receive from the business, not the overall profits. Profits remaining in the business are subject to corporation tax. Profits may be retained, or distributed to the owners as dividends. Companies are closely regulated in terms of reporting, and are required to file statutory accounts at Companies House. These records are available to the public.

Limited liability partnerships (LLPs) were introduced in April 2001. They are a hybrid between a limited company and a partnership. The business owners making up an LLP are referred to as members. As with a limited company, the liability of each member is limited to the amount invested in the business. LLPs have similar reporting restrictions to limited companies, in that accounts must be filed on a public register. However, the business is much less restricted in its internal organization, and there is no requirement for formal articles of association.

The tax advantages of one business structure over another will depend on the proportion of profits that are retained in the business as opposed to being distributed to the owners, and the tax and National Insurance rates in force. Any form of limited liability causes the business to lose the right to privacy about its financial affairs, due to reporting regulations.

Joint venture practices have arisen from large group practices, inspired by similar business moves among opticians. Each joint venture practice is a separate legal business, but benefits from a reliable source of capital and a central business management structure.

ETHICS

RCVS Guide to Professional Conduct

The Royal College of Veterinary Surgeons is the governing body of the veterinary profession. It acts as a regulator to the profession, undertaking the statutory responsibilities set out in the Veterinary Surgeons Act 1966. These include maintaining a register of veterinary surgeons eligible to practise in the UK, and regulating veterinary education and professional conduct.

The guide is divided into three main sections:

- Responsibilities of a veterinary surgeon – covering the key responsibilities of veterinary surgeons to their patients, clients, public and professional colleagues, as well as their responsibilities under the law.
- The guidance – this section provides general guidance on areas such as fees, disclosure of information, practice standards, running the business, and complaints.
- Annexes – giving more detailed guidance on specific issues such as 24-hour cover, consent forms, prescribing of medicines, and other areas of concern.

The full text of the Guide can be viewed on line at www.rcvs.org.uk.

VPMA code of ethics

The Veterinary Practice Management Association has a code of ethics for its members. This is reproduced in Box 21.1.

Ethical behaviour of members of the practice

All members of the practice should behave ethically in their day-to-day work, not only in matters fundamental to the veterinary profession, such as animal welfare, but also in general human terms, such as behaving with honesty, respect and integrity.

Box 21.1 VPMA code of ethics

I pledge that I will:

- Maintain and promote the profession of veterinary practice management;
- Seek every possible opportunity to enhance my personal experience, skill and expertise in the profession of veterinary practice management;
- Seek and maintain an equitable, professional and co-operative relationship with fellow members of the Veterinary Practice Management Association and with my colleagues in my business and professional life;
- Fulfil my obligations and responsibilities to the best of my ability to enable my employer and colleagues to deliver the highest possible standards of service to our clients and their animals within the guidelines set down in the current RCVS Guide to Professional Conduct;
- Pursue my profession in veterinary practice management with honesty, integrity and industry, placing the emphasis of my efforts on the highest possible standards of service to my employer(s);
- Ensure the confidentiality of any information relating to the business or personal affairs of my employer(s) and the clinical or other details of their clients and patients, except as may be required or compelled by appropriate law or other regulation;
- Protect any of my employer's property under my control and acknowledge that all information gathered, maintained or produced within the practice is the exclusive property of the practice owner(s) and will not be reproduced, shared or distributed outside the practice without the owners' consent.

A guide to professional conduct for veterinary nurses is available on the RCVS website. It covers aspects of veterinary nursing such as:

- general standards
- acknowledgement of limitations
- relationships with veterinary colleagues
- conscientious objections
- confidentiality
- health and safety
- promotion of products or services.

Standards of ethical behaviour required of practice staff can be included in contracts of employment and staff handbooks, and may even form part of the practice mission statement. These may cover issues such as confidentiality and dealings with clients and colleagues.

CHAPTER CONTENTS

Resistance to employing managers 239

Spreading the load 240

Does your veterinary practice need a practice manager? 241

The pitfalls 243
- Avoiding the pitfalls – the owner's point of view 244
- Avoiding the pitfalls – the manager's point of view 244

Well, who should do the managing? 244

22

Who should do the managing?

Resistance to change, not uncommon in veterinary practice, also spills over into the field of practice management. It has been difficult for many owners and partners to see the need for, or advantages of, employing a full- or part-time manager. This situation is changing as the business of veterinary practice becomes more complex and profits more difficult to make. The Quo Vadis Survey of 1998 published a table showing the employment of veterinary practice managers in the UK. This is shown in Figure 22.1. It can be seen from the table that the employment of practice managers increased in proportion to size of the veterinary practice, with 42% of practices with six or more veterinary surgeons employing a person to whom they had given the title of 'practice manager'. In a survey carried out in July 2001 by the *Veterinary Business Journal*, 45% of veterinary practices were recorded as employing a practice manager.

RESISTANCE TO EMPLOYING MANAGERS

Understandably, owners of veterinary practices have been wary of handing over much of their practice management to a hitherto unknown quantity, but the veterinary world in the twenty-first century is much more aware of the need for good management and the employment of dedicated general or specialist managers. However, there is still reluctance and resistance, for both genuine and perceived reasons, to the

Size of practice (no. of vets)	% of practices with a full-time manager	% of practices with a part-time manager	% of practices with no manager
1–2	11	8	80
3–5	20	15	64
6+	42	14	43

Figure 22.1 Employment of Veterinary Practice Managers in the UK (from Quo Vadis Survey 1998).

employment of practice managers. Some of the reasons are:

- The practice is too small – it does not warrant the employment of a full-time or even part-time manager and could not afford one.
  This may be a very justifiable reason, and as long as the practice is being well managed, employing a specific individual as the practice manager may not be necessary.
- A manager would be too expensive.
  It is a common perception that all a manager will do is cost you money, both in their own salary and the improvements and changes they would wish to make in the practice. It could of course be argued that a manager would make savings in the practice which would easily pay for their salary, and that many of the changes would be very necessary, e.g. the implementation of health and safety regulations.
- Other practice staff share the management – therefore a manager is not needed.
  If this is the case, and the staff responsible for different aspects of management are well trained and managing well, a manager is not needed.
- The owner/partner would lose control.
  This is an unjustified fear. The owner or partner, of course, still has the final control of the business. Employing a manager involves setting up an effective communication system so that owners/partners are kept well informed about management issues and always have the opportunity for significant input. In this way they retain overall control but are relieved of the day-to-day management issues.
- The owner/partner wants to keep in touch with the business.
  There is no reason whatsoever why the owner or partner should not still be in close touch with the business if they have good communication with their manager. They will not lose touch if they have regular management meetings, are kept informed by their practice manager, and continue to take an active interest.
- The practice manager would have too much power.
  This will only be the case if the owner allows it. From the moment a decision is made to employ a manager, lines of authority must be established to ensure the powers the manager has. Their job description should show very clearly what is their remit and what is not. If this is done carefully and thoroughly and there is good communication between owner and manager there should be no 'power struggles'.

SPREADING THE LOAD

One of the simplest and easiest ways to assess the need for a practice manager or other management help is to identify the management roles within the practice and then look at who currently carries them out. Figure 22.2 gives an example of the sort of exercise which could be carried out.

List all the management tasks which need to be carried out in your practice. This includes those which are currently carried out, those which should be but are not, and your wish-list of management tasks you would like carried out in the future. Next to the list under the headings of Who Does It Now?, complete the first four columns, recording which members of the practice are responsible for the different management tasks. This exercise in itself provides you with a good analysis of how management is carried out (or not) in your practice. It may well highlight quite a large number of tasks which are not yet carried out, or perhaps show how much management particular members of support staff are involved in. In a practice which does not have a manager it is likely that the table will show just how much management the senior partner/owner has to do on top of their clinical responsibilities.

Now complete the last three columns, recording who you would ideally like to carry out the practice management tasks. This exercise should provide you with good job analyses for the partner, members of support staff, or perhaps a part- or full-time practice manager. In essence these columns are the beginnings of job descriptions for management roles within the practice.

At the end of the exercise, if you are a veterinary surgeon you should be asking yourself the following questions:

- How many management tasks do I carry out?
- How many management tasks do I delegate to admin/support staff?
- How many management tasks are not carried out?
- Am I happy with the amount of management I am doing? Is it too much?
- Am I doing it well?
- Do I have enough time to do it?
- Should I be delegating some management tasks?
- Who should be responsible for the tasks at present not being carried out?

If you are a practice manager carrying out this exercise you should be asking yourself the following questions:

- How many management tasks do I carry out?
- How many management tasks do the partners carry out?
- Should I be taking on some of their management tasks?
- Who should be responsible for the tasks at present not being carried out?
- Will I have enough time to take on more management tasks?
- Should I be delegating some of my management tasks to support staff?
- Who should I delegate them to?

All practices are different. The way management is organized is a very individual process. However, by answering these questions the veterinary surgeon or practice manager should have a very much better idea of how to organize the management, assess the need for a dedicated manager or the delegation of tasks to others.

DOES YOUR VETERINARY PRACTICE NEED A PRACTICE MANAGER?

There are a number of factors to be considered by owners/partners who are assessing the need for a practice manager. Their decision is going to depend on the size of practice as well as the type, the existing management role of partners and staff, and the future plans for the practice, but the most important questions which need to be asked are:

- What tasks are you going to delegate?

  Be sure you are quite clear what tasks you will be delegating to the manager and that their job description details all the roles you expect them to carry out.

- Could you delegate these tasks to other members of staff rather than a practice manager?

  Be certain that it is better to delegate the tasks to a dedicated practice manager rather than distribute them to other members of staff.

- Do you need a part-time or a full-time manager?

  You may only need a part-time manager; assess the workload carefully before appointing a full-time person. If however you are contemplating expanding/developing the practice this may be the ideal time to employ a full-time manager to help you achieve this.

TASK	WHO DOES IT NOW?				WHO WOULD YOU LIKE TO DO IT?		
	Partner	P. Manager/ Administrator	Support staff	No-one	Partner	Support staff	Practice Manager
Personnel management							
Recruitment							
Job descriptions							
Contracts employment							
Discipline							
Training							
Payroll							
Appraisals							
Rotas							
Grievances							
Induction training							
Computer management							
Troubleshooting							
Websites							
Report generation							
Software assessment							
Hardware assessment							
Training							
Financial management							
Accounts							
Performance monitoring							
Banking							
Cash flow							
Stock control							
Drug purchase							
Insurance							
Financial planning							
Provision of financial information							
Insurance company meetings							
Accountant meetings							
Bankers' meetings							
Health and safety management							
Legislation awareness							
COSHH							
Risk assessments							
Fire regulations							
First aid							
Waste disposal							
SOPs							

Figure 22.2 Assessment of management tasks carried out in your practice.

TASK	WHO DOES IT NOW?				WHO WOULD YOU LIKE TO DO IT?		
	Partner	P. Manager/ Administrator	Support staff	No-one	Partner	Support staff	Practice Manager
Service and marketing management							
Dev. of new services							
Practice promotion							
Client newsletter							
Client brochure							
Open days							
Marketing planning							
Advertising							
Media liaison							
PR							
General office management							
Client accounts							
Debt control							
General purchasing							
Protocols							
Client complaints							
Equipment purchase							
Practice policies							
Internal communications							
Staff manual							

Figure 22.2 (Continued).

- What degree of responsibility will you give the manager?

  It is important to allow the manager to manage, and not be constantly looking over their shoulder. Be very clear from the outset and state in the job description areas of responsibility so that the manager knows what they are and are not responsible for.

- Who will be responsible for 'managing' the manager?

  The manager cannot exist in isolation. The owner or one of the partners must take responsibility for him/her, and for liaison.

THE PITFALLS

There are pitfalls for both employer and employee when it comes to employing a practice manager. It is important to establish at the outset that all the partners actually want a practice manager; if there is resistance to the appointment take care, as those individuals who are not comfortable about it have the potential to be obstructive and make the manager's life very difficult.

Both partners and manager must be very clear regarding the constraints of the job so that misunderstandings are avoided: hence the need for a very clear and detailed job description.

Sometimes partners experience difficulty 'letting go' of tasks which they have done for many years. This may be hard for them, but it is even harder, and very frustrating, for the new manager.

It takes time for a new manager who has not come from the veterinary industry to learn about 'the business of veterinary practice'. Partners and staff need to appreciate this and be patient.

The manager must be allowed to manage. This is what you are paying them for, and what they are qualified to do. Owners and partners should let the manager be a manager, but have regular meetings to discuss management issues.

Avoiding the pitfalls – the owner's point of view

- Be sure you and/or the partners really need a manager.
- Be sure you and/or the partners really want a manager.
- Be sure you know what they will be doing.
- Establish lines of authority and do not undermine the authority of the manager.
- Provide a comprehensive job description.
- Don't move the goalposts once you have appointed your manager.
- Allow the manager to manage, but be sure that you also 'manage' the manager.
- Communicate with the manager on a very regular basis.
- Listen to the manager's advice. This does not mean you have to take it.
- Remember that you are delegating the management of the practice, not the ownership – you remain in control.

Avoiding the pitfalls – the manager's point of view

- Make sure you have a comprehensive job description.
- Make sure you understand where your responsibilities lie and do not lie.
- Make sure you communicate with the owner/partners on a regular basis.
- Listen to the owner's/partners' advice. They have been running the practice a lot longer than you have.
- Remember that the owner/partners will always have the final say; you are there to manage and advise.

WELL, WHO SHOULD DO THE MANAGING?

The fact is that in many respects it doesn't actually matter who does it, as long as it is done well. Perhaps a bold statement, but the message is that what is really important is that veterinary practices are managed, efficiently, effectively and professionally. The way the management is organized and the management structure adopted are going to depend on the nature and culture of the practice. If you ask any veterinary practice manager what their role is, they will give you a unique job description, because no two managers in veterinary practice will carry out the same role.

However, practices which have chosen to employ a dedicated practice manager will undoubtedly have seen the benefits of a professional and experienced approach to practice management.

CHAPTER CONTENTS

Management training 245

Management roles 246

The effective use of staff 246

Adaptation to change 247

Specialization 247

Diversification 247

Reviewing and revising practice policy and procedure 248

Strategic planning 248

23

Where do we go now?

The last few years have seen significant changes in the veterinary profession, with the result that good management has become even more important.

Changes in the pet population, a more demanding public and increased veterinary competition in a shrinking market, together with increased legislation, the downturn in farming and the uncertainty on dispensing, reflected by the Marsh Report of 2001, have all contributed to a need for professional practice management.

Veterinary practice management is facing many challenges at the beginning of the twenty-first century. Will it be ready to meet them? The answer is yes, but a qualified yes, because success will depend on a number of important factors.

MANAGEMENT TRAINING

Whether a practice is managed by a practice manager, owner, or partner, the person/s responsible for management will require good management training if they are to carry the practice through the next 5–10 years. It is much more difficult today to 'just pick up' the administrative or management skills required to manage a small business, although in the past this sufficed for many of those managing veterinary practices.

Management training comes in many forms, from a University MBA qualification to a Diploma or Certificate in Management Studies, or a business studies course at a local college.

All courses have their place, but very few are specifically designed for the management of veterinary practices. Increasingly it is argued that this really does not matter a great deal. After all, managers are trained to manage a 'business', whether it be a factory, shop, hotel, restaurant or veterinary practice. The 'business' of veterinary practice, just like that of the factory, must be acquired on the job and any good manager should be very capable of this. It is of course reassuring if the manager comes to the practice with the double qualification of veterinary and management knowledge.

The Veterinary Practice Management Association, whose aim is to encourage quality management in veterinary practice, awards the Certificate of Veterinary Practice Management (CVPM) to those managers who complete the Association's exam and portfolio requirements. This qualification is seen by the Association as the 'Gold Standard' for veterinary practice management and a guide to the employer as to the standard and competence of the manager. The Association has also devised and provided, through local colleges, a course leading to the Veterinary Practice Administration Certificate qualification. This is aimed at providing supervisors and administrators in veterinary practice with the tools to perform their administrative role to the high standards required by veterinary practice.

MANAGEMENT ROLES

The role of practice management is constantly changing as veterinary practice develops. There is still a place for the individual in practice who is responsible for all the management tasks, and who delegates where possible and appropriate to other members of staff. However, as individual veterinary practices increase in size and more corporate and multi-site practices emerge, this kind of management role becomes increasingly difficult to fulfil.

For these large practices, specialist management has to be the way forward, with financial, human resource, technical, marketing and strategic managers each having responsibility for a group of practices and reporting back to a practice owner/director. Corporate practices offering venture capital opportunities to veterinary surgeons have attempted to remove the burden of management from the practice stakeholder, and to a large extent have achieved their aim. However, the veterinary surgeon in a venture capital situation still has a team of staff to organize and manage, and at the end of the day the business can succeed or fail on his/her ability to manage a team of veterinary surgeons and nurses.

Management roles can only become more onerous as the world of business and veterinary practice becomes more complex. BSAVA Practice Standards requirements are increasingly demanding and it is the manager's responsibility to ensure a practice fulfils and complies with them. Employment and health and safety legislation continually increase in volume and complexity. Managers will have to contend with partnership negotiations in an uncertain financial world, as well as the new limited liability partnerships.

In the same way, marketing management is becoming more and more important as veterinary competition increases. The manager must have a very good grasp of marketing strategy and be able to put this into practice skilfully.

THE EFFECTIVE USE OF STAFF

The effective use of staff is one of the important keys to a successful future. Never before have there been such opportunities to make the maximum use of well-trained staff. This is especially applicable to veterinary nurses, who are now highly trained, more than willing to take on the clinical responsibilities afforded them by Schedule 3, as well as the management of nursing teams and the organization of nurses' clinics. The veterinary nurse has the capability of relieving the veterinary surgeon of many of the more routine daily tasks, freeing them to concentrate on more interesting and more financially productive work. Nurses' clinics can, if well run, increase sales and bond clients to the practice.

Support staff have a pro-active role to play in promoting practice services and products, and should be recruited to fill this role; they are no longer 'just receptionists' answering the telephone and making appointments.

The veterinary surgeons must also play their part by actively promoting other practice services and nurses' clinics, as well as helping to bond clients to the practice.

It is the manager's responsibility to make the best use of their staff, to delegate wherever possible and constantly train and develop staff potential. It is also the manager's responsibility to instil in staff the fact that veterinary practice is a business like any other, with competition and market forces affecting it, and which is required to make a profit if it is to survive. Effective use of staff means not only that they carry out their roles to the optimum but that they understand the basic concepts of a business.

ADAPTATION TO CHANGE

We have to adapt to survive, and veterinary practice is very rapidly learning this. According to Fort Dodge Indices (FDI) figures, 2001 saw a slowdown in turnover growth, and a decrease in active as well as new clients. More veterinary practices are competing for fewer clients, and this situation seems set to increase over the next few years.

Managers must find ways of adapting to these changing circumstances. Each practice must be continually aware of its marketplace, monitoring trends and changes in client needs and demands and supplying those new needs and demands at competitive prices. Clients are becoming more sophisticated and critical of their pets' veterinary care, and we must meet these issues head on. No longer can a practice afford to provide mediocre pet care and hope to survive.

If the outcome of the Marsh Report and Competition Commission investigation results in the veterinary surgeons' income from dispensing being reduced, there will have to be a greater emphasis placed on income from fees. Fee charging is probably one of the areas that veterinary surgeons find the most difficult to change, unlike most, if not all, of the other professions, where generally fees are their only income and they are far from shy when it comes to fee setting.

The veterinary surgeon is no longer the sole provider of veterinary information. Vast amounts of clinical information are available through internet websites and are often quoted back to the veterinary surgeon during a consultation.

We must also adapt to twenty-first century technology, making available our practice information on websites, contacting clients via e-mail and sourcing information and training from the internet.

It is not just the clients who have increasing demands; staff too require better working conditions, longer holidays and more free time for outside activities. Legislation has gone a long way to achieve this for employees, but part-time working requirements, maternity and paternity leave, early retirement and work breaks will require managers to re-think working rotas and schedules to meet these changing needs.

SPECIALIZATION

Already veterinary practices are turning towards specialization. An increasing number of veterinary surgeons are taking certificates and looking to become specialists in their particular fields. Many practices offer referral facilities, and some practices are solely referral practices. Some of these specialists, such as cardiologists and radiologists, occupy definite niches in the veterinary market; while behaviour, homeopathy, alternative medicine and acupuncture are all examples of the new specializations in the veterinary marketplace. Other practices have seen an opportunity to specialize in night clinics and emergency cover for groups of veterinary practices.

DIVERSIFICATION

In an attempt to generate more income, some practices have expanded to encompass veterinary-associated enterprises such as kennelling, grooming, dog training and pet shops. There is a need for these associated services, but practices will have to consider the balance between their clinical and non-clinical services, drawing a very clear line between the two.

REVIEWING AND REVISING PRACTICE POLICY AND PROCEDURE

Never has it been more important to constantly review and revise policies and procedures in the veterinary practice. Survival means finding the right mix of client care, staff, pricing, marketing, information technology, and so on. All the systems which have been put in place need to be reviewed on a very regular basis to check if they are working successfully and producing the results you require. If the review highlights problem areas, policies and procedures need to be revised accordingly. Failure to review, measure and revise can put the success of the practice in jeopardy.

STRATEGIC PLANNING

Every practice needs to have a strategy for survival in the twenty-first century and it is the manager's role to draw up and implement this strategy. Some of the bases include:

- What will you do if another practice moves into the area?
- What will you do if there is a serious recession?
- What will you do if the pet population continues to decrease?
- What will you do if your nearest competitor reduces the cost of vaccinations?

These are just a few of the sort of questions you need to be addressing and answering, in the hope of course that you will not have to implement many of the strategies.

Good management is about planning for the present and for the future. We know what is happening today, and hopefully we are dealing with our business in the knowledge that our plans are being implemented to cope with today's problems and issues. But what about tomorrow? This is what we should now be planning for, with at least one-year and five-year plans so that we are fully prepared for the future.

Appendix: useful contacts

Advisory, Conciliation and Arbitration Service
Ross House, Kempston Way
Suffolk Business Park
BURY ST EDMUNDS
Suffolk IP32 7AR.
Tel: 01284 774500
Website: www.acas.org.uk

British Veterinary Association
7 Mansfield Street
LONDON W1G 9NQ.
Tel: 0207 636 6541
Fax: 0207 436 2970
Website: www.bva.co.uk
E-mail: bvahq@bva.co.uk

British Veterinary Hospitals Association
Oak Beck Veterinary Hospital
Oak Beck Way, Skipton Road
HARROGATE
North Yorkshire HG1 3HU.
Tel: 01423 561414
Fax: 01423 521550
Website: www.bvha.org.uk
E-mail: info@bvha.org.uk

British Veterinary Nursing Association
Level 15, Terminus House
Terminus Street
HARLOW
Essex CM20 1XA.
Tel: 01279 450567
Website: www.bvna.org.uk
E-mail: bvna@bvna.org

British Small Animal Veterinary Association
Woodrow House
1 Telford Way
Waterwells Business Park
QUEDGELEY
Gloucestershire GL2 4BA.
Tel: 01452 726700
Website: www.bsava.com
E-mail: adminoff@bsava.com

Chartered Institute of Personnel and Development
CIPD House
Camp Road
LONDON SW19 4UX.
Tel: 020 8971 9000
Website: www.cipd.co.uk

Courts Service Website
Website: www.courtservice.gov.uk

Department of the Environment, Food and Rural Affairs
Helpline: 08459 33 55 77
Website: www.defra.gov.uk

Department of Trade and Industry
1 Victoria Street
LONDON SW1H 0ET.
Tel: 020 7215 5000
Website: www.dti.gov.uk

Health and Safety Executive
Infoline: 08701 545 500
Website: www.hse.gov.uk

H M Customs and Excise
Adviceline: 0845 010 9000
Website: www.hmce.gov.uk

HSE Books
PO Box 1999
SUDBURY
Suffolk CO10 6FS.
Tel: 01787 881165
Website: www.hsebooks.co.uk

Information Commissioner (formerly the Data Protection Registrar)
Wyecliffe House, Water Lane
WILMSLOW
Cheshire SK9 5AF.
Tel: 01625 545 745
Website: www.dataprotection.gov.uk
E-mail: mail@dataprotection.gov.uk

Inland Revenue
St Mungo's Road
Town Centre
Cumbernauld
GLASGOW G70 5TR.
Tel: 01236 736121
Website: www.inlandrevenue.gov.uk

Office of Fair Trading
Fleetbank House
2–6 Salisbury Square
LONDON EC4 8JX.
Tel: 0845 7224499
Website: www.oft.gov.uk
E-mail: enquiries@oft.gov.uk

Peoples Dispensary for Sick Animals
Head Office
Whitechapel Way
Priorslee
TELFORD
Shropshire TF2 9PQ.
Tel: 01952 290999
Website: www.pdsa.org.uk

Royal College of Veterinary Surgeons
Belgravia House
62–64 Horseferry Road
LONDON SW1P 2AF.
Tel: 0207 222 2001
Fax: 0207 222 2004
E-mail: admin@rcvs.org.uk
Website: www.rcvs.org.uk

Royal Society for the Prevention of Cruelty to Animals
Head Office
Causeway
HORSHAM
West Sussex RH12 1HG.
Tel: 01403 264181
Website: www.rspca.org.uk

Society of Practising Veterinary Surgeons
Briery Hill Cottage
Stannington
MORPETH NE61 6ES.
Website: www.spvs.org.uk
E-mail: office@spvs.org.uk

Telecoms Advice Website
Website: www.telecomsadvice.co.uk

Trading Standards
Website: www.tradingstandards.gov.uk

Veterinary Defence Society
4 Haig Court
Parkgate Industrial Estate
KNUTSFORD
Cheshire WA16 8XZ.
Tel: 01565 652737

Veterinary Helpline
Tel: 07659 811 118

Veterinary Practice Management Association
60 Stanley Street
Rothwell
KETTERING
Northants NN14 6EB.
Tel: 07000 782324
Website: www.vpma.co.uk
E-mail: secretariat@vpma.co.uk

Veterinary Surgeons Health Support Programme
Tel: 01926 315 119

Index

Notes

1. *Page numbers in* italics *refer to figures, tables and information boxes.*
2. *The following terms have been used in this index:*
 'practice' refers to 'veterinary practice'
 'versus' refers to a comparison in the text.

A

ACAS website, current employment legislation, 75
Accident book, 217
Accounting, 151–152
 auditing, 50
  see also Auditing
 audit logs, 197
 balance sheets, 139–141
  see also Balance sheets
 basics, 136
 budgeting objectives, 151–152
 computerized reports/budgets, 189
 computer software, 188
 financial goals, 151
 increasing profits, 154, *154*
 profit and loss account, *136*, 136–139
 responsibilities, 26
 worked examples, *145*
 see also Financial accounts
Accounting Rate of Return (ARR) *see* Return on capital employed (ROCE)
Accounts, interpretation of, 141–145
 acid test, 143
 cost of drugs/disposables, 142
 current ratio, 142–143
 debtor days, 143–144
 expenses, 142
 gearing, 143
 gross profit percentages, 142
 net profit percentage, 142
 previous year comparisons, 142
 return on capital employed, 144
 return on equity, 144
 salaries/locum fees, 142
 stock days, 143
Acupuncture, 6
Administrators, *versus* managers, 24
Admissions, client care standards, 113
Advertising, 129
 ethics, 129
 jobs, 63–64
  what to say, 63–64, *64*
  where to advertise, 64
Advisory, Conciliation and Arbitration Service, contact details, 249
Age discrimination, 76
Alternative veterinary medicine, 6
Anaesthetic gases, risk assessment, 216
Animals, computerized records, 186–188
Annual performance appraisals, 104, *108–109*
Annual profit, capital investments, 157
Annual veterinary fees, 11
Anti-surge electrical extension cable, computer safety, 195
Appointment bookings
 client care standards, 113
 computerized, 187–188
Appraisals, 87, 102–105
 annual performance, 104, *108–109*
 five golden rules, 103–104
 interview, 104–105
 process, 104, *110*
 self-appraisal form, 104, *107*
 setting up, points to remember, 105
 timing, 103
 who appraises whom?, 102–103, *103*
 written record, 104
Archiving records, 201
Assets, valuation, 139–140
Association of British Veterinary Acupuncturists (ABVA), 6
Auditing, 48–51, *51*
 accounts, 50, 197
 clients, 50
 clinical standards, 48
 future plans, 50–51
 internal systems, 49–50
 marketing/sales, 49
 premises, 48
 public relations/communication, 49
 services, 48
 staff, 49
 stock, 49–50, 162, 167

B

Balance sheets, 139–141
 capital, 141
 current liabilities, 141
 currents assets, 139
 fixed assets, 139
 goodwill, 140–141
 long-term liabilities, 141
Bankers Automated Clearing Service (BACS), 189
Banking, Internet, 189
Billing, calculation, 187
Bonded clients, marketing principles, 121–122
Bookings, client care standards, 113
Bottom up budgeting, 154
 effect on fee setting, 176
Bovine Spongiform Encephalitis (BSE) *see* BSE
Brainstorming sessions
 partners, future planning, 53
 staff, SWOT analysis, 51
British Animal Nursing Auxiliaries Association (BANAA), 7
British Small Animal Veterinary Association (BSAVA)
 contact details, 250
 foundation, 2
 practice standards requirements, 246
British Veterinary Association (BVA), 69
 Code of Practice on Medicines, 231
 contact details, 249
 practice survey, 149
British Veterinary Hospital Association (BVHA), 4
 contact details, 249
British Veterinary Nursing Association (BVNA), 7–8
 contact details, 249
Brochures, marketing the practice, 132
BSE, impact on practices, 2, 9, 12
Budgeting, 152
 computers, 189
 legislation impact, 13
 objectives, 151–152
Budgeting for capital expenses, 156–159
 factors to consider, 156
  see also Capital investment
 net present value, *158*, 158–159
 payback period, 157, *157*
 return on investment, 157–158, *158*
Budgeting for cash, 154–156
 avoiding sudden dips, 156
 cashflow forecast, 154–156, *155*
 VAT, 155
Budgeting for profit, 152–154, *154*
 bottom up strategy, 154
  effect on fee setting, 176
 expenses, 153–154
 planning income, 152–153
 staff input, 152
 top down strategy, 154
 turnover, 152–153, *153*
Buildings, 3–4
 meeting client needs, 112
 see also Premises management
Buildings and contents insurance, 234
Building work, minimizing disruption, 207
Business ethics, 19, 237–238
Business management, application to practices, 19
Business planning, 47–55
 assessing current situation, 47–52
  auditing, 48–51
  see also Auditing
  SWOT analysis, *51*, 51–52, *52*
 future goals, 52–55
  successful planning, 53–55, *55*
 SMART objectives, 54

C

Candidate profiling
 assessment form, 66–67, *74*
 personal qualities, 63, *72*
 skills, 63, *72*
Capital, balance sheets, 141
Capital expenses, budgeting for, 156–159
 see also Budgeting for capital expenses
Capital gains tax, 235
Capital investment
 effect on current services, 158–159
 financing expenditure, 159
 legal causes, 156
 objectives, 156
 payback period, 157, *157*
 viability calculations, 156–159
Case volume
 management accounts, 150
 turnover, 152
Cashflow
 auditing, 50
 forecast, 154–156, *155*
Certificate in Veterinary Practice Management (CVPM), 24, 28, 246
Change, management, 90–92
 adaptation to, 247
 barriers, 90–91
 incremental/major, 90
 new ways of working, 91–92
 steps for success, 91
Chartered Institute of Personnel and Development, contact details, 250
Client care, 6–7, 8, 111–118, *113*
 achieving excellence, 118
 assessing/maintaining, 114–116
 client feedback, 114–116, 131
 client requirements, 111–112
 complaints *see* Complaints
 managers' responsibilities, 27, 111
 providing good care, 112–114
 results of good/bad care, 112
 staff feedback forms, 116, *117*
 staff responsibilities, 58, 113
 standards, 112–114
Clients
 billing, 187
 computerized records, 186–188
 difficult *see* Difficult clients
 existing, marketing principles, 121–122
 income analysis, 150
 increasing expectations/demands, 129, 247
  TV influence, 9, 11
 new, marketing principles, 121–122
 newsletters, 132
 practice structure, 8–9
 surveys, 114–116
 turnover, management accounts, 151
Climate Change Levy, 207, 235
Clinical meetings, 89
 product range reduction, 164
Clinical protocols, 187
Clinical records, computerized, 186–187
Clinical services, 6–7
 marketing, 127–128
 personal promotion, 132–133
 pricing, 171–172
  see also Fee setting
 sales method, 123–124
Clinical waste
 COSHH regulations, 220
 legal requirements, 220
Communication, 85–90
 client care standards, 114
 computers, 190
 importance, 90
 monitoring regulations, 190, 206–207
 responsibility for, 90
 stock control, 169–170
 where?, 86–90
 who, when, what?, 86
Community liaison, marketing, 131
Competition for clients, 14
Complaints, 114
 dealing with them, 116–117
Computer banking, 156, 189
Computerized practice management system (PMS), 186
 contingency plans, 195–197, *198*
 cost, 194–195
 hardware specification, 193
 operating systems, 193
 practice needs, 191
 software requirements/compatibility, 192–193
 software security, 196
 suppliers, 192
 support and training, 194
 system manager, 196
 system monitoring, 196
 see also Computers in practices
Computers in practices, 13, 186–191, *187*
 accounting software, 188–189
 anti-theft security, 196
 client/animal records, 186–188
 damage prevention, 196
 data back-up, 195
 Data Protection Act, 186, 197, 200–201
 Display Screen Regulations, 194, 197, 212, 219
 fraud awareness, 196–197
 hacking risk, 196
 Health and Safety regulations, 194
 legislation, 197
 location/space considerations, 193–194
 Portable Electrical Appliance regulations, 196
 power supply, 195–196
 sabotage risk, 197
 stock control, 161, 162, 189
 system choice/evaluation, 191–195
  see also Computerized practice management system (PMS)
 theft of consumables, 197
 uses/limitations, 185–186
Constructive dismissal, 79
Consumer credit licences, 204
Contingency plans, computer safety, 195–197, *198*
Continuing Professional Development (CPD)
 Internet/CD Roms, 14, 190–191
 record cards, 100, *101*
Contract of employment, 67–68
 ethical behaviour standards, 67
 what to include, 67–68
Controlled drugs, 226–227
Control of Substances Hazardous to Health (COSHH), 13, 170, 220–221
 anaesthetic gases, 216
 assessing actual risk, 221
 hazard definition, 220
 paperwork, 221
 risk assessment, 220–221, *222*, *223*
Corporate Practice Enterprises, 5, 6, 15
 management roles, 20–21, *22*
  future, 246
Corporation tax, 236
Cost centre analysis, fee calculation, 178, *178*
Cost cutting, report parameters, 151
Cost of drugs/disposables, percentage of turnover, 142
Cost of sales, profit and loss account, 137–138, *138*
Cost price changes
 effect on profits, 174–175, *175*
 responses, 175, *175*
Courts Service website, 250
Credit control, 201–204, 204
 allow clients help, 203
 causes of problems, 201
 client care standards, 114
 consumer credit licences, 204
 county court action, 204
 debt collection agencies, 203–204
 displaying payment policy, 202
 displaying prices, 202
 make paying easy, 202–203
 prompt billing, 203
 quick follow-up, 203
 surgeons rights, 203
 writing off debts, 204
  VAT relief, 204
Current liabilities, balance sheets, 141
Current ratio, interpreting accounts, 142–143

Customer service *see* Client care
HM Customs and Excise, contact details, 250

D

Data back-up, 195
Database, marketing uses, 133
Data Protection Act, 186, 197, 200–201
  data subjects rights, 200–201
Debt collection agencies, 203–204
Debt control *see* Credit control
Debtors, relation to turnover, 137, *137*
Delegation, 39–42
  effective use, 40–41
  managers problems, 40
  need for, 40
  responsibilities if it goes wrong, 41–42
Departmental meetings, 89, *89*
Department of Trade and Industry (DTI)
  contact details, 250
  current employment legislation, 75
Depreciation
  capital investments, 157
  expenses, 138–139
Desktop publishing software, marketing uses, 188
Diet, stress response, 44
Difficult clients
  dealing with them, 117–118
    staff training, 118
  hidden agenda, 118, *118*
Disability discrimination, 76
Discharging, client care standards, 113
Disciplinary procedure, 68–69, *69*
  gross misconduct, 68
  interview, 68–69
  legal advice, 69
  misconduct, 68
Discounting, 181–182
  basic rules, 181–182
  effect on mark-up percentages, 173, *173*
  extra product incentives, 182
  impact assessment, 181–182
  making normal price clear, 182
  practice policy, 182
  reasons for, 181
Discounts, 167–169
Discrimination, 75–76
Dismissal
  constructive/unfair, 79
  employment law, 78–79
  justifiable reasons, 79
  minimum period of notice, 79
Dispensary manual, 228, *229*
Dispensing, 225–231
  batch numbers, 228–229
  fees, 175–176
  further information, 231
  health and safety, 228
  labelling of medicines, 228
  medicine containers, 229–230
  prescribing cascade, 230
    owner consent forms, 230
    written records, 230
  repeat prescriptions, 230
  returned medicines, 230–231
Dispensing review, 175, 225
  implications for practices, 247
  recommendations, 225–226
Display Screen Regulations, 194, 197, 212, 219
Diversification, 247–248
Drugs *see* Medicines

E

Electrical safety, regulations, 218
Electricity at Work Regulations (1989), 218
E-mail, 190
  discussion groups, 190, 191, 203
  internal, 86
Emergency service, 6
  client care standards, 114
Employer's liability insurance, 234
Employment Bill (2001) proposals, 77
Employment law, 75–79
  current legislation information, 75
  discrimination, 75–76
  dismissal, 78–79
  family emergencies, 77
  maternity rights, 76
  minimum period of notice, 79
  national minimum wage, 77–78
  part-time workers, 77
  redundancy, 78
  working parents, 77
  working time regulations, 78
Energy saving
  habits, 208
  hardware, 208–209
Environmental health officers, 212
Environment regulations, 217
  drug storage, 227
Equal pay, 76
Equine flu vaccination, Jockey Club regulations, 188
Ethical behaviour, 237–238, *238*
European Working Time Directive, 78
Exercise, stress response, 44
Existing clients, marketing principles, 121–122
Expectant mothers, health and safety regulations, 217–218
Expenses
  accountancy fees, 138
  budgeting for profit, 153–154
  controllable/uncontrollable costs, 153
  depreciation, 138–139
  fixed/variable costs, 153
  insurance costs, 138, *138*
  percentage of turnover, 142
  per surgeon, 149
  profit and loss account, 138–139
  see also Capital investment
External stressors, 43
Extra product incentives, 182

F

Face-to-face questionnaires, 115
Facilities regulations, 217
Family emergencies, right to time off, 77
Farm animals, health plans, dispensing review recommendation, 225
Farming crisis, impact on practices, 2, 4, 12
Farm visits, client care standards, 113–114
Federation of Small Businesses (FSB), 69
Fees, 171–183
  annual expenditure, 11
  auditing, 50
  calculation, 187
  dispensing/injections, 175–176
  effect of price changes, 180–181, *181*
  income analysis, 149
  managing increases, 179
    gradual *versus* single, 179, *179*
  minimizing complaints, 183
  monitoring of, 179–180
  pricing, 171–172
  relation to turnover, 137, *137*
  setting of *see* Fee setting
  shopped/non-shopped items, 172
  surveys, 171
  turnover, 152
  value for money, 172
Fee setting, 176–180
  calculation strategies
    cost centre analysis, 178, *178*
    cost plus percentage, 177–178
    last year's plus a percentage, 177
    market driven, 178
  fundamental basis, 177
  need for agreement, 178–179
  practice fee culture, 176
  pricing systems, 176–177
  variable pricing structure, 176–177
    drawbacks, 177
  visit fees, 177
Female veterinary surgeons, impact on practice structure, 15
Financial accounts
  computers, 189
  figures for management accounts, 149
  net profit percentage, 142

Financial accounts (*contd*)
  reasons for, 135–136
  understanding, 135–145
  see also Accounting; Accounts, interpretation of
Financial planning, 147–159, 152
Financial reports, 151
Financing expenditure, 159
  hire purchase, 159
  leasing, 159
  outright purchase, 159
Fire Officer, 216
Fire Precautions Act (1971), 216
Fire Precautions Regulations (1999), 216
Fire safety regulations, 216
First aid box, HSE recommendations, 217
First aid regulations, 216–217
  accident book, 217
  practice responsibilities, 217
Fixed costs, 153
Fixed-price fees, 176–177
Food-producing animals, prescribing cascade, 230
Foot and Mouth Disease (FMD), impact on practices, 2, 4, 9, 12
Fort Dodge Animal Health, practice turnover, 122
Fort Dodge Indices (FDI), 149, 247
  average transaction fees, 150
Fraud, computer, 196–197
Fraud prevention, audit logs, 197

G

General management, responsibilities, 25
General Sales List (GSL) medicines, 125, 226
  mark-up percentages, 173
Goodwill, balance sheets, 140–141
Graduates, expectations/ambitions, 5, 14–15
Gross misconduct, disciplinary procedure, 68, *69*
Gross profit percentages, 142
Guide to Professional Conduct (RCVS, 2000), 231, 237
  writing off debts, 204

H

Hacking, risk in practices, 196
Handout questionnaires, 115
Hazard definition, 213
  COSHH, 220
Hazard identification, 220
Head of department meetings, 88
Head receptionist, sample job description, *70*
Health and safety, 211–223
  auditing, 49
  computers, 194
  employees' responsibilities, 213
  employers' responsibilities, 26, 211–212, 213
  enforcing bodies, 212
  legislation, 13, 211–212
  pharmacy and dispensing, 228
  practice policy writing, 213
  risk assessments, 215–220
    see also Risk assessments
Health and Safety at Work Act (1974), 211
Health and Safety at Work Regulations (1992), 211
Health and Safety Commission (HSC), 212
Health and Safety Executive (HSE), 212
  contact details, 250
    website, 212, 221
  first aid box recommendations, 217
  InfoLine, 221
  inspectors' rights, 212
  publications, 221
    contact details, 250
  'Tackling work-related Stress', 219
Healthcare programmes, marketing, 128
Health insurance, 234
Health plans, farm animals, dispensing review recommendation, 225
Helplines *see* Veterinary Helpline
Herbal medicines, 6
Hire purchase, capital investment, 159
HM Customs and Excise, contact details, 250
Holistic veterinary medicine, 6
Homeopathic medicine, 6
Housekeeping regulations, 217
House visits, client care standards, 113–114
Human resource management, 57–74, 81–92
  communication, 85–90
  discipline, 68–69
  employee management software, 190
  recruitment, 61–68
    see also Recruitment
  responsibilities, 25–26
  staff expectations, 59–60, *60*
  staff requirements, 58–59, *60*
  teamwork, 81–85
  training/appraisals, 93–110
    see also Appraisals; Training

I

Importance *versus* urgency, 36–37, *37*
Income analysis, 148, *148*
  categorizing work, 149–150
  figures for management accounts, 149–150
Income budgeting, 152–153
Income Protection insurance (IP), 234
Income taxes, 235–236
Independence *versus* teamwork, *82*
Induction training
  first day, 94–95
    paperwork, 94, *95*
    timetable, 94–95, *95*
  health and safety, 221
  programme, 95–96
    observation list, 96, *96*
Infectious diseases, discovery, 1
Informal communication, 86
Information Commissioner, 200, 201
  contact details, 250
    website, 201
Information technology, uses/limitations in practices, 185–198
  see also Computers in practices
Initial job skills training, 96–97
Injection fees, 175–176
Inland Revenue, 135
  contact details, 250
    website, 236
  see also Taxes
Insurance
  buildings and contents, 234
  employer's liability, 234
  health, 234
  locum, 234
  motor, 234
  partnership protection, 234–235
  pet, 128
  private medical, 234
  professional indemnity, 234
  public liability, 233
Insurance management
  auditing, 50
  consulting financial advisors, 234–235
  statutory requirements, 233–235
Insurance premium, tax, 235
Internal e-mail, 86
Internal memos, 86
Internal stressors, 43
Internet, 206
  Continuing Professional Development, 14
  pet supplies, 13, 14
  practice website, 129–131
  use in practices, 13–14
  see also Website
Internet banking, 189
Interviewing, 64–66
  candidate acceptance, 67
  candidate assessment, 66–67, *74*
  procedure, 64–66
  sample questions, *73*
  selection process, 64

structure, 66
Inventory control systems, 161
see also Stock control
Investment *see* Capital investment
Invoicing, RCVS guidelines, 178
Ionizing Radiations Regulations (1999), 216
IT management
auditing, 49
responsibilities, 26–27
see also Computerized practice management system (PMS)

J

Job advertising, 63–64
Job descriptions, 61–62, *70*, *71*, 104, *106*
hours of work, 62
lines of authority, 62
location, 62
main duties, 62
practice manager, 243
role/responsibilities, 61–62
skills required, 62
title, 62
training provision/requirement, 62
Jockey Club, equine flu vaccination regulations, 188
Joint Venturing Schemes, 5, 15, 237
management practice, 20–21, *22*

L

Large animal visits
client care standards, 113–114
sliding fee scales, 177
Large practices
present-day management, 20, *21*
traditional management, 17, 18, *18*
Leaflets, marketing, 132
Learning styles, 96
Leasing, capital investment, 159
Legal advice, 69
Legislation
computers in practices, 197
impact on budgets, 13
impact on practice structure, 13
increased staff demands, 247
product pricing, 173
stock control, 170
Limited companies, 237
Limited Liability Partnership Act (2000), 5–6
Limited liability partnerships (LLPs), 237
Litigation, 14
Locum insurance, 234
London Veterinary College, foundation of, 1
Lone workers, health and safety regulations, 218
Long-term liabilities, balance sheets, 141

M

Maintenance contracts, office equipment, 205
Maintenance work, minimizing disruption, 207
Management *see* Practice management
Management, of change *see* Change, management
Management accounts, 147–159
average transaction fee, 150
case volume, 150
client turnover, 151
converting data into useful information, 148, *148*
cost of data/information, 148
figures from financial accounts, 149
figures from income analysis, 149–150
moving annual total, 148
need for, 147
specific income groups, 150
staff feedback reports, 151
staff ratios, 150
tailoring reports, 151
what to include, 149
see also Accounts, interpretation of
Management of Health and Safety at Work Regulations (1999), 211, 212
fire safety, 216
lone workers, 218
new/expectant mothers, 217–218
stress, 219
young persons, 218
Management skills, 16
self-management *see* Self-management
time management *see* Time management
Manpower Survey (RCVS, 1998), 7, *7*
Manual handling, health and safety regulations, 219
Manual Handling Operations Regulations, 212, 219
Manufacturer discounts, 167–169
calculation, 168–169
optimization, 167, *168*
Marketing, 119–133
clinical database use, 188
Data Protection Act, 201
definition, 119
ethics, *121*
features and benefits, 122–123
general principles, 121–124
management responsibilities, 27
objectives, 124
planning aspects, 122, 124, *125*, *126*
practice attitudes, 120, *121*
products, 124–127
professions, 120–121
reasons for, 120–121
versus sales, 119–120
services, 127–128
so what? test, 122–123, *123*
Marketing indices, 188
Marketing tools, 129–133
advertising, 129
client feedback, 131
client newsletters, 132
community liaison, 131
database, 133
leaflets, 132
media, 131
personal promotion, 132–133
practice brochure, 132
wall-mounted displays, 131–132
website, 129–131
Mark-ups
definition, 174
versus margins, *174*
product pricing, 173–174
Maternity rights, 76
Media
free advertising, 131
impact on practices, 12–13
Medicines
archiving records, 201
classification, 226–227
dispensing review recommendation, 226
dispensing *see* Dispensing
displaying, 227–228
personnel, 228
prescribing cascade, 230
stock control, 228
storage and management, 226–228
conditions/objectives, 227
storage in cars, 227
waste disposal, 231
Medicines Regulations, prescribing cascade, 230
Meetings, 87–90
making effective use of, 38, 87
planner, *87*, 87–88
structure/procedure, *89*, 89–90
Mental fitness, 42
Menu pricing fees, 176–177
Misconduct, disciplinary procedure, 68, *69*
Mobile phones, 206
Mothers, new/expectant, health and safety regulations, 217–218
Motivation, teamwork, *84*, 84–85
Motor insurance, 234
Moving annual total (MAT)
data presentation, 148
manufacturer discount calculation, 168–169
Multi-site practices, 6
present-day management, 20, *21*

N

National Insurance contributions (NIC), 236
National minimum wage, 77–78
Net present value (NPV), investment viability, *158*, 158–159
Net profit
  percentage, 142
  per partner, 149
  profit and loss account, 139
New clients, marketing principles, 121–122
New mothers, health and safety regulations, 217–218
Newsletters, marketing tools, 132
Newspaper articles, impact on practices, 12
Noise at Work Regulations (1989), 218
Non-food animals, prescribing cascade, 230
Non-shopped fees, 172
Notice boards, 86
Nurses *see* Veterinary nurses (VN)

O

Objectives, 53
Office equipment, 204–205
  care, 204–205
    delegation, 205
  suppliers/consumables list, 205
Office management, 199–209
  credit control, 201–204
  office equipment, 204–205
  premises, 207–209
  record keeping, 199–201
  security, 209
  telecommunications, 205–207
  see also individual areas
Office of Fair Trading (OFT)
  contact details, 250
  POM pricing investigation, 174, 175
Office of Gas and Electricity Markets (OFGEM), website, 208
One to one communication, 86
  services promotion, 132–133
Operation booking, client care standards, 113
Outright purchase, capital investment, 159
Ownership of practices, 5–6, 236

P

Pagers, 206
Pareto's rule, stock control application, 162
Partnership protection insurance, 234–235
Partnerships, 236–237
  formation of, 5
Partners' meetings, 88
Part-time workers, employment law, 77
Passive practice, marketing, 120
Pay as you earn (PAYE), 235
  employee benefits, 236
  records, 201
Payback period, investment viability, 157, *157*
Payment policy, 202–203
Pensions, 233–235, 235
  stakeholder, 235
Peoples Dispensary for Sick Animals (PDSA), 176
  contact details, 250
  practice ownership, 5, 236
Performance monitoring
  management accounts, 147
  report parameters, 151
Permanent Health insurance (PHI), 234
Personal Pension plans, 235
Personal Protective Equipment Regulations, 212, 218
Pet-aid schemes, 176
Pet-care products, 13
  marketing, 127
Pet food, marketing, 127
Pet Healthcare Clinics, nurses, 8
Pet industry, 13
Pet insurance, marketing, 128
Pet owners, influence on practice structure, 11–12
Pet travel scheme, positive effects, 152
Pharmaceutical waste
  COSHH regulations, 220
  disposal regulations, 231
Pharmacy, 225–231
  cost reducing, dispensing review recommendation, 225
  health and safety, 228
  personnel, 228
Pharmacy and Merchants List (PML), 125, 226
  dispensing review recommendation, 225
  farm medicine marketing, 126
Pharmacy Only Medicines (P), 226
Photographic records, 187
Physical fitness, 42
Planning for the future, 248
Portable Electrical Appliance regulations, 197, 218
  computers, 196
Practice as a business, 19
  marketing strategy, 128–129
  performance report parameters, 151
Practice brochure, marketing, 132
Practice Health Plans, consumer credit licence, 204
Practice management, 17–22
  20th century, 17–18, *18*
    reasons for success, 18
  21st century, 19–22
    increased burden, 19–20, *20*
  future prospects, 245–248
    management roles, 246
    reviewing policies/procedures, 248
    strategic planning, 248
  spreading the load, 240–241, *242–243*
    do you need a manager?, 241–243
  Veterinary Nursing Degree, 29
  who should do it?, 239–244
Practice management system (PMS), computerized *see* Computerized practice management system (PMS)
Practice managers, 8, *8*, 23–29
  administrators *versus*, 24
  assessing the need for, 240–241, 241–243, *242–243*
  client care responsibility, 111
    dealing with complaints, 116–117
    dealing with difficult clients, 117
  evolution, 17
  implementing change, 90–92
  management skills, 16
  meetings
    departmental, 89, *89*
    heads of departments, 88
    managing partner, 88
  other titles used, 24
  performance assessment, 33
  pitfalls of employing, 243–244
    avoiding them, 244
  present-day, 23–24
  qualifications/experience, 24, 28
  resistance to employment of, 239–240
    common reasons, 240
  roles/responsibilities, 24–27, 32, *32*
    changes, 28–29
  salary survey, 27–28, *28*
  self-management *see* Self-management
  time management *see* Time management
Pregnant Workers Directive (EU), 76
Premises management, 207–209
  building/maintenance work, 207
  utilities, 207–209
    habits, 208
    hardware, 208–209
Prescribing cascade, medicines, 230
Prescription fees, 176
Prescription only medicines (POM), 125, 226
  display regulations, 227–228
  independent review of dispensing (2001), 225
  marketing, 125–126

mark-up percentages, 173
OFT pricing investigation, 174
Prescriptions, dispensing review recommendation, 225
Present-day practice management, 19–22
increased burden, 19–20, *20*
Pressure Systems Safety Regulations (2000), 219
Pricing
fees/products, 171–183
effects of changes, *180*, 180–181
see also Fee setting; Products, pricing of
minimizing complaints, 183
Private medical insurance, 234
Pro-active practice
changes, 92
marketing, 120
Products
marketing, 124–127
personal promotion, 132–133
pricing, 172–175
assessing cost price, 172–173
cost price changes, 174–175, *175*
effect of changes, *180*, 180–181
factors affecting, 171–172, 171–183
mark-ups, how much?, 173–174
minimizing complaints, 183
percentage mark-up, 172, *172*
profit margins, 174
versus mark-ups, *174*
see Products, pricing of
range refining, 164–165
methods, 164
sales method, 123–124
Professional indemnity insurance, 234
Profit and loss account, *136*, 136–139
cost of sales, 137–138, *138*
expenses, 138–139
net profit, 139
turnover, 137, *137*
Profit and loss budget, 154–156
cash flow forecast, 154–156, *155*
Profit margin
definition, 174
versus mark-ups, 174
product pricing, 174
Profits
budgeting for, 152–154
effect of price changes, *180*, 180–181
Provision and use of Work Equipment Regulations (1998), 212, 219
Public liability insurance, 233

Q

Questionnaires *see* Surveys
Quo Vadis Survey (1998), 4, 7, *7*
practice managers, 8, *8*, 239, *240*

R

Race discrimination, 76
Radiation Protection Advisor (RPA), appointing of, 216
Radiation Protection Supervisor (RPS), appointing of, 216
Reactive practice
changes, 92
marketing, 120
Reception area, meeting client needs, 112–113
Receptionists meetings, 88
Recommended retail price, 173
Record keeping, 199–201
archiving, 201
Data Protection Act, 200–201
filing systems, 200
statutory minimum requirements, 199
Recruitment, 61–68
archiving records, 201
costs, 61
Recruitment procedures, 61–68
advertising jobs, 63–64
candidate profiling, 62–63, *72*
interviewing, 64–66
job description, 61–62
see also individual areas
Redundancy, employment law, 78
Redundancy Payments Act (1965), 78
Registered Animal Nursing Auxiliaries (RANA), 7
Register of Companies, 135
Relaxation, stress response, 44
Reporting of Injuries, Diseases and Dangerous Occurrences (RIDDOR)
archiving records, 201
employers' obligations, 201
first aid, 216–217
Retailing principles, 127
Return on capital employed (ROCE)
accounting, 144
investment viability, 157–158, *158*
Return on equity (ROE), accounting, 144
Return on investment (ROI) *see* Return on capital employed (ROCE)
Risk assessments, 212, 213–220
definition of risk, 213
paperwork, 215–220
procedure, 214–215
risk rating chart, 213–214, *214*
single general form, 214–215, *215*
Royal College of Veterinary Surgeons (RCVS)
contact details, 250
website, 237
directory of practices, 129
ethical advertising, 129
fees, 153
foundation, 1
Guide to Professional Conduct (2000), 231, 237
writing off debts, 204
invoicing guidelines, 178
Manpower Survey (1998), 7, *7*
POM display recommendations, 227–228
Veterinary Helpline, 16
Royal Pharmaceutical Society of Great Britain (RPSGB), medicine containers, 229–230
Royal Society for the Prevention of Cruelty to Animals (RSPCA)
contact details, 250
practice ownership, 5, 236

S

Sabotage risk, computers, 197
Safety regulations, 217
see also Health and safety
Salary survey, VPMA, 27–28, *28*
Sales, 119–133
discounting *see* Discounting
effect of price change, *180*, 180–181
income analysis, 149
management responsibilities, 27
versus marketing, 119–120
products *versus* services, 123–124
turnover budgeting, 153
Security
computer theft prevention, 196
legislation, 209
office management, 209
potential threats, 209
Self-appraisal form, 104, *107*
Self-assessment tax return, 235
Self-investment pension plans (SIPPs), 235
Self-management, 31–45
achieving job satisfaction, 31–34
determination of responsibilities, 31–32, *32*
future plans, 34
health, 42–45
performance assessment, 32–34, *33*
time, 34–42
see also Time management
Services *see* Clinical services
Sex discrimination, 75–76
Shopped fees, 172
Sliding fee scales, multiple large animal procedures, 177
Small animals
product marketing, 126–127
visits, client care standards, 113–114
Small Claims Court, 204
website, 204
Small practices
present-day management, 20, *20*
traditional management, 17, 18, *18*

SMART objectives
business planning, 54
time management, 36
Society of Practising Veterinary Surgeons (SPVS)
contact details, 250
e-mail discussion groups, 190, 191
practice survey, 149
Software *see* Computerized practice management system (PMS)
Sole traders, 236
Specialization, 6, 14, 247
Special offers, assessing true value, 169
SPVS *see* Society of Practising Veterinary Surgeons (SPVS)
Staff, 7–9
attitude towards clients, 117–118
client care, 58, 113
communication, 114
costs, 57–58
effective use of, 246–247
ethical behaviour, 237–238
expectations, 59–60, *60*
importance, 57–58
increasing demands, 247
practice requirements, 58–59
product/service promotion, 132–133
qualities, 58–59
requirements, 58–59, *60*
skills, 59
source of income, 58
training *see* Training
see also Support staff
Staff meetings, 88
Staff newsletters, 86
Staff queries, making time for, 37
Staff ratios, management accounts, 150
Stakeholder pensions, 235
Standard Operating Procedures (SOPs), 216
drug storage/dispensing, 228
Statutory Maternity Pay (SMP), 76, 77
Statutory Paternity Pay (SPP), 77
Statutory requirements, 233–238
insurances, 233–235
pensions, 235
Stock control, 161–170
auditing, 49–50, 162, 167
communication, 169–170
computers in practices, 161, 162, 189
current situation, 162–163
cost, 163
losses, 163
usage/sales, 162–163
what's in stock?, 162
cutting losses, 167
damage checking, 167
factors influencing system, 161
legislation, 170
medicines, 228
optimizing discounts, 167–169
ordering strategies, 165–167, *166*
Pareto's rule, 162
planning, 162
re-order levels, 165
re-order quantity, 165–166
rotation, 167
strategies, 164–170
maximum stock levels, 165
order timing/quantities, 165–166
range control/rationalization, 164–165
targets, 163–164
minimizing cost, 164
price, 163–164
quantity, 163
Stocktaking, 162
Strategic planning, 248
Stress, 42–45
causes, 43
classic signs, 43–44
dealing with it, 44–45
health and safety regulations, 219
impact on practice structure, 15–16
what is it?, 43
Structure of practices, 1–9, 236–237
components, 3
factors affecting change, 11–16, *12*
external factors, 11–14
internal factors, 14–16
future, *3*
history, 1–2
past, *2*
Support staff, 7–8
client care and communication, 8
standards/expectations, 114
effective use of, 247
impact on practice structure, 15
increased demand, 7
reorganizing numbers, 151
Surcharges, 182–183
reasons for, 182
what do they achieve?, 182–183
Surveys
client care, 114–116
planning/designing questionnaires, 115–116
VPMA salary survey, 27–28, *28*
Swine fever, impact on practices, 2
SWOT analysis, *51*, 51–52, *52*

T

'Tackling work-related Stress', HSE managers' guide, 219
Targets, 53–54
Task assessment
importance and urgency, 36–37, *37*
time management, 35–38
Tax-efficient borrowing, 156
Taxes, 235–236
archiving records, 201
on goods and services, 235
on income, 235–236
see also Inland revenue
Team briefings, 87
Teamwork, 81–85
advantages, 85
behaviour, 83
building a successful team, 84
difficult member(s), 85
versus independence, *82*
leadership, 84
motivation, 84–85, *85*
practice team, *83*
reasons for failure, 85
skill/personality mix, 82–83, *83*
Technology, impact on practice structure, 13–14
Telecommunications, 205–207
Internet/e-mail, 206
mobile phones, 206
out of hours services, 206
pagers, 206
Telecoms Advice website, 205, 250
telephone systems, 205–206
call management, 206
see also E-mail
Telecommunications Regulations (2000), 190, 197, 206–207
Telephone calls
client care standards, 113
making effective use of, 38
Telephone questionnaires, 115
Television programmes *see* TV programmes
Theft, computer, prevention, 196
Time-based fees, 176–177
Time management, 34–42
common time wasters, 37–38
creating time for, 38–39
current use of time, 35
delegation, 39–42
see also Delegation
improvements, 36–37
incoming tasks, 36
keeping it up, 39
personal issues, 34–39
routine tasks, 36
signs of poor management, 34–35
SMART objectives, 36
task analysis, 35–36
time logs, 35, *36*
Time theft, computer use, 197
Top down budgeting, 154
Total stock cost, 164
Trading Standards, contact details, 251
Traditional practice management, 17–18, *18*
reasons for success, 18
Training
advantages, 93
computerized practice management system, 194
dealing difficult clients, 118
do's and don'ts, 102

evaluation, 100
first aid, 216
health and safety, 218, 221
individual plans, 100
induction, 94–96
see also Induction training
initial job skills, 96–97
competence checklist, 97, *97*
learning styles, 96
management, 245–246
future needs/goals, 245–246
monitoring, 100, *101*
obstacles, 97–98
on-going development, 97
plan, 98, *99*
process, 94
reviewing, 101–102
Training programme development, 98–102
aims, 98
design considerations, 98–100
needs, 98
Turnover, 137, *137*
average per surgeon, 149
effect of price changes, *180*, 180–181
Fort Dodge Animal Health data, 122
percentage breakdown, 142
TV programmes
impact on practices, 12
increased client expectations/demands, 9, 11
Two-tier treatment system, 14
Types of practice, 4–5

U

Unfair dismissal, 79
Uninterruptible Power Supply (UPS), computer safety, 195
Urgency *versus* importance, 36–37, *37*
Useful contacts, 249–251
Utilities management, 207–209
reducing consumption, 208–209

V

Vaccination reminders, clinical database use, 188
Value for money, perceptions, 172
Variable costs, 153
VAT, 235
accounting basics, 136
archiving records, 201
budgeting for cash, 154–156
VAT relief, bad debts, 204
Veterinary Business Journal, 4
Veterinary Computer Users group (VCU), e-mail discussion groups, 190, 191
Veterinary Defence Society (VDS), 14
contact details, 251
professional indemnity insurance, 234
Veterinary fees, annual expenditure, 11
see also Fees
Veterinary Helpline, 16, 251
stress help, 45
Veterinary hospitals, 4
Veterinary knowledge, 14
Veterinary Medicines Directorate (VMD), dispensing review recommendation, 225
Veterinary nurses (VN), 7–8
effective use of, 246
guide to professional conduct, 238
meetings, 88
sample job description, *71*
Veterinary Nursing Degree, practice management as part of, 29
Veterinary Practice Administration Certificate, 246
Veterinary Practice Management Association (VPMA), 8, 69
code of ethics, 237, *238*
contact details, 251
e-mail discussion groups, 190, 191
foundation, 16
management training, 246
salary survey, 27–28, *28*
Veterinary surgeons, 7
average turnover, 149
effective use of, 247
expenses, 149
income, percentage of turnover, 142
spreading management load, 240–241, *242–243*
Veterinary Surgeons Health Support Programme, 45, 251
Visiting arrangements, client care standards, 113–114
VPMA *see* Veterinary Practice Management Association (VPMA)

W

Wall-mounted displays, marketing, 131–132
Website, 190
accessibility, 130
content, 130–131
maintenance, 130
marketing tool, 129–131
setting-up, 129–130
webcams, 190
Wholesaler discounts, 167
Working parents' rights, 77
Working time regulations, 78, 219–220
Work load, effect of price changes, *180*, 180–181
Workplace health, safety and welfare, 217
Workplace Regulations, 212
Workplace Regulations (1992), 217
Work-related stress, health and safety risk, 15–16
Writing off debts, 204

Y

Young persons, health and safety training, 218
Young Workers Directive, 78